GENETIC SCREENING
Programs, Principles, and Research

Committee for the Study of
Inborn Errors of Metabolism
Division of Medical Sciences
Assembly of Life Sciences
National Research Council

NATIONAL ACADEMY OF SCIENCES
WASHINGTON, D.C. 1975

NOTICE: The project which is the subject of this report was approved by the Governing Board of the National Research Council, acting in behalf of the National Academy of Sciences. Such approval reflects the Board's judgment that the project is of national importance and appropriate with respect to both the purposes and resources of the National Research Council.

The members of the committee selected to undertake this project and prepare this report were chosen for recognized scholarly competence and with due consideration for the balance of disciplines appropriate to the project. Responsibility for the detailed aspects of this report rests with that committee.

Each report issuing from a study committee of the National Research Council is reviewed by an independent group of qualified individuals according to procedures established and monitored by the Report Review Committee of the National Academy of Sciences. Distribution of the report is approved, by the President of the Academy, upon satisfactory completion of the review process.

Supported by the National Science Foundation
Contract NSF-C310, Task Order No. 245

Library of Congress Cataloging in Publication Data

National Research Council. Committee for the Study of Inborn Errors of Metabolism.
Genetic screening: programs, principles, and research.

"Supported by the National Science Foundation contract NSF-C310, task order no. 245."
1. Metabolism, Inborn errors of. 2. Medical screening. I. Title. [DNLM: 1. Mass screening. 2. Metabolism, Inborn errors—Diagnosis. 3. Phenylketonuria—Diagnosis. WD205.P5 N277g]
RC620.5.N34 1975 616.3'9'042 75-5790

Available from

Assembly of Life Sciences, National Research Council
2101 Constitution Avenue, N.W., Washington, D.C. 20418

Printed in the United States of America

Preface

The Committee hopes that the report will be read with profit by all persons concerned with teaching preventive medicine or engaged in its practice. The audience we hope to reach includes health professionals in various disciplines and interested consumers, as well as the many other persons engaged in work related to the preservation of health, such as economists and other social scientists, lawyers, educators, and policymakers.

Screening, the systematic search in populations for persons with latent, early, or asymptomatic disease, has been going on for many years and has come to be regarded as an appropriate and useful medical practice. The successes and failures of numerous programs have been analyzed sufficiently so that plans for screening for new disorders can be drawn up within the context of established procedure.

Screening programs for genetic diseases and characteristics, however, have multiplied rapidly in the past decade, and many have been begun without prior testing and evaluation and not always for reasons of health alone. Changes in disease patterns and a new emphasis on preventive medicine, as well as recent and rapid advances in genetics, indicate that screening for genetic characteristics will become more common in the future. These conditions, together with the mistakes already known to have been made, suggested the need for a review of current screening practices that would identify the problems and difficulties and give some procedural guidance, in order to minimize the shortcomings and maximize the effectiveness of future genetic screening programs.

Such a review was undertaken by the Committee for the Study of Inborn Errors of Metabolism, commissioned by the Division of Medical Sciences of the National Research Council in response to a letter addressed to the President of the National Academy of Sciences by the Chairman of the Social Issues Committee of the American Society of Human Genetics. The letter requested an investigation into the origins, history, and current standing of screening for phenylketonuria (PKU) and into the effectiveness of its treatment. The Committee was charged to conduct such a survey of PKU and, in addition, to extend its purview to encompass screening for other genetic diseases and characteristics as well. This aim was interpreted broadly to include a study of the relations between genetics and preventive medicine. The questions to be answered were to what degree genetics has played a part in preventive thinking and practice and how the relationship should be fostered and extended.

The Committee held a series of meetings and workshops. Various Committee members and staff prepared papers. Experts in economics, ethics, genetics, health education, the law, medicine, political science, psychology, and public health were consulted; for certain purposes, professionals were employed to gather and analyze data. A description of the Committee's work and a list of all contributors appear in Appendix A.

The report is presented in eight parts, beginning with the Committee's recommendations. The recommendations are followed by an introductorv section, in which the prospects for screening are reviewed with reference to both current health practices and advances in genetics, and in which a definition of screening is provided. Part III reviews history of screening for phenylketonuria in the United States, embracing medical, social, and legal experiences and summarizes the lessons to be derived from them. Part IV presents a survey of experiences with screening for a variety of genetically determined diseases and characteristics. In addition, the use of genetic registries and family screening is reviewed. Part V reviews the principles of health behavior and presents the results of studies of attitudes toward screening and other preventive health care expressed by physicians and by patients and screenees. The study of physicians' attitudes was commissioned by the Committee. Part VI includes discussion of legal, ethical, and economic principles in screening, together with suggestions for future research. Part VII provides procedural guidance for health authorities planning new screening programs or the improvement of old. It is to be emphasized that these precepts flow not only from interpretations and analysis of data collected by the Committee but also from the views of participants and practitioners in screening programs now in progress. They are thus not derived from "expert" opinion alone. This part of the report is intended to serve as a guide for persons actively involved with genetic screening. It is therefore self-contained and can be read and used separately.

Part VIII consists of appendixes. It contains agendas and lists of participants in the meetings (Appendix A: Work of the Committee); a glossary of genetic terms that appear frequently in the text (Appendix B: Glossary); history of the early phases of screening for PKU in the United States [Appendix C: Historical Aspects (Socioeconomic and Legislative) of the PKU Screening Program in the United States]; statements by the American Academy of Pediatrics on Phenylketonuria (Appendix D: Statements by the American Academy of Pediatrics on Screening); a statement by the American Academy of Pediatrics on mandatory screening (Appendix E: American Academy of Pediatrics Statement on Compulsory Testing of Newborn Infants for Hereditary Metabolic Disorders, 1967); a statement by the American College of Obstetricians and Gynecologists on Maternal PKU (Appendix F: American College of Obstetricians and Gynecologists: Maternal Phenylketonuria); and tables summarizing interviews with public health authorities and a questionnaire used in a study of physicians' attitudes (Appendix G: Data on Physicians' Knowledge and Attitudes).

The report also contains two very important appendixes on foreign experience (Appendix H: Screening for PKU in the United Kingdom; and Appendix I: Screening Practices in Canada). The organization of screening in these two countries is ahead of that in the United States. These appendixes are important reading for anyone interested in the question of how genetic screening might be improved in the United States. The Committee's recommendations do not flow from these foreign models because the Committee felt that, to be constructive, its recommendations had to build upon the structure currently operating in this country. Therefore, they have been included as separate appendixes, rather than incorporated into the body of the report.

BARTON CHILDS, *Chairman*
Committee for the Study of Inborn
Errors of Metabolism

ARTEMIS P. SIMOPOULOS, *Project Director*
Acting Executive Secretary
Division of Medical Sciences
Assembly of Life Sciences

COMMITTEE FOR THE STUDY OF INBORN ERRORS OF METABOLISM

BARTON CHILDS, M.D., *Chairman*; Professor of Pediatrics, The Johns Hopkins University School of Medicine, Baltimore, Maryland

ROBERT A. BURT, J.D., Professor of Law and of Law in Psychiatry, The University of Michigan, Ann Arbor, Michigan

ALEXANDER M. CAPRON, LL.B., Assistant Professor of Law, University of Pennsylvania Law School, Philadelphia, Pennsylvania

JOSEPH D. COOPER, Ph.D., Professor of Political Science, Howard University, Washington, D.C.

CHARLES J. EPSTEIN, M.D., Professor of Pediatrics and Biochemistry, University of California, San Francisco, California

DONALD S. FREDRICKSON, M.D., President, Institute of Medicine, National Academy of Sciences, Washington, D.C.

NEIL A. HOLTZMAN, M.D., Associate Professor of Pediatrics, The Johns Hopkins University School of Medicine, Baltimore, Maryland

CYRUS LEVINTHAL, Ph.D., Professor of Biology, Columbia University, New York, New York

ORLANDO J. MILLER, M.D., Professor of Human Genetics and Development and of Obstetrics and Gynecology, Columbia University College of Physicians and Surgeons, New York, New York.

ARNO G. MOTULSKY, M.D., Professor of Medicine and Genetics, University of Washington School of Medicine, Seattle, Washington

ROBERT F. MURRAY, JR., M.D., Professor of Pediatrics and Medicine, Howard University College of Medicine, Washington, D.C.

IRWIN M. ROSENSTOCK, Ph.D., Chairman, Department of Health Behavior and Health Education, The University of Michigan School of Public Health, Ann Arbor, Michigan

DAVID ROSENTHAL, Ph.D., Chief, Laboratory of Psychology, National Institute of Mental Health, Rockville, Maryland

GERALD ROSENTHAL, Ph.D., Director, National Center for Health Services Research, Health Resources Administration, Rockville, Maryland

WILLIAM J. SCHULL, Ph.D., Professor of Population Genetics, Graduate School of Biomedical Sciences, University of Texas Health Science Center, Houston, Texas

CHARLES R. SCRIVER, M.D., C.M., Professor of Pediatrics, McGill University, Montreal Children's Hospital Research Institute, Montreal, Canada

Staff

ARTEMIS P. SIMOPOULOS, M.D., *Project Director;* Acting Executive Secretary, Division of Medical Sciences, Assembly of Life Sciences, National Research Council

Acknowledgments

The Committee is most grateful to the following persons, who provided material for or prepared a number of significant sections of this report:

Artemis P. Simopoulos, M.D., Project Director and Acting Executive Secretary of the Division of Medical Sciences, Assembly of Life Sciences, National Research Council, who prepared papers that were incorporated into Part III, Chapters 2 and 3, and who also prepared Table 5-1, Part IV, "Survey of State Screening Programs for Inborn Errors of Metabolism"; Marilyn Jahn, M.S., of the University of Pennsylvania, who performed the field study of PKU legislation; Elena O. Nightingale, M.D., Ph.D., National Academy of Sciences Resident Fellow, who compiled the tables that comprise Appendix C; and Norman Fost, M.D., Department of Pediatrics, University of Wisconsin School of Medicine, who contributed Part VI, Chapter 11, on the ethical aspects of genetic screening; Felicity Skidmore, of the University of Wisconsin, who assisted in the organization and editing of the report; and Allyn M. Mortimer and Jill Perrott, of the Division of Medical Sciences, who helped assemble the report and assisted with typing, verification of references, and proofreading.

Contents

I

RECOMMENDATIONS

GENERAL

1. *Genetic screening, when carried out under controlled conditions, is an appropriate form of medical care when the following criteria are met:*

a. There is evidence of substantial public benefit and acceptance, including acceptance by medical practitioners.

b. Its feasibility has been investigated and it has been found that benefits outweigh costs; appropriate public education can be carried out; test methods are satisfactory; laboratory facilities are available; and resources exist to deal with counseling, follow-up, and other consequences of testing.

c. An investigative pretest of the program has shown that costs are acceptable; education is effective; informed consent is feasible; aims of the program with regard to the size of the sample to be screened, the age of the screenees, and the setting in which the testing is to be done have been defined; laboratory facilities have been shown to fulfill requirements for quality control; techniques for communicating results are workable; qualified and effective counselors are available in sufficient number; and adequate provision for effective services has been made.

d. The means are available to evaluate the effectiveness and success of each step in the process.

2. *Screening for phenylketonuria should be continued, and additional studies directed to its improvement should be supported.* Although hind-

sight reveals that screening programs for phenylketonuria were instituted before the validity and effectiveness of all aspects of treatment, including appropriate dietary treatment, were thoroughly tested, current assessment reveals that case finding methods are reasonably efficient, the means for moving from test to definitive management are adequate, and the appropriate dietary treatment is harmless and effective. Experiences in screening for phenylketonuria, both favorable and adverse, constitute a valuable resource for guidance in the design and operation of future programs. It is important that these experiences be kept in mind and used where appropriate.

ORGANIZATIONAL

3. *Responsibility for the organization and control of genetic screening programs should be lodged in some agency representative of both the public and the health professions.* This is necessary because of the public nature of genetic screening and its use of public facilities. It is also essential because such screening carries some potential for invasion of privacy, "labeling," breach of confidentiality, and psychological abuse. The agency might take its authority from local or state government or from regional representation of a federal program.

4. *Public representation is necessary both in determining that a new screening program is clearly in the public interest and also in the design and operation of any such program.* This is because genetic screening is likely to affect, for one test or another and perhaps for many, every member of the population.

5. *Screening agencies should consult regularly with local medical societies, stimulating their cooperation and participation.* This is important in order to give genetic screening the maximum public and professional acceptance.

6. *The aims of genetic screening should be clearly formulated and spelled out by the initiators of any screening program and should be publicly articulated with precision and candor.* Thus there will be no possibility of a mistaken impression that the program is intended to be an instrument of discrimination or is devoted to any "eugenic" cause.

7. *Some degree of standardization of screening projects is desirable.* Demographic diversity, inequality of financial and educational resources of the various states, and the individuality of initiators of screening projects all lead to variation in the design, quality, and cost of screening programs. Standardization might be achieved by some national agency that could act as a clearinghouse for ideas and techniques, set standards, and exert quality control.

8. *Regional programs with laboratories and other facilities based on population numbers rather than political subdivisions should be developed to make screening services of high quality available equally to all.* Such programs would avoid the low priority currently given to genetic screening in states of low population density and low budget and would prevent the hardship otherwise suffered by the relatively few persons in such states to whom screening would be beneficial.

9. *In the future, genetic screening should be regarded as one among several preventive health measures and its development should take place in the context of the evolution of health care in general.* New projects should be dictated by general principles governing genetic screening rather than by pressures originating in the special qualities of particular diseases.

EDUCATIONAL

10. *It is essential to begin the study of human biology, including genetics and probability, in primary school, continuing with a more health-related curriculum in secondary school because*

a. In the absence of sufficient public knowledge of human biology and genetics, the difficulties of arousing concern over genetic diseases cannot be overcome, since even longstanding attempts to educate the public regarding traditional preventive health measures have had variable success.

b. In the short run, the educational aspects of genetic screening must consist of special campaigns devoted to each program. Sufficient knowledge of genetics, probability, and medicine leading to appropriate perceptions of susceptibility to and seriousness of genetic disease and of carrier status cannot be acquired as a consequence of incidental, accidental, or haphazard learning.

11. *Screening authorities could improve the effectiveness of public education by studying and employing methods devised and tested by professional students of health behavior and health education.* The use of the mass communication media and other techniques to change attitudes and behavior has not been particularly successful, partly because of failure to follow the appropriate precepts.

12. *Continuing education courses for physicians should place emphasis on human genetics and particularly on the practical application of population genetics. In medical schools the study of genetics should be included in courses of epidemiology and preventive medicine, as well as*

in courses of medicine, pediatrics, and obstetrics. Such emphasis would raise the level of genetic knowledge of physicians and would increase their orientation toward preventive medicine so that they would be able to take an active role in genetic screening.

13. *Schools of medicine, public health and hygiene, and allied health sciences, as well as universities, should receive support for programs to set standards and train persons to inform and counsel participants in screening programs.* Such counselors are already in short supply.

LEGAL

14. *Participation in a genetic screening program should not be made mandatory by law, but should be left to the discretion of the person tested or, if a minor, of the parents or legal guardian.*

15. *Identifying information obtained through genetic screening should not be made available to anyone other than the screenee except with the permission of the screenee or, in the case of a minor, with the permission of the parents or legal guardian.*

16. *Screening authorities should consult regularly with lawyers and other persons knowledgeable in ethics to avoid social consequences of screening that may be damaging.* These take the form of invasion of privacy, breach of confidentiality, and other transgressions of civil rights, as well as psychological damage resulting from being "labeled" or from misunderstandings about the significance of diseases and carrier states. The usefulness of or need for legislation to protect the participants in screening programs from such dangers should be reviewed from time to time.

17. *For states considering legislation mandating genetic screening, the Committee recommends examination of a law creating a Board on Hereditary Disorders such as that proposed by the Council of State Governments' Committee on Suggested State Legislation.*

RESEARCH

18. *Research in genetic screening should be governed by the rigorous standards employed in laboratory investigation.* Special efforts should be made to evaluate all aspects, even of routine procedures, and the social and ethical ramifications of screening in the lives of the persons tested should be investigated. So far, experience in genetic screening is insufficient to foresee and to forestall all possible untoward side effects. Accordingly, it should be approached in an experimental mood. At present, it is

impressions that prevail, rather than data collected and analyzed according to scientific rules.

19. *It is important that screening be used to study the natural history of genetic disorders for which there is no treatment at this time.* Such research, in which the object of screening is to discover the full range of expression of the disease, will further the development of new methods of treatment and can provide the control data needed to evaluate proposed treatments. Particular effort must be exerted to protect individuals identified by such screening against the psychological and social hazards that attend all screening programs, but whose impact may be enhanced by the lack of an effective treatment.

20. *Research should be supported in adapting discoveries of new genetic characteristics for screening purposes.* This research includes increasing the number and quality of tests, reducing their cost, building regional networks of laboratories and other facilities to broaden and improve service, and designing simple, inexpensive, and effective treatments for newly discovered diseases. The acquisition of genetic knowledge is proceeding exponentially, and much of it is germane to the aims of genetic screening.

21. *Research to discover polymorphic alleles occurring in high frequency should receive more substantial support.* Certain common alleles have been shown to be associated with disease, and it is predictable that many more will also be implicated.

II

INTRODUCTION

1 Prospects for Genetic Screening

DEFINITION

Genetic screening may be defined as a search in a population for persons possessing certain genotypes that (1) are already associated with disease or predispose to disease, (2) may lead to disease in their descendants, or (3) produce other variations not known to be associated with disease. The persons in the first category are indentified so that medical management may be provided. The second group is discovered so that reproductive options may be discussed. Both these categories are also counted for epidemiologic studies establishing incidence or prevalence figures. The third category gathers information for research purposes—that is, for the study of the genetic constitutions of populations.

For the sake of brevity, all three types of screening will be referred to from time to time simply as genetic screening. (A glossary of technical terms that appear frequently in the text may be found in Appendix B.)

Genetic screening is being pursued in the United States today and seems likely to expand, evolving in response to changes in genetics and medicine as they occur. This evolution is properly subject to some direction to see that the aims are constantly adjusted to the current state of knowledge and techniques as well as to the needs and receptivity of the people who are the objects of the screening. The major question addressed in this report, therefore, is: In what directions should screening proceed, and with what safeguards and provisos?

MODERN MEDICAL PRACTICE

There is general agreement that health care in the United States is undergoing radical change. Social progress, in the form of improvements in nutrition, sanitation, housing, and education, together with advances in medical technology, has brought about a significant decline both in infant mortality and in premature death at other stages of life. This fall in mortality has had two principal effects. First, there have been shifts in the patterns of diseases affecting both young and old, more anomalies and genetic conditions among the surviving young, and more chronic diseases among the old. Second, the increased numbers of persons of middle and old age who no longer die of diseases that have been eradicated constitute a growing pool of potential patients for those who treat the infirmities of old age.

Specifically, these trends mean a high incidence among patients in children's hospitals of disease transmitted by mendelian inheritance or due to chromosomal aberrations, as well as malformations and other disorders of more uncertain genetic derivation.[1-3] They also mean that, among adult patients, chronic debilitating diseases of middle and late age whose causes, although poorly defined, include an important "constitutional" or hereditary component[4,5] are increasingly common. Table 1-1 reveals the contribution of genetic diseases to the census of several children's hospitals.

Few estimates have been made of the incidence of genetic disease and disability in the population at large. Studies carried out in Northern Ireland and in British Columbia indicate that about 6% of persons born in those areas suffer some form of serious genetic disease at some time of life.[6,7] These figures include single-gene disorders, chromosomal aberrations, and malformations; they take in only severely handicapping diseases in which the genetic contribution is clear, while omitting most of the disorders that cause premature death in adult life and whose genetic origins we are only now beginning to appreciate. Thus they probably

TABLE 1-1 Relative Frequency of Causes of Diseases among Hospitalized Children (in Percent)

Study	Single Gene	Chromo-somal	Gene-Influenced	Unknown	Nongenetic
Montreal[1]	6.8	0.4	22.3	6.7	63.7
Baltimore[2]	6.4	0.7	31.5	8.2	53.2
Newcastle[a, 3]	8.5	2.5	31.0	17.0	41.0

[a]Mortality.

understate by a wide margin the true impact of genetic variation on the physiologic adjustment of human beings, which is still incalculable.

The management of all these hereditary disorders, both in early life and later, is complicated and demands facilities, money, and human energy—underlining the urgent need to discover their causes so as to design ways to treat them effectively and economically, to minimize their adverse effects, and, where possible, to prevent them altogether.[8]

The complexity of technique, as well as the cost, of the care of patients requiring hospitalization is well known to all; the former continues to proliferate and the latter to grow at a dismaying rate. Medical schools and teaching hospitals have responded to this intensification of care by training specialists capable of performing the requisite surgical artistry, of solving intricate diagnostic puzzles, and of managing often tricky, sometimes life-long, treatments. But since it is clear that hospitalized patients are a minority of the sick and that all but a small portion of health care is directed at ambulatory patients, new methods for primary care are also evolving, taking the form of comprehensive care clinics, prepaid group health plans, and health maintenance organizations intended to make health supervision available to all.[5,9] These mechanisms are shaped by the aims of providing early treatment of incipient disease, of offering education and counseling to patients and families in adapting to medical adversity, and of taking positive steps to prevent disease and enhance well-being. Medical education is responding with a renewed emphasis on the training of primary physicians and by creating new schools to train auxiliary medical personnel to meet these goals.[10,11]

An important outcome of these efforts to spread primary medical and health care (and possibly also the spur that initiated them) is a growing public perception of medical care as something to which everyone has a right. This awareness is manifest in action leading to federal legislation for universal health insurance and other forms of government support for health programs.

ADVANCES IN HUMAN GENETICS

The exuberant growth of knowledge of human genetics has been both a cause and a result of some of the changes in medicine already outlined—a cause because it has supplied the conceptual approach to the clarification of many newly described diseases, and an effect because the changing patterns of disease have made hereditary problems more visible and their elucidation more urgent.

The discovery of new inborn errors of metabolism and the resolution of syndromes into component disorders, each taking its origin from mutant genes occupying a single locus, are proceeding exponentially, and there appears to be no reason why the discovery and description of such disorders should not continue at a brisk rate for the foreseeable future. Indeed, our rapidly growing knowledge of enzymatically controlled metabolic pathways suggests that there is a vast reservoir of gentically determined metabolic variations yet to be discovered.

For many of the conditions already known, usually inherited as recessives, the enzyme whose activity is reduced has been determined and, in most, the heterozygote can be distinguished from the homozygote by means of tolerance tests or by direct enzyme assay.[12] Most dominantly inherited conditions, on the other hand, have resisted biochemical characterization, but for a few (C_1 esterase inhibitor* and some of the unstable hemoglobin variants are examples) there is evidence of altered activity of an enzyme or other protein that results in disease in heterozygotes. Many clinically indistinguishable phenotypes have been shown to be heterogeneous by demonstration of a deficiency in activity of quite different enzymes, indicating genetic as well as phenotypic heterogeneity. In addition, differences in electrophoretic and other physical properties of the affected protein have been demonstrated in unrelated persons; this implies allelic diversity, which means that the same disorder is the result of different mutations in different persons. For some of these inborn errors, relatively simple tests suitable for mass screening for homozygotes, for heterozygotes, or for both, are available.

In contrast, other kinds of phenotypes whose biochemical attributes are unknown and that are commonly inherited as dominants have also been described, and the heterogeneity of these syndromes is demonstrated by showing the similarity of clinical expression within families, as opposed to differences among unrelated families.[13] Here the decision as to whether the differences can be assigned to more than one allele or to genes at different loci is more difficult. Again, there is no reason to suppose we are any nearer the end in establishing a complete list of these conditions than we are in the description of the recessive inborn errors.

The advances in biochemistry that are responsible for the discovery of the inborn errors of metabolism have also been employed to advantage in studies that are beginning to uncover both the quality and the quantity of heritable human variation, whether related to disease or not. Such studies have revealed that while assiduous effort will usually be rewarded by the discovery of rare mutant genes with frequencies of 0.1% or less for nearly all existing loci, common representatives, or alleles with frequencies of 1% or more, are found for perhaps 30% of loci.[14,15] Be-

* A defect in C_1 esterase inhibitor production results in angioneurotic edema.

cause the methods used for such detection underestimate the true extent of this variability, or polymorphism, reasonable extrapolations suggest that there are common variants for more than half the human gene loci and that each person might be heterozygous for at least 7% of them and perhaps for as many as 20%. These assessments are made by analysis of the physical properties of enzymes or other protein products of the genes and have nothing to do with their meaning, if any, for health or disease. On the other hand, some of the common protein variants (glucose-6-phosphate dehydrogenase A^- and some hemoglobins are examples) are directly implicated in diseases, and although the contribution of others to human variation is not obvious, it is a reasonable inference that many of them do contribute to individual differences and that some will be found to be associated with, and perhaps to predispose to, disease.[16,17] Further, since these are the common variant alleles in the gene pool, if they are involved in disease at all, it will be with common diseases, particularly those in which a genetic component exists but is not yet defined—the so-called multifactorial disorders.

Advances in cytogenetics are keeping pace with those in other fields. New techniques have made it possible to identify each chromosome and, in severe aberrations, to correlate the clinical features with the cytologic change.[18] It has also promoted a burst of activity in the assignment of gene loci to specific chromosomes and in sorting out the spatial relationships of one locus to another.[19] Here, too, chromosomal variations are being discovered whose clinical effects, if any, are uncertain. Like some of the polymorphic genes, some of these variations may, given appropriate conditions of environment and experience, lead to nonadaptive function or behavior.

THE IMPACT OF GENETICS ON MEDICINE

These advances in genetics have some substantial conceptual implications for medicine, both in introducing new thoughts about old diseases and in suggesting new ways to deal with them.

Although most inborn errors of metabolism are rare, generally varying downward in frequency from 1/10,000, their heterozygote or carrier frequencies are not, varying from 1/1,000 to several percent. This introduces the problem of rather large numbers of people with a significant probability for mating with another carrier, such mating leading to a risk of 1 : 4 of producing an afflicted child. If the intent is to detect all patients with such diseases in order to decide whether to treat them, or in order to prevent their conception or birth, then very large numbers of persons must be examined in order to find the few who are carriers.

A Definition of Genetic Disease

In general, the carriers of those mutant genes that in homozygotes are associated with inborn errors of metabolism show no overt expression of the disease or any other obvious nonadaptive effect, and some of these genes are sufficiently common as to be numbered among the polymorphic alleles that may be presumed to underlie much normal human variation. On the other hand, as we have seen, in quantitative tests of gene action, values for the heterozygotes fall somewhere between those of normals* and the homozygotes. That is, the heterozygotes are not normal with respect to that particular gene, since they can be distinguished from persons presumed to possess only the normal genes; but neither are they diseased since in tests of qualities everyone would agree represent disease the heterozygotes are not distinctive. This is presumably due to those regulatory processes, or homeostatic powers, of the body that preserve physiologic equilibrium in the face of threats of special conditions or experiences. These capabilities for adjustment, however, can be exceeded. Thus, the heterozygous parent of a phenylketonuric child can be induced to show some of the biochemical manifestations of that disease by doses of phenylalanine that the possessor of two normal alleles could metabolize with ease, and the latter could be made phenylketonuric by even larger amounts of phenylalanine, which would overwhelm even his capacity to dispose of it. Thus all disease may be represented as the result of pressures that have overpowered the mechanisms of adjustment, and the genetic contribution to any disease will be in the direction of more or less resistance to the pressures, depending upon the qualities of the gene or genes most directly involved.

According to this definition, on the one hand, the whole species may be genetically incompetent to maintain its state of favorable adaptation in the face of some threats—for example, extreme dietary deficiency of essential amino acids and vitamins—while, on the other hand, some persons possessing a particular genotype, even a single mutant gene, may be destroyed by conditions that to most genotypes are common experience. In addition, such is the variability of homeostasis that the same mutations may be associated in different individuals with a range of manifestations varying from normal to death. This variability is sometimes neglected, especially when ascertaining causes by some biochemical marker, so that treatment may be instituted when it is not necessary. It should be noted that this definition does not state that genes *cause*

* By "normal" is meant the most common genotype found in the population, the genotype that maximizes the adaptability of the individual to a particular environment or to a particular environmental agent or does not produce disease.

diseases, but rather that the actions of the genes have been insufficient to maintain equilibrium in the face of special experiences. If these provocative conditions are generally prevalent, as for example a common dietary component, the genetic origin of the disorder will be more evident since all members of families who possess the relevant genotype will show at least some of the effects; but if the precipitating conditions prevail only occasionally, the disease will appear sporadically and its genetic origin may be overlooked.

The discovery in individuals of mutant genes that lead to disease in the face of occasional, but discretely defined, menacing conditions elucidates what was called "idiosyncrasy" in the medical literature of the past. The discovery of other mutants in individuals suffering chronic disorders whose environmental origins appear to be both manifold and diverse gives precision to such designations as "host factors," "constitutional predisposition," or "diathesis." It is no doubt dangerous to generalize in the present state of ignorance, but it may turn out that, in general, idiosyncracies will be shown to be the result of mutants at single loci that cause a deficiency in activity of some protein specified by the gene, while the "diatheses" or "constitutional predispositions" will often be seen to be the result of genes that by themselves produce only minor or moderate change in function, but that, acting in concert with one or several others in a climate of repeated or persistent exposure to adverse conditions, allow that slow erosion of physiologic adjustment that culminates early or late in the overt signs and symptoms of chronic disease.

The effects of chromosomal aberration are no less variable than those of mutant genes. Some are associated with grotesque distortion of development; others appear to lead, under appropriate but still undefined circumstances, to nonadaptive behavior; while others do nothing at all, or what they do falls within the definition of normal.

Medical Management

The traditional medical response to disease consists of treatment where possible and prevention whenever it can be accomplished. The former consists of some corrective action directed to the cause or, if that is not possible, of management and support in the form of ameliorative procedures or advice and help in adjusting to the condition. Prevention depends upon knowing the conditions that precipitate the disease and eradicating or avoiding them. Genetic diseases are no less susceptible to these approaches than others, but the specific forms of both treatment and prevention are a little different.

Treatment directed to the cause of a genetic disease involves addition of that which is lacking, or removal of that which is injurious. This differs from the care of nongenetic diseases in that genetic disease usually persists, although not always with the same intensity, throughout life. When the pathogenesis of the disorder is not known, or when it consists of some form of irreversible developmental distortion, the physician must fall back upon those forms of management that relieve symptoms or improve social adjustment. Treatment is also in a sense preventive, since many genetic disorders (having their onset during some phase of maturation) may, if untreated, end up in gross developmental aberration, if not in death. This underlines the necessity of identifying affected persons at birth, or, at any rate, before the onset of such unfavorable events.

Prevention of genetic diseases takes two forms. The first is straightforward and consists of finding susceptible persons in order to teach them to avoid specific conditions that are known to precipitate the manifestations. For some the adjustment is rather uncomplicated, involving only taking medication or avoiding certain drugs or dietary components; but for some disorders the necessary design for life may be much at variance with prevailing customs or with the entrenched habits of the family in which an affected baby must be raised. In addition, the knowledge of the predisposition may itself prejudice development, engendering a climate sure to fulfill dire predictions or creating those feelings of separateness and oddity that are so damaging to health and maturation. The second form of prevention consists of attempts to forestall the birth of affected persons, either through the agency of abortion after antenatal diagnosis, or by providing a couple contemplating childbearing with information as to the susceptibility of their offspring and as to the odds for having an affected child, so that they may make an informed decision. Thus, preventive measures may be as demanding of the physician's time, energy, and tact as treatment.

Genetics and Preventive Medicine

The number of genetic diseases, predispositions, carrier states, and other conditions that can be detected by tests adaptable to widespread screening is growing apace and will continue to do so. Further, the means to treat effectively or to prevent many such disorders also are accumulating, though at a slower rate.

On the medical side, the new emphasis on primary care and prevention to be carried out by family practitioners and allied health personnel, in comprehensive care clinics, group practice settings, and health maintenance organizations, will create an improved setting for the accomplishment of screening aims.

Should increased emphasis on prevention of disease and the promotion of good health ever become more than a pious hope, then analysis of each individual genotype will be an essential prelude to guidance toward and away from particular conditions known to enhance or to threaten the individual's adaptive state. Such an approach is somewhat at variance with current preventive medicine in which rules of avoidance or moderation are recommended for everyone. The genetic view, which predicts that not everyone is equally susceptible to all threats, suggests that nonsusceptibles should be spared the fearful anticipation of events that never materialize and the onerous requirement to abide by rules that are, for them, irrelevant.

Universal rules of preventive medicine would be more to the point in the underdeveloped areas of the world where health is measured by the availability of necessities. In those countries people are subject to selective forces that act on the genetic incapacity of the whole population to survive in the face of the lack of basic nutrients or overwhelming exposure to pathogenic organisms and parasites; individual genetic variations have less quantitative importance. But in societies of abundance, differential selection acts through the agencies of individual habits and ways of living, as well as through pollutants, drugs, chemical additives, and special occupational exposures almost too numerous to count. If one were to make universal preventive rules to cover such a multitude of threats, the life of asceticism such instructions would dictate would offer little fulfillment, and in any case human nature would cause them to be little honored. But to point out to a specific person the conditions under which his particular endowment may fail to protect him from impairment of his health offers some chance of rational behavior on his part.

That now is a good time to consider so radical a change in the traditions of medical care is attested to not only by the advances in genetics and changes in patterns of health care but also by the accelerating public awareness of the costs of after-the-fact medical attention and the increasing demand for medical care as a right.

Obstacles to Be Overcome

This merger of genetic and medical capabilities cannot, however, be expected in the immediate future. Experience suggests that most practicing physicians are not prepared for it, either in knowledge of genetics or by traditional modes of practice. Nor have the proponents of the missions of public health and preventive medicine given much attention to the study of genetics or to genetic screening. Public education in biology does not provide the persons who are the objects of screening programs with sufficient information of genetics to participate knowledgeably. Furthermore, the experiences of the past (exemplified in programs of screening for phenylketonuria and sickle cell disease and trait that are described later in this report) attest to the need for study, not only of screening methods and logistics, but of the many social, ethical, educational, and legal questions that are only now being raised. Some of these questions are quite novel and are not commonly considered in ordinary office practice. They concern legal rights and whether new statutes are needed to protect them; confidentiality and dissemination of information about people's genetic constitution; and new ethical issues in the doctor–patient relationship, and particularly in the ways physicians use or misuse techniques and knowledge that give them extraordinary new power for good and harm.

As further screening tests become available, their benefits must be demonstrated in well-designed and controlled studies before they become widely employed and integrated into public health programs or routine office procedure. Nor should each new test be studied and employed without reference to others, since screening for genetic diseases and variations will not be limited to the detection of one or two or a few genetic characteristics. Rather, programs should be designed so that new tests, no matter what their number, can be added as they are tried out and are shown to have benefit. Genetic theory suggests that the human genotype contains tens of thousands of loci and that mutants must exist for most or all of them. *The limit for characteristics to be screened will be set, therefore, by the usefulness of the knowledge gained, the costs of obtaining it, and its impact on the persons tested rather than by the number of tests that can be devised.*

Screening and the "Perfectibility" of Man

It may be appealing to some to think that genetic knowledge could be used, through selective breeding, reproductive manipulation, genetic engineering, and the like, to improve the heritable quality of the human species and that genetic screening might be one of the means to this end. In fact, none of these possibilities is likely soon to be accomplished, nor is genetic improvement likely to become a legitimate goal of screening or of other applications of genetic knowledge. There is now a considerable body of literature pressing for public debate of the aims and methods of the new eugenics with the intention of testing these ideas in the moral climate of the day so that they cannot be sprung on an uninformed and dazzled public. However, there is a strong countervailing inertia in the conservatism of medical practitioners and many other members of society who tend to be wary of designs for human "improvement."

A more subtle threat exists in the erroneous idea that screening or genetic knowledge could be used in some way, not so much to improve the species, but to make the outcome of every pregnancy a perfectly healthy baby, or to eliminate all disease, or to make everyone "normal." These aims can never be realized, but given currency in the public mind such ideas could lead to a constricted view of normality and a loss of respect for genetic and phenotypic diversity. Further, such aims could tend to impose a sense of restricted choice on the public, when in fact the purpose of screening and the uses of all genetic knowledge should be to increase options and make choices informed and free of the constraints of ignorance.

REFERENCES

1. Scriver, C. R., J. L. Neal, R. Saginur, and A. Clow. The frequency of genetic disease and congenital malformation among patients in a pediatric hospital. Can. Med. Assoc. J. 108:1111–1115, 1973.
2. Childs, B., S. M. Miller, and A. G. Bearn. Gene mutation as a cause of human disease, pp. 3–14. In H. E. Sutton and M. I. Harris, eds. Mutagenic Effects of Environmental Contaminants. New York: Academic Press, 1972.
3. Roberts, D. F., J. Chavez, and S. D. Court. The genetic component in child mortality. Arch. Dis. Child. 45:33–38, 1970.
4. Glazier, W. H. The task of medicine. Sci. Amer. 228:13–18, 1973.
5. White, K. L. Life and death and medicine. Sci. Amer. 229:22–33, 1973.
6. Stevenson, A. C. The load of hereditary defects in human populations. Radiat. Res. Suppl. 1:306–325, 1959.
7. Trimble, B. K. The amount of hereditary disease in human populations. Personal communication.
8. Thomas, L. Commentary: The future impact of science and technology on medicine. Bioscience 24:99–105, 1974.
9. Wilson, V. E. HMOS: Hopes and aspirations. J. Med. Educ. 48(Suppl.):7–10, 1973.
10. Millis, J. S. A Rational Public Policy for Medical Education and Its Financing. New York: The National Fund for Medical Education, 1971.
11. Challenor, B. D., J. Wicks, and G. I. Lythcott. Community medicine: An evolving discipline. Ann. Intern. Med. 76:689–695, 1972.
12. Brock, D. J. H., and O. Mayo, eds. The Biochemical Genetics of Man. New York: Academic Press, 1972.
13. McKusick, V. A. Mendelian Inheritance in Man. 3rd ed. Baltimore: Johns Hopkins Press, 1971.
14. Harris, H., and D. A. Hopkinson. Average heterozygosity per locus in man: An estimate based on the incidence of enzyme polymorphisms. Ann. Hum. Genet. 36:9–20, 1972.
15. Harris, H., D. A. Hopkinson, and E. B. Robson. The incidence of rare alleles determining electrophoretic variants: Data on 43 enzyme loci in man. Ann. Hum. Genet. 37:237–253, 1974.
16. Neel, J. V., and W. J. Schull. On some trends in understanding the genetics of man. Perspect. Biol. Med. 11:565–602, 1968.

17. Childs, B., and V. M. Der Kaloustian. Genetic heterogeneity. N. Engl. J. Med. 279:1205–1212, 1267–1274, 1968.
18. Hamerton, J. L. Human Cytogenetics. Vol. I, General Cytogenetics; Vol. II, Clinical Cytogenetics. New York: Academic Press, 1971.
19. McKusick, V. A., and G. A. Chase. Human genetics. Ann. Rev. Genet. 7:435–473, 1973.

III

SCREENING FOR PHENYLKETONURIA

Assessment of the successes and failures of screening for phenylketonuria (PKU) was one aspect of the Committee's charge. Several meetings, therefore, were devoted to interviews with officials of state health departments and physicians in treatment centers associated with them, experts in screening methods, and the director and other staff members of the Collaborative Study, a group of centers that are pooling their resources in an effort to obtain statistically significant answers to questions still outstanding with respect to PKU.

To learn more about the history of the social aspects of these programs, including the role of local chapters of the Association for Retarded Children in pressing for legislation, and the part played by state health officials and the local medical societies, a sociologist was employed by the Committee to visit 12 states (selected according to variations in demographic and economic characteristics) and interview legislators, public health people, and physicians involved in local programs; the results are tabulated in Appendix C. In addition, the role of the Children's Bureau was investigated by interviews with appropriate staff and by a review of the minutes and transactions of meetings (see also Chapter 3).

In the United States, 43 states have passed laws mandating screening for PKU. In order to study these laws in detail, each state was asked to submit its statute together with its regulations. In addition, regulations were obtained from states that do not have statutes.

The data collected and the conclusions and recommendations of the Committee, together with appropriate references to the literature, are presented in this Part.

2 Historical Experience of Screening for PKU

Phenylketonuria (PKU) is sought in more individuals in the United States than any other obvious genetic disorder.* Some 90% of all newborns are now screened (see Appendix C). Since 1963, 43 states have passed laws requiring or recommending PKU screening in newborns. These programs were undertaken with the following assumptions:

- that untreated PKU results in severe mental retardation
- that restriction of dietary intake of phenylalanine prevents the development of retardation in infants with PKU, provided treatment is started soon after birth and
- that PKU can be detected in the newborn

In this section the evidence regarding these assumptions is analyzed. As will quickly become apparent, screening for PKU was begun with only a partial understanding of the disease and its prognosis. Nevertheless, screening has produced many benefits, including some increase in our understanding of the disorder.

* Screening for PKU has been going on in the United Kingdom longer than in the United States. One member of the Committee, therefore, spent 2 months visiting centers and investigating programs in England, Scotland, and Ireland. These programs are in many respects superior to those in the United States, one reason being that they operate under a National Health Service, which facilitates the communication among different components of the health delivery system. A description of the PKU screening system in the United Kingdom appears as Appendix H.

RETARDATION AND PHENYLKETONURIA

An Apparent Association

The association of phenylketonuria with mental retardation was discovered by Fölling in 1934.[1] Shortly thereafter, Jervis surveyed 20,300 institutionalized retardates in the United States and found 0.8% to have phenylketonuria.[2] Although it is clear that phenylketonuria is associated with mental retardation, the treatment of PKU has been challenged on the grounds that the IQ of such patients is often normal even without treatment.[3] However, evidence for this view is difficult to find. For example, it has been estimated that fewer than 10% of untreated phenylketonurics have IQ's over 50, and recent surveys of nonretarded populations have discovered only five individuals with PKU who have IQ's above 75 among 358,797 screened.[4,5] Of these, three were mentally abnormal[6] and the other two were found in an institution for the mentally ill.[4] In an exhaustive literature search, Hsia[7] found reports of 23 individuals meeting the diagnostic criteria for PKU who have IQ's over 70. Only three of these had IQ's over 100. However, reports of more than 2,000 retarded phenylketonurics appeared. Thus, while an occasional individual with PKU has been found who is not retarded, sufficient data are available to reject Bessman's contention[3] that "many people with normal intelligence have now been discovered who have blood concentrations of phenylalanine in the range found in patients with severe retardation."

The criteria used to diagnose PKU in the surveys of older children and adults were a positive urine $FeCl_3$ test or a blood phenylalanine of 20 mg% or more, or both. Serum phenylalanine in the normal population is approximately 2 mg%. The risk of retardation in individuals with persistent moderate elevations, between 6 and 20 mg%, is much less than among those with higher elevations.[8-11] Thus, hyperphenylalaninemia is not synonymous with retardation.

Phenylalanine Restriction to Prevent Retardation

In patients with phenylketonuria, phenylalanine hydroxylase (the enzyme that catalyzes the synthesis of tyrosine from phenylalanine) is defective.[12] As a consequence, phenylalanine accumulates, although some is diverted to other pathways. Tyrosine deficiency develops unless adequate amounts are provided in the diet.

The pathogenesis of the resulting mental retardation is not understood. Increased concentrations of phenylalanine or its metabolites interfere with the transport and metabolism of several other amino acids. The resulting imbalances undoubtedly contribute to structural and functional changes in the central nervous system.[13] In view of the multiple reactions involved, there are many opportunities for modification of the effects of the enzyme deficiency. Thus, it is not surprising that different degrees of retardation, even among siblings, have been reported.[14,15]

In the mid-1950's it was reported that diets low in phenylalanine could reverse the major biochemical abnormalities associated with PKU.[16,17] Although short-term studies in which therapy was directed at either providing tyrosine[18] or reducing phenylalanine metabolites[19]—without lowering the phenylalanine level—proved successful chemically, they were not pursued to determine their effect on mental development after the low-phenylalanine diet became available.

Removal of phenylalanine from casein hydrolysates was accomplished relatively inexpensively by passage over charcoal, and a commercial preparation was made available in the United States by 1958. As for the age to begin treatment, Knox and later Baumeister agreed that results were best when the diet was started no later than 20 weeks of age.[4,20]

When started later, there was a great variation in IQ and virtually no correlation between the age at which treatment was begun and the IQ attained. Knox also suggested that initiation of therapy after 3 years of age was "without impressive change in mental and neurological status."[13]

If, in order to be effective, treatment must be undertaken in the first few months of life, then biochemical diagnosis is required, since, with the exception of eczema and odor (which are not always present), the clinical findings of PKU are seldom evident before 1 or 2 years of age. Detection of all infants at risk requires biochemical screening of all newborn babies. Restricting biochemical studies only to the newborn infants of families with previously affected children would result in the discovery of only a small proportion of all babies born with the disorder.[22]

THE DEVELOPMENT OF MASS SCREENING

When phenylalanine restriction was first reported to be of apparent benefit, the only feasible screening test for PKU was the urine ferric chloride test, used by Fölling in discovering the disorder. This test measures phenylpyruvic acid and not phenylalanine. A positive test is the result of deamination of phenylalanine by a transaminase whose activity is often low or absent in the neonatal period. In addition, phenylpyruvic acid is relatively unstable, and the test is most accurate when performed on fresh urine.[23] Because of the shortcomings of the urine test, the Children's Bureau Technical Committee on Clinical Programs for Mentally Retarded

Children concluded, in 1959, that there was no test suitable for populationwide screening that combined the advantages of ease, low cost, and sensitivity.* Despite these reservations, however, the Children's Bureau recommended that the ferric chloride test become part of routine testing in clinics, hospitals, and doctors' offices.[25]

Initial Trial of the Guthrie Test

In 1961 Guthrie reported a microbiological assay for blood phenylalanine adaptable to mass screening.[26] In 1962 the Children's Bureau approved a proposal submitted by Guthrie[27] "to demonstrate the value of a simple blood phenylalanine screening method to test specimens collected, as part of regular hospital routine, from infants born in hospitals."

State health department laboratories were to choose hospitals to be included in the study and to conduct the test in the state laboratory. Infants who were discharged before the third day and nonwhite infants (in whom the risk of PKU was considered to be much lower) were not to be included. In order to determine whether any infants were missed by the first test, mothers were given a filter-paper collecting unit at the time the first test was obtained in the hospital. They were asked to soak the paper with urine from a wet diaper when the infant was 3 weeks old and mail it to the laboratory. Blood and urine phenylalanine were both determined by the bacterial inhibition assay developed by Guthrie.

Twenty-nine states eventually contributed data on a total of 404,568 infants. Among the 275 infants whose first test showed an elevated phenylalanine, 37 were confirmed to have phenylketonuria. One infant whose initial test was read as negative was found to have a blood phenylalanine of greater than 20 mg% at 4 weeks of age on a specimen sent in by a private physician. This baby had been tested originally on the third day of age. Only 261,344 urine samples were returned and no additional cases were discovered as a result of the urine test. However, 4 of the 37 babies with PKU had negative urine tests. Thus, since the urine test was shown to produce false negative results, the true sensitivity of the Guthrie method could not be established by the field trial, and it was concluded that a follow-up blood test was needed.[27]

Two of the thirty-seven babies who proved to have PKU were screened on the second day of life and had minimal elevation (6-8 mg% on the first test). Of the remaining 35, 8 were screened on the third day and only one of these had an initial blood level of greater than 20 mg%. In

* One year later the Ministry of Health in the United Kingdom came to the opposite conclusion and recommended routine screening of urine of infants aged 4–6 weeks by a modified ferric chloride method.[24]

contrast, of the 26 phenylketonurics initially screened on the fourth day or later, 14 had initial serum phenylalanine levels of greater than 20 mg%. Thus, the earlier in the newborn period that the test was performed, the lower the concentration of blood phenylalanine. In the report, Guthrie and Whitney[27] stated, "It is undoubtedly possible that there may be a period during the first few hours of protein feeding when any assay might fail to detect an infant with PKU."

Pressures for Screening

Most states involved in the Guthrie field trials continued to screen, and an increasing number of states established programs. By 1964, four states had laws requiring screening of infants for PKU.[25]

In 1963 the National Association for Retarded Children (NARC), a group consisting of parents of retarded children and interested health professionals, recommended "that State Associations emphasize the urgency of testing all newborns for metabolic disorders, including PKU" and that they "bring the NARC policy position to the attention of state and local health officers" and "to the attention of the Presidents of the State Medical Societies and solicit their support." While it did not recommend mandatory screening, it pressed "for legislation . . . that would direct the State Board of Health to make recommendations for appropriate screening tests as they are developed and accepted."

On September 30, 1964, the Children's Bureau urged "the screening of all newborn infants for PKU on a routine basis."[28] In October 1964, NARC strengthened its stand and went "on record as recommending mandatory legislation for the screening of PKU."[29,30] Two members of the Public Health Services Committee of NARC sat on the Technical Committee on Clinical Programs for Mentally Retarded Children of the Children's Bureau.[25,30]*

Questions Not Answered at the Inception of Mass Screening

When mass screening began in the United States in 1962, a number of questions relating to prognosis for phenylketonuria with and without treatment were still unanswered:

1. *What proportion of infants with persistent phenylalanine elevations were at risk for retardation?*

* The information gathered on the social aspects of the history of PKU legislation, including the role of the medical profession, is tabulated in Appendix C, Tables C-1 through C-3.

In 1964 the assumption was made that every baby in whom the blood phenylalanine was persistently above normal (4 mg%) had PKU.[27,31] Using this criterion, the original field trial in this country gave an "unexpectedly high" yield of cases.[27]

It soon became apparent that not all infants with persistent elevations were destined to become retarded. Several infants whose screening test results were only moderately elevated (less than 20 mg% of phenylalanine) were found to have older siblings, born before any screening tests were available, who had elevations of similar magnitude but were not retarded.[32] Approximately two thirds of all infants with elevated phenylalanine levels on both screening and follow-up tests have only moderate elevations[33] and are not at risk for retardation secondary to their hyperphenylalaninemia.

2. *Does restriction of phenylalanine early in life prevent retardation in infant with* PKU?

If all of the infants with persistent but moderate elevations of serum phenylalanine (less than 20 mg%) were included among those treated for PKU, on the belief that they would become retarded, then the treatment would appear to benefit a large proportion without having any real effect on those destined to develop retardation. It seems quite likely that infants not at risk for retardation were treated for PKU in the first few years of the screening programs. Their inclusion thus made the evaluation of therapy tenuous.[34]

Relatively few infants placed on a diet in the first 3 months of life had reached an age, at the time of the Guthrie field trial, when their ultimate intellectual achievement could be predicted. In a perceptive review published in 1964 Kleinman concluded that a longer follow-up was needed to determine the ultimate effects of phenylalanine restriction on intellectual function. He wrote[4]:

> Developmental tests of infants and young children emphasize sensory and motor capacities while intelligence tests in later childhood involve verbal and conceptual skill. . . . These factors limit not only the diagnostic power but also the predictive power of development and intelligence tests.

In studies that compared the IQ's of subjects treated early with those of their unaffected siblings, the scores were seldom obtained at the same chronological age; usually the treated subjects were younger. In almost all published studies the psychologist was aware of the treatment status of the child being tested; in addition, since tests were performed at frequent intervals, the possibility of a practice effect was raised.[3]

3. *At what level should the blood phenylalanine be maintained (by*

dietary regulation) in order to provide optimal physical and mental growth in infants and children with PKU?

Dietary deficiency of phenylalanine in treated phenylketonurics was well documented in 1966.[35] In 1968 Hackney *et al.* found impaired physical development if the serum phenylalanine frequently dropped below 1.5 mg% during the first 6 months and suggested that mental development might be impaired by "overtreatment."[36]

Thus, screening was started, frequently under mandatory laws, when questions regarding diagnosis, prognosis, and optimal management were unanswered. With screening organized along state lines, patients were usually referred to centers within the state for confirmation and management. Consequently, except in the most populous states, few clinics accumulated a large enough number of patients to carry out any systematic study that would yield statistically valid answers in a relatively short period of time.

4. *Can the low-phenylalanine diet be terminated after most brain growth is completed?*

The low-phenylalanine diet severely restricts the foods PKU children can eat. Not infrequently PKU youngsters about the time they enter school demand additional foods and often resort to stealing, imposing a significant stress on the family. It is important, therefore, to know how long dietary treatment should be continued.

Finding the Answers

Criteria for Diagnosis As it became apparent that variant forms of hyperphenylalaninemia were not associated with retardation, diagnostic criteria became more stringent. Since the late 1960's accepted criteria are a blood phenylalanine of 20 mg% or more, a tyrosine of less than 5 mg%, and a positive response to a phenylalanine challenge after the low-phenylalanine diet has been started.[37] With these criteria, it is doubtful that PKU is being overdiagnosed. The incidence of PKU discovered as a result of screening in 16 states between 1968 and 1970 was 5.4 per 100,000 infants screened[38] (see also Appendix C, Table C-5). This figure agrees remarkably well with the estimates extrapolated from the prevalence of PKU among the mentally retarded in the prescreening era[2,4] (see p. 24, above).

Based on the infrequency of normal intelligence in untreated phenylketonurics, it is doubtful that more than 5% of infants meeting these stringent criteria would escape some degree of retardation without treatment.[5] This small group cannot be distinguished by any biochemical test currently available as part of the diagnostic routine.

Assessing the Effectiveness of Therapy: The Collaborative Study of Children Treated for Phenylketonuria At a meeting of the Children's Bureau Technical Committee on Clinical Programs for Mentally Retarded Children in September 1964, Dr. Richard Koch raised the possibility of a collaborative study of children with PKU. The issues would never be resolved "in any one individual clinic," Koch said, "because each individual who became a sort of pioneer in this field came into it with very distinct viewpoints and great feelings. To ameliorate these disparate points of view, it seemed to me that we had to have some people who felt one way meet with people who felt another way, so that we could come to a middle channel."[39]

In 1965 the Committee on the Handicapped Child of the American Academy of Pediatrics concluded that[40]

> much more data, taking into account all the known variables must be accumulated and carefully analyzed before any definitive statements can be advanced regarding the precise value of diet in preventing or ameliorating phenylketonuria. This will require some considerable time. A collaborative study to evaluate management of this disease would be valuable.

By the late 1960's it appeared likely that early administration of the low-phenylalanine diet could prevent marked retardation, but whether it permitted the highest level of intelligence anticipated for a child (based on the intelligence of his sibs and parents and a number of socioeconomic factors) remained unclear.[41]

The Children's Bureau provided funds for a Collaborative Project in 1966, but it was not until the end of 1967 that the project actually began. The study was designed to answer two questions[42]:

> What are the effects of diets restricted in phenylalanine on the physical, cognitive, and psychosocial development of PKU children? If dietary therapy is completely effective, then PKU children treated prospectively from near birth should be comparable with their non-PKU siblings and other normative samples on variables tested. If dietary therapy is completely ineffective, then PKU children treated prospectively from near birth should be comparable with untreated PKU siblings, on variables tested. An important secondary question is: does dietary control of serum phenylalanine at low versus moderate levels result in different outcomes? If so, then PKU children treated prospectively at these two levels should be significantly different on variables tested.

Nineteen centers, each located in a state that conducted routine screening of newborns for PKU, collaborated, although three have since dropped out, largely because of inadequate funds. To be judged in need of treatment, babies must have at least two serum phenylalanine determinations at or above 20 mg% and two serum tyrosine determinations of below 5 mg%. In addition, they must respond to a challenge with phenylalanine, between 90 and 120 days after the tentative diagnosis, by an elevation of blood phenylalanine to greater than or equal to 20 mg% 72 hours after the start of the challenge. Treatment of those meeting all of the above criteria must begin immediately after the results of the phenylalanine challenge are known. Approximately 15% of babies meeting the initial two criteria do not give a positive response to the challenge. At the discretion of the local clinic director, these babies may be placed on regular diets. When this is done, levels over 20 mg% are seldom observed.

Infants who met the requirements for tentative diagnosis were assigned to one of two treatment groups. For those in the first group, the aim was to maintain blood phenylalanine between 1 and 5.4 mg% through dietary regulation. For those in the second, the aim was to maintain the serum phenylalanine between 5.5 and 9.9 mg%. The serum phenylalanine was monitored once a week in the first year of life and once a month thereafter. Although each center performed its own phenylalanine determinations, they were checked periodically by a serum reference laboratory. Psychologic evaluations, using standardized protocols, were performed at specified ages on all index patients and all siblings of the index patients were given the same tests at the same ages. The psychologist was unaware of the treatment status of the child and frequently did not even know that the child had phenylketonuria. All test results were reviewed by the project staff. Physical growth measurements, hemoglobin determinations, and EEG's were also carried out periodically in the index patients.

The assignment of index PKU children was completed on October 1, 1972. Of the 224 children originally enrolled, 153 remain active. Of the 71 inactive subjects, 40 were diagnosed as PKU variants. Of the remaining 31, 11 moved out of the area of a collaborative clinic, 2 died, 10 were dropped because of parental noncompliance, and 8 because their clinic dropped out of the project. As of January 1, 1974, there were 14,256 items of information required from the collaborators. Of this number, 13,899 had been provided to the central data bank, and only 123 were irretrievably lost.[43]

Once each year the medical director, nutritionists, psychologists, and, often, the nurses meet with the project staff to review the results of the study up to that time. When necessary, modifications in procedure are made.

Although the Collaborative Project is reluctant to draw conclusions regarding psychologic evaluations until all subjects have reached the age at which the last evaluation will be performed, the results thus far suggest that near normal IQ's are attained as a result of early treatment, that there is relatively little difference in physical and mental development between the two treatment groups, and that, despite the restriction of phenylalanine, the diet is adequate to ensure physical growth within the normal range of the American population.

Diet Termination At its annual meeting in 1973, the Collaborative Project agreed to evaluate the effects of termination of the low-phenylalanine diet in a controlled study. When the patients enrolled in the project reach 6 years of age, they will be allocated either to a termination group (in which phenylalanine restriction will gradually end) or to a diet continuation group. It is hoped that subjects will be maintained in their assigned groups until 10 years of age. Except for a small study recently completed at the Johns Hopkins Hospital, which showed no harmful effect of diet termination after 2 years of age,[44] this is the first randomized clinical trial in this area and, because of the numbers involved, it should provide information on whether it is possible to terminate the diet at 6 years of age.

Thus, while important questions regarding phenylketonuria were unanswered when screening began, screening itself, given the extraordinary organization of the Collaborative Project, facilitated the collection of data that would provide answers.

PROBLEMS REMAINING IN PKU SCREENING AND TREATMENT

Although, as already mentioned, the incidence of PKU revealed by screening agrees with estimates extrapolated from the prevalance of PKU among the mentally retarded, approximately 5–10% of PKU children are not discovered through screening.

The Guthrie field trial suggested that babies screened early might be missed. In addition, the follow-up employed for babies screened after 3 days of age was inadequate to determine whether some of those with negative tests initially might, in fact, have phenylketonuria.

Direct evidence that babies are being missed was obtained from a 1970 survey of state health departments and of physicians known to be caring for children with PKU. Twenty-three infants whose initial blood test for phenylalanine was negative but who were subsequently proven to have PKU with maximum blood phenylalanines in excess of 20 mg% were reported. The states or clinics reporting these false negatives reported, over the same time, 253 patients in whom the diagnosis of PKU was made as a result of screening. Therefore, approximately 92 percent of infants with PKU were discovered by screening.[38] In addition to false negatives found by the survey, one baby was missed by initial screening in Connecticut[45] and two were missed in the State of Washington by blood screening.[46] Nine of the babies who were missed by the first screening were discovered as a result of a second screen. The majority of the other false negatives were discovered in clinics because of their delayed development.[38]

In 12 states providing data, 44% of all infants tested for PKU were screened on or before day 3 and 25% on day 4. Of the false negatives, 65% were screened on or before day 3.[47] This suggests that the timing of screening tests is critical.

Timing and Number of Tests

The 1970 survey also revealed that approximately one quarter of the infants with PKU who were discovered by screening had initial levels of phenylalanine of 8 mg% or less and most of these had been screened on or before 3 days of age.[33] There is now good evidence that the blood phenylalanine concentration in infants with PKU is only minimally elevated, if at all, at birth and does not rise to greater than 20 mg% until the end of the first week.[33]

The rate of rise of blood phenylalanine levels in females with PKU appears to be slightly slower than in males during the first 4 days, so that there is a greater possibility of missing females than males if screening is done before the fourth day of life.[47] Protein intake also influences the rate of phenylalanine rise.

In their final 1964 recommendations, Guthrie and Whitney stated that "the specimens should be collected from the infants as late as possible, before discharge from the hospital. . . . A follow-up test of all infants using a second filter paper blood specimen obtained at four weeks of age is highly recommended."[27]

In 1965 the Committee on the Fetus and Newborn of the American Academy of Pediatrics published its recommendations[48]:

> A blood test for elevated concentration of phenylalanine performed no sooner than 24 hours after onset of milk feeding and prior to discharge is recommended for all newborn infants.
>
> A second blood test at four or six weeks of age is recommended for all infants. This will detect infants who had borderline or low plasma concentrations of phenylalanine in the first few days of life.

(See Appendix D for the full text of the recommendations.)

However, the lead commentary in *Pediatrics,* the journal of the American Academy of Pediatrics, in March 1967 noted that the second test in Massachusetts had resulted in only one new case in 277,664 late tests. The commentary went on, "it is difficult to believe that continuation of this part of the program is economically justified."[49]

Guidelines issued by the Maternal and Child Health Service of the Department of Health, Education, and Welfare in 1966 and again in 1971 suggest that a follow-up test at a later age for all "negative newborns is desirable."[50] In the revised version (1971) a blood test at 4–6 weeks was recommended in preference to a urine test, but the publication states that the urine test "is to be preferred over no follow-up testing."

In 1972 the American Academy of Pediatrics listed a second test for PKU as a recommended procedure on 1-month-old infants, although it did not stipulate whether a blood or urine test should be used.[51]

A second screening test never became widespread in the United States. In 1970 it was being employed in 5 states, and in none was it mandatory.[52] Furthermore, many infants receive their first screening test earlier than recommended. These errors of omission and commission cannot be justified either by data made available as a result of the initial trials or by later experiences. Infants are often discharged from the newborn nursery before 48 hours of age, and it is uncertain when or where they will receive follow-up care.* Under these circumstances, most states and hospitals choose to screen before nursery discharge, taking the relatively small chance that a baby with PKU will be falsely negative rather than the greater chance that no test will be performed if not done in the nursery. In a few rural states tests are done by a public health nurse after discharge from the nursery.[52]

A repeat screening test for PKU at 1 month of age is currently being considered by at least two states. Admittedly, the yield will be small[53]: If 10 percent of PKU's are missed by the first screen in a state with 100,000 live births per year, the second test would discover only 1 patient approximately every 2 years.

Economic factors played a role in the decision not to repeat the test routinely despite its benefits. One cost of testing is the follow-up of the false positive, and the age at which the test is performed can affect the magnitude of this cost. In the 1970 survey, for every PKU infant there were 19 whose initial screening test was positive but who did not have PKU. Ninety-five percent of these false positives had initial serum phenylalanine levels of 10 mg% or less.[33] Values of less than 10 mg% in infants with classical PKU seldom occur after 1 week of age. Thus, if screening were delayed, the upper limit of blood phenylalanine concentration not requiring follow-up could be raised and fewer infants with normal elevations of phenylalanine would require follow-up. The advantages and dis-

* This contrasts with the situation in the United Kingdom, where every baby is visited in the home by a health visitor within 14 days. If the baby leaves the nursery before 7 days of age, the health visitor performs a test for PKU.[24] (See Appendix H for more detail.)

advantages for three options concerning the timing of PKU screening can be summarized as follows:

Option	Advantage	Disadvantage
1. One test prior to nursery discharge.	Largest proportion of babies screened. Early initiation of treatment possible.	False negatives as a result of early discharges. Large number of false positives requiring follow-up. Nonhospital births not screened.
2. One test at 7–14 days of age.	False negatives unlikely. Lower limit of "abnormal" phenylalanine can be raised to reduce the number of false positives. Moderately early initiation of treatment possible.	Many babies will escape testing.
3. Option 1 plus a second test at 1 month of age (babies whose first test positive to be followed up immediately).	As in Option 1; reduction in false negatives.	Added cost.

The occurrence of false positive test results is higher in nonwhites than in whites. It is therefore sometimes suggested that nonwhites should be excluded from screening. Although PKU is found less frequently in nonwhites, it still occurs with an incidence of 4.6/100,000 nonwhite births in the State of Maryland, compared to an incidence in whites of 9.6/100,000 births. Thus, eliminating nonwhites from the populations screened would lead to significant numbers of undetected cases.[54]

Laboratory Performance

Interlaboratory variability was apparent in the Guthrie–Whitney field trial, which revealed that the incidence of presumptive positive blood tests varied from 1 in 918 to 1 in over 10,000.[27] Part of this could have been due to inexperience with the test as well as to differences in the age of the newborns screened. However, marked variation in the incidence of presumptive positives still existed in 1968 and 1970, ranging between 5 per 100,000 and 275 per 100,000 infants screened on the third day of life.[38]

That the source of this variability lies largely in the laboratories is suggested by a study of the accuracy of phenylalanine testing in health department laboratories in 18 states and the District of Columbia, conducted by the Center for Disease Control. Proficiency of some of the laboratories was low. For blood phenylalanine concentrations of 2–6 mg%, 11 of 24 laboratories overestimated the value by at least 2 mg% and 5 underestimated it by at least that much.[55] As this is the cutoff range that determines whether a follow-up will be requested, the inaccuracies can influence the rate of occurrence of false positives and false negatives. It was also found that commercial standards for phenylalanine sometimes contained concentrations significantly different from that stated.[56]

The situation in California, although extreme, is instructive in the problems of establishing effective quality control. Before a mandatory law was passed in 1965, the State Health Department planned to establish seven regional laboratories to evaluate the suitability of fluorometric assay for blood phenylalanine as a screening method. After the law was passed, regional labs were rejected because[57]

> Pathologists and the bioanalysts who operate laboratories in California argued very strongly that any lab that is licensed by the state is technically capable of performing the test, and that there is no over-riding interest in the state that could restrict the test to a limited number of laboratories.

Initially, 250 licensed laboratories indicated interest in performing the test. Approximately 200 were approved. Within a short time, on the basis of proficiency testing and reporting requirements, this number was reduced to 175. At the end of 1972 there were 161 approved laboratories. Proficiency testing is performed much less frequently today than in former years. The laboratories in California charged between $.90 and $15.00 for the test.[57] (See Appendix C, Table C-4.)

In infants screened after 4 days of life, the blood phenylalanine level is always high enough for any false negatives to be attributable to laboratory error. Before that time, false negatives may be due to blood levels that are still too low to be counted as elevated. In principle, the proportion of false negatives due to laboratory error in the early period can, however, be ascertained after the fact. Filter paper containing the blood specimen can be saved indefinitely without loss of phenylalanine, allowing repetition of the test using the same paper in any case when phenylketonuria is later diagnosed.

The larger the number of laboratories performing a given test, the greater the likelihood of variability and the more difficult it is to impose quality control. Guthrie urged regionalization of screening programs, including the amalgamation of the programs in several small states, in order to improve quality and efficiency.[58]

Monitoring of blood phenylalanine in phenylketonurics receiving a low-phenylalanine diet is a requirement of good management. If there is a wide range of variability among laboratories performing these determinations, then statements regarding optimal levels of blood phenylalanine are meaningless. Without accurate determinations, good management will be impossible.

Follow-up and Commencement of Treatment

There is some urgency in following up a positive screening test and establishing a definite diagnosis, because evidence suggests that infants started on treatment between 3 and 6 weeks of age have a poorer outcome than those treated earlier, although the outlook is still far better than for those treated later or not at all.[59]

The 1970 survey revealed that the mean time elapsed between the screening result and the decisive test was 25 days for all infants, and in 22.6% of cases, more than 30 days elapsed before the test was repeated. The interval differs significantly among states.[38] In a second study, which included 388 infants in whom a diagnosis of PKU was established, the mean interval was 12 days, but in 31 cases it took more than 30 days.[52] Presumably, infants with high levels on the initial screen received priority in follow-up over those who had only minimal elevations.

The reasons for delay can be appreciated by considering the steps between collection of the specimen in the nursery and institution of treatment. In most states specimens are sent, usually by mail, to a health department laboratory. In some instances, specimens are accumulated over a few days before being sent. Some hospitals perform their own screening tests, while others send the specimen to a private laboratory. If an infant is found to have an elevated phenylalanine level, the hospital or the physician is notified and must contact the family to arrange for a follow-up. If PKU is suspected as a result of the follow-up, the family physician is notified or, if there is none, contact with the family is made through the hospital in which the baby was born, the local health department, or directly. Arrangements must then be made for referral to a center for confirmatory studies. There is no published information on how frequently family physicians undertake to treat without referral. There are no statutes that prevent them from doing so.

Maternal Phenylketonuria

Examinations of over 100 offspring of untreated PKU mothers indicates that virtually every one is retarded, and congenital malformations may be present as well. These conditions are not dependent on the father's genotype and appear to result from toxicity of phenylalanine *in utero*.[11,60] There is some uncertainty as to the frequency with which women with blood phenylalanine levels of 10 to 20 mg% will give birth to retarded infants,[11,61,62] but the risk is higher than that for the general population. The problems that these findings pose for the management of females with PKU discovered by neonatal screening are enormous. Assuming that the low-phenylalanine diet can be terminated in late childhood without further risk of retardation in the patient herself, the following questions must be answered: (a) Should affected females remain on the low-phenylalanine diet through their childbearing years despite the great hardship of doing so? (b) Should these females come off the diet in late childhood but resume it before they plan to have children? Reimposition of the diet may be difficult and, as yet, there is no conclusive evidence that conception and normal gestation are possible while the woman is on a low-phenylalanine diet.[61] Single case reports of dietary treatment during pregnancy offer some promise.[63] (c) Should females with PKU forego having their own children?

A rather poignant example of the problem of maternal hyperphenylalaninemia and the putative hazard to the fetus emerged during the course of the Committee's work. A major drug company has recently received approval from the Food and Drug Administration to market a new type of artificial sweetener. The substance, aspartame, is a metabolizable peptide containing L-phenylalanine. It is not improbable that intrauterine hyperphenylalaninemia will be augmented in women homozygous for the PKU or hyperphenylalaninemia alleles. In this situation this new environmental agent will be a distinct hazard to the normal development of the few babies born to homozygous mothers. It has been shown, however, that the heterozygote will not develop hyperphenylalaninemia when exposed to the sweetener even in large doses.

Massachusetts and Maryland screen pregnant women for PKU since women currently of childbearing age were not screened as infants. The American College of Obstetricians and Gynecologists recently recommended screening of pregnant women who are retarded or who have a family history of PKU or retardation.[64] (See Appendix F.)

Low-Phenylalanine Diets and Other Therapy

Lofenalac is the only commercially available low-phenylalanine preparation manufactured in the United States. While it is well suited for infants with PKU, its residual phenylalanine content and low protein/calorie ratio restrict the amounts of other foods that older PKU children can take. In Europe and the United Kingdom commercial preparations are available that are more suitable to the needs of older children than Lofenalac. Should it prove unsafe to terminate the low-phenylalanine diet in later childhood, there will be a great need for such products in this country. In addition, they would be much more palatable to women of child-bearing age should phenylalanine restriction prove effective in preventing retardation in the offspring of hyperphenylalaninemic women.

In 1969 Mead Johnson began development of such a product but they have not yet perfected it. In reply to an inquiry of this Committee, Dr. H. P. Sarett, Vice-President, Nutritional Science Resources, Mead Johnson, commented that a serious problem in its development is " 'stealing' considerable segments of time from other major responsibilities" of nutritional research and development. He goes on to comment:

> . . . we spent a lot of time, money and effort on rare disorders, but it's almost impossible to continue to do this. If other rare disorders require dietary management, it would be out of the question for us to donate the time and expense of carrying out the research, developing a formula, providing the formula, and monitoring its use. However, we would be glad to consider doing this, if it were properly subsidized by a government agency.

Thus, for PKU and other inborn errors for which treatment might be possible, reliance on private industry may prove an obstacle.

The use of B-2-thienylalanine to block phenylalanine absorption from the intestine was suggested by Lines and Waisman.[65] This compound is a competitive inhibitor of phenylalanine uptake. With it, higher amounts of phenylalanine might be used in the diet. However, no controlled studies have been performed to indicate whether it is safe or beneficial.

Tyrosine supplements, with or without phenylalanine restrictions, have been recommended. The effect of alterations in the ratio of phenylalanine to tyrosine in the body fluids on mental development deserves further study.

At present, enzyme replacement therapy for PKU does not appear feasible, but systematic investigation of the use of exogenous enzymes is beginning.[66,67]

SUMMARY

Although elevations of blood phenylalanine above 4 mg% are not always associated with mental retardation, persistent elevations above 20 mg% with normal or low tyrosine levels in infants on normal diets almost always are. Reduction of the serum phenylalanine by initiation of the low-phenylalanine diet in the first month of life can prevent retardation. Given a reliable screening test of blood phenylalanine level, all infants with PKU ingesting normal amounts of milk can be detected after 7 days of age.

Current practice in the United States, in which most screening is performed at 3 days of age, results in failure to detect 5–10% of babies with PKU.

A low-phenylalanine diet is known to be necessary for several years after diagnosis, if mental retardation is to be avoided. It is still unknown exactly how long such restriction should continue. There is little doubt, however, that high blood phenylalanine levels in pregnant women will cause retardation in all their offspring.

REFERENCES

1. Fölling, A. Uber Ausscheidung von Phenylbrenztraubensaure in den Harn als Stoffwechselanomalie in Verbindung mit Imbezillität. Hoppe-Seyler's Z. Physiol. Chem. 227:169–176, 1934.
2. Jervis, G. A. The genetics of phenylpyruvic oligophrenia. (A contribution to the study of the influence of heredity on mental defect.) J. Ment. Sci. 85:719–762, 1939.
3. Bessman, S. P. Legislation and advances in medical knowledge—acceleration or inhibition? J. Pediat. 69:334–338, 1966.
4. Kleinman, D. S. Phenylketonuria. A review of some deficits in our information. Pediatrics 33:123–134, 1964.
5. Cunningham, G. C. Phenylketonuria testing—Its role in pediatrics and public health. CRC Crit. Rev. Clin. Lab. 2:45–101, 1971.
6. Levy, H. L., V. Karolkewicz, S. A. Houghton, and R. A. MacCready. Screening the "normal" population in Massachusetts for phenylketonuria. N. Engl. J. Med. 282:1455–1458, 1970.
7. Hsia, D. Y-Y., M. E. O'Flynn, and J. L. Berman. Atypical phenylketonuria with borderline or normal intelligence. Amer. J. Dis. Child. 116:143–157, 1968.
8. Hsia, D. Y-Y. Phenylketonuria and its variants. Prog. Med. Genet. 7:29–68, 1970.
9. Berman, J. L., and R. Ford. Intelligence quotients and intelligence loss in patients with phenylketonuria and some variant states. J. Pediat. 77:764–770, 1970.
10. Levy, H. L., V. E. Shih, V. Karolkewicz, *et al.* Persistent mild hyperphenylalaninemia in the untreated state. A prospective study. N. Engl. J. Med. 285: 424–429, 1971.
11. Perry, T. L., S. Hansen, B. Tischler, F. M. Richards, and M. Sokol. Unrecognized adult phenylketonuria. Implications for obstetrics and psychiatry. N. Engl. J. Med. 289:395–398, 1973.
12. Jervis, G. A. Phenylpyruvic oligophrenia deficiency of phenylalanine-oxidizing system. Proc. Soc. Exp. Biol. Med. 82:514–515, 1953.
13. Knox, W. E. Phenylketonuria, pp. 266–295. In J. B. Stanbury, J. B. Wyngaarden, and D. S. Fredrickson, eds. The Metabolic Basis of Inherited Disease. 3rd ed. New York: McGraw-Hill, 1972.
14. Perry, T. L., S. Hansen, B. Tischler, R. Bunting, and S. Diamond. Glutamine depletion in phenylketonuria. A possible cause of the mental defect. N. Engl. J. Med. 282:761–766, 1970.
15. Koch, R. Personal communication, 1973.

16. Bickel, H., J. W. Gerrard, and E. M. Hickmans. Influence of phenylalanine intake on the chemistry and behaviour of a phenylketonuric child. Acta Paediat. 43:64–77, 1954.
17. Armstrong, M. D., and F. H. Tyler. Studies on phenylketonuria. I. Restricted phenylalanine intake in phenylketonuria. J. Clin. Invest. 34:565–580, 1955.
18. Snyderman, S. E., P. Norton, and L. E. Holt, Jr. Effect of tyrosine administration in phenylketonuria. Fed. Proc. 14:450–451, 1955 (abstract).
19. Meister, A., S. Undenfriend, and S. P. Bessman. Diminished phenylketonuria in phenylpyruvic oligophrenia after administration of L-glutamine, L-glutamate or L-asparagine. J. Clin. Invest. 35:619–626, 1956.
20. Baumeister, A. A. The effects of dietary control on intelligence in phenylketonuria. Amer. J. Ment. Defic. 71:840–847, 1967.
21. Knox, W. E. An evaluation of the treatment of phenylketonuria with diets low in phenylalanine. Pediatrics 26:1–11, 1960.
22. Kirkman, H. N. Enzyme defects. Prog. Med. Genet. 8:125–168, 1972.
23. Centerwall, W. R., R. F. Chinnock, and A. Pusavat. Phenylketonuria: Screening programs and testing methods. Amer. J. Publ. Health 50:1667–1677, 1960.
24. Holtzman, N. A., and B. H. Starfield. Detection and management of phenylketonuria in the United Kingdom. (Appendix H.)
25. Simopoulos, A. P. The Role of the Children's Bureau in the Development of the PKU Program. Paper prepared for the Committee, 1973.
26. Guthrie, R. Blood screening for phenylketonuria. (Letter to the Journal) JAMA 178:863, 1961.
27. Guthrie, R., and S. Whitney. Phenylketonuria. Detection in the Newborn Infant as a Routine Hospital Procedure. U.S. Dept. Health, Education, and Welfare, Children's Bureau Publ. No. 419. Washington, D.C.: U.S. Government Printing Office, 1965.
28. U.S. Department of Health, Education, and Welfare. PKU Blood Screening in Hospitals. Washington, D.C.: U.S. Dept. Health, Education, and Welfare, Sept. 30, 1964.
29. Legislation for Mandatory Screening for Phenylketonuria (PKU) Recommended by NARC's Board of Directors. National Association for Retarded Children, Inc., Weekly Action Rep. No. 58, January 4, 1965.
30. Simopoulos, A. P. The Role of the National Association of Retarded Children in the Development of PKU Legislation and Screening. Paper prepared for the Committee, 1973.
31. Koch, R. Pediatric aspects of phenylketonuria, pp. 8–20. In The Clinical Team Looks at Phenylketonuria. U.S. Department of Health, Education, and Welfare, Welfare Administration, Children's Bureau. Washington, D.C.: U.S. Government Printing Office, 1961.
32. Berman, J. L., G. C. Cunningham, R. W. Day, R. Ford, and D. Y-Y. Hsia. Causes for high phenylalanine with normal tyrosine. In newborn screening programs. Amer. J. Dis. Child. 117:54–65, 1969.
33. Holtzman, N. A., E. D. Mellits, and C. H. Kallman. Neonatal screening for phenylketonuria. II. Age dependence of initial phenylalanine in infants with PKU. Pediatrics 53:353–357, 1974.
34. Birch, H. G., and J. Tizard. The dietary treatment of phenylketonuria: Not proven? Dev. Med. Child. Neurol. 9:9–12, 1967.
35. Rouse, B. M. Phenylalanine deficiency syndrome. J. Pediat. 69:246–249, 1966.

36. Hackney, I. M., W. B. Hanley, W. Davidson, and L. Lindsao. Phenylketonuria: Mental development, behavior, and termination of low phenylalanine diet. J. Pediat. 72:646–655, 1968.
37. Holtzman, N. A. Screening for phenylketonuria and its problems, pp. 263–267. In A. G. Motulsky and F. J. G. Ebling, eds. Birth Defects. Proceedings of the Fourth International Conference, Vienna, Austria, 2–8 September, 1973 (International Congress Series No. 310). Amsterdam: Excerpta Medica Foundation, 1974.
38. Holtzman, N. A., A. G. Meek, and E. D. Mellits. Neonatal screening for Phenylketonuria. I. Effectiveness. JAMA 229:667–675, 1974.
39. Koch, R. Personal communication, 1974.
40. Committee on the Handicapped Child, AAP. Statement on treatment of phenylketonuria. Pediatrics 35:501–503, 1965.
41. Holtzman, N. A. Dietary treatment of inborn errors of metabolism. Annu. Rev. Med. 21:335–356, 1970.
42. Williamson, M. Collaborative Study of Children Treated for Phenylketonuria: I. Study design and description of the sample. Personal communication, 1974.
43. Collaborative Study of Children Treated for Phenylketonuria. Preliminary Report Number 7. Tenth General Medical Conference. Aspen, Colorado, 1974.
44. Holtzman, N. A., E. D. Mellits, and D. W. Welcher. A controlled evaluation of diet termination in phenylketonuria. Manuscript in preparation.
45. Mahoney, M. J. Personal communication, 1974.
46. Scott, R. Personal communication, 1974.
47. Holtzman, N. A., A. G. Meek, E. D. Mellits, and C. H. Kallman. Neonatal screening for phenylketonuria. III. Altered sex ratio. Extent and possible causes. J. Pediat. 85:175–181, 1974.
48. Committee on Fetus and Newborn, AAP. Screening of newborn infants for metabolic disease. Pediatrics 35:499–501, 1965.
49. Gerald, P. S. Commentary. The dangers of a successful PKU program. Pediatrics 39:325–326, 1967.
50. U.S. Department of Health, Education, and Welfare. Recommended Guidelines for PKU Programs for the Newborn. Public Health Service Publ. No. 2160. Rockville, Md.: U.S. Department of Health, Education, and Welfare, 1971.
51. American Academy of Pediatrics. Standards of Child Health Care. Evanston, Ill.: American Academy of Pediatrics, 1972, p. 23.
52. Holtzman, N. A. Unpublished information. Personal Communication, 1974.
53. Buist, N. R. M., G. R. Brandon, and R. L. Penn, Jr. Follow-up screening for phenylketonuria. (Letter to the Editor) N. Engl. J. Med. 290:577–578, 1974.
54. Holtzman, N. A., A. G. Meek, and E. D. Mellits. Neonatal screening for phenylketonuria. IV. Factors influencing the occurrence of false positives. Amer. J. Publ. Health 64:775–779, 1974.
55. Ambrose, J. A. Report on a cooperative study of various fluorometric procedures and the Guthrie bacterial inhibition assay in the determination of hyperphenylalaninemia. Health Lab. Sci. 10:180–187, 1973.
56. Ambrose, J. A. Report on a study of commercial lyophilized sera for use as reference controls for the amino acid analyzer and the manual fluorometric phenylalanine procedure. (Unpublished, 1970.)
57. Cunningham, G. Personal communication, 1972.
58. Guthrie, R. Personal communication, 1973.

59. Kang, E. S., N. D. Sollee, and P. S. Gerald. Results of treatment and termination of the diet in phenylketonuria (PKU). Pediatrics 46:881–890, 1970.
60. Howell, R. R., and R. E. Stevenson. The offspring of phenylketonuric women. Social Biol. 18:S19–S29, 1971.
61. Levy, H. L., and V. E. Shih. Maternal phenylketonuria and hyperphenylalaninemia. A prospective study. Pediat. Res. 8:391, 1974 (abstract).
62. Hansen, H. Risk of fetal damage in maternal phenylketonuria. J. Pediat. 83: 506–507, 1973.
63. Farquhar, J. W. Baby of a phenylketonuric mother. Inferences drawn from a single case. Arch. Dis. Child. 49:205–208, 1974.
64. Maternal phenylketonuria. Amer. Coll. Obstet. Gynecol. Tech. Bull. No. 25, December 1973.
65. Lines, D. R., and H. A. Waisman. Renal amino acid reabsorption in hyperphenylalaninemic monkeys infused with beta-2-thienylalanine. Proc. Soc. Exp. Biol. Med. 134:1061–1064, 1970.
66. Bergsma, D., Ed. Enzyme Therapy in Genetic Diseases. Baltimore: Williams & Wilkins, 1973.
67. Holtzman, N. A., G. F. Bell, M. J. Krantz, H. H. Liv, and Y. C. Lee. Enzyme replacement therapy: Directing exogenous enzyme to the liver. Pediat. Res. 8:382, 1974 (abstract).

3 The Development of Legislation and Regulation for PKU Screening

It has been suggested[1,2] that the adoption of statutes in nearly all the states requiring screening for PKU and other rare (and, to the average layman or legislator, obscure) inborn metabolic errors is explained by the existence of a high-powered campaign coordinated by national voluntary organizations and the Children's Bureau of the Department of Health, Education, and Welfare. Thus it may seem surprising to discover that the state statutes on metabolic testing of newborns do not all derive from a single legislative model. The state variations are not so startling, however, in light of the usual modes and pressures of legislative activity and of the particular facts of the PKU lobbying effort, which was national in scope but local in execution. In this chapter we explore the history of PKU legislation and analyze a number of significant factors about the statutes.

The PKU screening statutes were adopted in a rush in the mid-1960's. After the first steps taken by Massachusetts in 1963, and by Rhode Island, Louisiana, and New York in 1964, the majority of states adopted laws in 1965, with a number of others following suit in the next 2 years. Most states undertook to draft laws of their own, although communication among lawmakers and lobbying groups on a regional and national level led to some common elements and legislative patterns in the statutes. In some cases all or part of one state statute can be seen to have been borrowed by others or by the draftsmen of "model" statutes.

LOBBYING

The National Association for Retarded Children

Americans tend to express their humanitarian and philanthropic interests through voluntary organizations, particularly in the health and welfare fields.[3] Thus, in light of the acute lack of community services for retarded children and the deplorable conditions in many state institutions, it is not surprising that parents of retarded children banded together to form local units concerned with improving the lot of the mentally retarded. This grassroots movement coalesced into the National Association for Retarded Children (NARC) in 1950, stimulated in part by the opportunity to gain a platform at the Midcentury White House Conference on Children and Youth and in part by indications of potential federal funding of mental retardation programs.[4]

The Association, on both national and local levels, was developed largely by parents of retarded children who felt neglected by professionals (Appendix C, Table C-1). While physicians played some role in the NARC, they did so largely because of personal, family experience with mental retardation. By 1963, when the NARC was considering PKU legislation, its Public Health Services Committee consisted of twelve physicians (one with a PhD as well), two registered nurses, and one person holding a PhD. But these were unusual physicians, who certainly did not agree with organized medicine's opposition to mandatory screening (Appendixes C and E).

In October 1963, the NARC Board of Directors adopted a policy statement prepared by the NARC Public Health Services Committee: "Rather than seek specific mandatory legislation for screening for separate metabolic defects . . . NARC should press for legislation in each State that would direct the State Board of Health to make recommendations for appropriate screening tests as they are developed and accepted."

In October 1964, NARC's Public Health Services Committee reviewed the results of PKU screening in the United States in light of an additional year of experience and presented to the NARC Board of Directors a resolution "that the NARC upon the recommendation of its Committee on Public Health Services go on record as recommending mandatory legislation for the screening of PKU." On October 11, 1964, this resolution was accepted as NARC's official policy, despite the fact that both the American Academy of Pediatrics and the American Medical Association were against mandatory screening. The NARC went even further and suggested a model law.

Massachusetts, which had adopted a mandatory law in 1963,* already had achieved nearly 100% screening of newborns for PKU. It was not surprising that Massachusetts was first. The Director of the State Health Department in Massachusetts, Dr. Robert A. MacCready, was the chairman of NARC's Public Health Services Committee, of which Dr. Robert Guthrie was a member, and Dr. Guthrie's research for the development of the PKU screening test had in fact been supported by the NARC.

In its Weekly Action Report of January 4, 1965, NARC carried the September 30, 1964, publication of the Children's Bureau indicating the number of hospitals that did PKU screening, including copies of the state laws pertaining to PKU as of January 1965, and documenting that only 20% of newborn babies were being screened. The Association concluded then that the only way to get all newborns screened on a routine basis was through mandatory legislation. A later newsletter presented the state laws on PKU as of November 1966 with the following preface:

> How the goal of screening all infants is attained is a decision to be made in each State. Some States have achieved the desired program by means of legislation; others, by action of the State health department. In many States bills pertaining to screening are pending in the State legislature.

Lobbying efforts on behalf of PKU screening legislation were carried on by the state Associations for Retarded Children (ARC's) in most states. The impact of ARC pressure, of a state's participation in the trial of the Guthrie test, and of special factors (for instance, legislators who had retarded children) is conveyed by Table C-1 in Appendix C, which reports some of the data derived from the sociohistorical survey of twelve representative states.

In the case of PKU legislation, whatever opposition there was came from organized medicine—which was then fighting a battle against what it saw as a host of laws (particularly federal legislation on medical payments for indigents and the elderly) that threatened to dictate to physicians how to practice their profession (Appendix E). In the face of the parents' claims that screening could prevent mental retardation that caused suffering and cost the government a great deal, the medical opposition apparently had little impact on legislators.

The question of statutory formulation became a matter of borrowing

* At the time that the NARC acted on October 11, 1964, Rhode Island had a similar statute (effective May 5, 1964), and Louisiana had a longer mandatory statute (effective July 29, 1964). The process of borrowing and adoption of statutes is discussed more fully in the next subsection.

elements of existing statutes that dealt with the subject in a manner compatible with the state's general practice. In some states, the department of public health is a large operation, highly respected and with much autonomy; such departments were likely to be told by the legislature to attack the problem of phenylketonuria as they thought best. Statutes in other states, in which the general pattern of delegation of authority in the jurisdiction was less free, set out duties in much more detail. The ARC lobbyists, sensitive to local variations and personalities, adapted themselves to this legislative background. Urged on, rather than controlled, by their National Association, the local ARC supporters of PKU screening were satisfied with a variety of statutes.

The Children's Bureau

While the Children's Bureau of the Department of Health, Education and Welfare had sponsored the initial field trials of Guthrie's inhibition assay test in 1962–1963, there is no evidence that the Bureau supported the enactment of legislation in the states for PKU screening. The Bureau was, of course, aware of the lobbying efforts, not least because two members of its Technical Committee on Clinical Programs for Mentally Retarded Children at this time were also members (one, Dr. Richard Koch, was Vice Chairman) of NARC's Public Health Services Committee. The evidence it gathered in 1964–1966 on the extent of voluntary screening in hospitals and its lists of state statutes were also used by the NARC lobbyists as the major exhibits in the campaign for mandatory laws, as was the Bureau information sheet published on September 30, 1964, "PKU Blood Screening in Hospitals," which urged the screening of all newborn infants for PKU on a routine basis.

The Children's Bureau did not, however, officially join in the effort to get legislation passed, as can be seen from its October 25, 1965, *Report on State Laws Pertaining to PKU Screening*:

> The setting up of a State program for screening of all newborn infants is not necessarily contingent upon a legislative requirement. In some of the States with nonmandatory laws and in some States without a legal requirement, good screening programs are in operation. On the other hand, in some States which now have laws, implementation is a problem. The Children's Bureau believes that emphasis should be placed on the development of screening programs. It is unfortunate that public concern with legislation on this subject has created the impression that, unless a State has a law, it cannot have a program. Parent organizations and other interested groups should work with State Health Departments in developing programs to insure screening of all newborn infants in every State.

LEGISLATION

The Relationship among the Statutes

The various PKU statutes differ substantially in length and specificity.* An illuminating contrast is provided by Utah, which gets by with a one-sentence law, and Tennessee, whose statute runs to ten separate sections (some of which consist of multiple sentences or subsections). Not surprisingly, the short statutes vest a great deal of discretion in the state's public health department to determine the number and type of tests required; in some cases even the judgments on whether to have tests and whether to make them mandatory are left up to the department. Some of the longer statutes (for example, Arkansas, California, and Oklahoma) also create highly discretionary arrangements, but most of them are more specific on such questions as the test to be given and when, the duties of the testers, and the responsibilities of state health officers for such further activities as research or treatment.

The actual borrowing of language is easiest to see in the shorter statutes. Massachusetts' pioneering 1963 effort was picked up intact by Rhode Island; in New Hampshire it was modified by deleting the religious limitation on the parental right to object; and in North Dakota the wording was modified somewhat and a sentence was added requiring that positive diagnoses be reported to the state department of health.

The Massachusetts statute was also indirectly influential in many other states because it was relied upon by the National Association for Retarded Children in drawing up the model law for mandatory PKU testing that it promulgated in October 1964. The NARC model statute, which was adopted immediately in New York and then in largely the same form in Alabama, Connecticut, Kansas, Kentucky, and Minnesota, speaks in terms of a duty imposed on various persons "to cause to have administered to every . . . infant" a test for phenylketonuria. The NARC version also requires "such other tests for preventable diseases" as prescribed by the state's health department, but this broader version of screening was not incorporated by the states using the NARC model, except Kentucky (which did not mention PKU but only "a test for inborn errors of metabolism") and Minnesota ("other inborn errors of metabolism causing mental retardation," in addition to PKU).

* States with short statutes include Alabama, Connecticut, Florida, Georgia, Hawaii, Iowa, Kentucky, Massachusetts, Montana, New Hampshire, New York, North Dakota, Ohio, Pennsylvania, Rhode Island, South Carolina, Utah, and Wisconsin. States with lengthier statutes include Arkansas, California, Colorado, Idaho, Nebraska, Oklahoma, Tennessee, Texas, Virginia, Washington, and West Virginia.

The longer statutes seem to be largely patchwork affairs. For example, the "education" clause of the law adopted in 1963 in Oregon (before testing became mandatory there in 1965) was incorporated virtually whole cloth by Illinois, Indiana, Kansas, and Oklahoma in 1965, and partially by New Mexico in 1966. Similarly, other identical clauses appear in various statutes; Illinois and Kansas both have "registry" provisions, Oklahoma borrowed the "accepted medical practice" wording from Massachusetts, but within a nonmandatory framework, and so forth. In at least one case, a long statute was borrowed almost intact—the 1965 Texas act, which tracks the 1964 Louisiana law very closely. The borrowing of statutory patterns has a definite regional flavor, but not exclusively so.

Analysis of the Statutes

Those points on which the PKU statutes differ and on which some states have taken an unusual stance are illustrative of the policy choices facing the legislators. Thus, it is worthwhile to analyze the statutes on a number of significant points. The analysis is set forth in tabular form in Table 3-1; the reference in all cases is to the current PKU screening statute, since a number of states have amended their laws (moving, for example, from voluntary to mandatory programs) since they were adopted a decade ago.

Activities Mandated The most general way of categorizing the PKU laws is according to the degree of state activity they mandate. Most of the statutes either make testing mandatory or give administrators the power to require tests when they believe them to be justified. In addition to testing, there are three indications of the degree of state involvement: the promotion of research and education, the establishment of a registry, and the support of treatment of affected children. The first of these, while important, need not reflect a very active state program; the emphasis on education in many of the statutes probably resulted from a recognized need for a "public relations" effort on the state's part to inform physicians about the disease and to enlist their cooperation in testing all newborns. (The variation among states is reflected in Question 5 in Table 3-1.) The second, establishment of a registry, indicates a greater degree of state activity. In a few states (e.g., Illinois and Kansas), statutes actually require that a registry be established; in a number of other cases, however, such a registry may result from the required reporting to some state official of all (or all positive) test results (this point is reflected in Question 10 in Table 3-1). Finally, a statutory requirement of treatment provided by the state is probably the most significant indication of state involvement. Since the purpose of PKU testing is to prevent mental retardation by early detection and treatment of the condition, it is perhaps ironic that none of the states mandate treatment. Some states do clearly anticipate that the state health department will actively encourage and assist physicians and parents (Illinois, Kansas, Louisiana, Nebraska, Texas, Virginia, and Washington are good examples; see Question 11 in Table 3-1).

Mandatory Participation The heart of the statutes is, of course, their requirement of testing the infant for PKU. When the statutes are spoken of as "mandatory," it is in reference to testing. (Note, however, that despite their mandatory language, only six of the statutes specify a penalty for violation; see Question 7 in Table 3-1.) Any interests invaded by the laws, accordingly, would seem to be those of the parents and child—in privacy, autonomy, and well-being. Yet it was physicians, not parents, who opposed the laws. (See also Appendix C, Tables C-1 through C-3.)

Two factors explain this paradox. First, many of the laws place their legal requirements on the physicians or other health personnel (see Question 6 in Table 3-1). Even when the parent is responsible for reporting the test, it will still have to be performed by health personnel. Thus, it is really the conduct of physicians that is being controlled by the mandatory statutes; rather than being left to their judgment, under the common law of malpractice, the performance of the test is required by statute. Second, even where there is no mandatory statute, there will still probably be a strong impetus for the parent to have the child tested; and for a physician to fail to offer the test, even in the absence of a statutory requirement—the situation today in Arizona, Delaware, Mississippi, North Carolina, Vermont, Wyoming, and the District of Columbia (which have no statutes), and in Washington (whose statute makes screening voluntary)—would subject him to a malpractice judgment if the child had undetected PKU.

Parental Objection One difference between a mandatory law and reliance on the common law is that in the latter situation a physician would need parental consent before performing the test. In fact, many of the PKU statutes that are mandatory contemplate such consent by indirection; five of the forty-three states with mandatory statutes provide that screening will not be performed if the parents object, and another thirty-one permit parental objection if made on religious grounds (Question 2 in Table 3-1). Unfortunately, the Committee's study revealed that parents are frequently not informed of the test or of their right to object; parents may first learn of the test after the blood sample has been taken, or not at all.

Quality Control One of the major problems in PKU screening, as mentioned earlier, has proven to be the uneven quality of the laboratory testing. Aside from a few states with centralized, state-operated facilities, most samples are analyzed in private laboratories. Even though this is currently the case, all the statutes (except that of Nevada, which does not mention the state health department) vest broad powers in the public health officials to draw up necessary rules and regulations pertaining to the tests (see Question 9 in Table 3-1). In conjunction with their general authority to license and regulate laboratories, these powers would seem to permit more active and rigorous monitoring of lab performance than is currently the case.

Diseases Screened for Interviews with legislators and review of hearing transcripts indicate that most public officials, and indeed most of the lobbyists and others involved in the process, thought of the legislation in terms of mental retardation and not genetic principles. None of the statutes mention genetics. The provisions in Alaska and California come the closest, and speak of "heritable disorders leading to mental retardation." The Idaho statute speaks of "preventable diseases," and most of the other 17 statutes that go beyond PKU itself speak in terms of "metabolic errors," often modified by "which can be prevented" or "which lead to mental retardation."

The expansion of testing beyond phenylketonuria is left to the judgment of the state health departments in 20 states (see Question 1 in Table 3-1). In addition, the Maryland statute enacted in 1973 establishes a Commission on Hereditary Disorders (see Note 1 to Table 3-1), and in at least one state (Massachusetts) the health department has expanded screening beyond PKU, despite its lack of statutory mandate for this step.

Analysis of the Regulations

As stated in the preceding section, most state statutes make provision for the health department to promulgate regulations concerning PKU testing. In addition, some states without statutory mandated screening have regulations covering their voluntary programs. As with the statutes, there is great diversity in the detail with which the program is spelled out by the regulations. In some cases, the regulations are only a few pages long; at the other extreme, the Connecticut regulations fill an entire binder and even go into such detail as diet.

No attempt will be made here to examine all the differences in state department of health regulations. Many of these are as much a reflection of idiosyncracies in state administrative practices as an indication of different views surrounding PKU. For example, the reason quality control of private laboratories is not part of the Wisconsin PKU statute or regulation is simply that Wisconsin already had detailed legislation for approval of private laboratory examinations made for public health purposes (§14B.15 Wisc. statutes).

The state regulations covered fall into a number of patterns (Table 3-2). The most general distinction, as with the statutes, is the extent of state involvement in the PKU testing and treatment process. Comparison of the New York and Oregon regulations is instructive in this regard.

The New York regulations prescribe a specific PKU test to satisfy the testing requirement of §2500-a of the Public Health Law. This is the Guthrie Inhibition Assay Procedure. No state services are provided either in the form of treatment kits or screening itself. Results are not forwarded to state officials; they are forwarded to the hospital, but this is solely so that the results can be recorded on the infant's chart. While the state Commissioner of Health does "designate" acceptable laboratories, the procedures for acceptance are not set out. Neither does the State involve itself in any but this initial screening. The regulations do not make follow-up tests, consultation for treatment, or special treatment kits the responsibility of the state.

In Oregon, on the other hand, both an initial and a follow-up screening are required, and the State provides testing materials for both. While a private laboratory may theoretically be licensed to process the tests, only the State laboratory actually undertakes testing (at least through 1969). A booklet describing the Oregon program issued by the State Board of Health points out that "our experience has indicated that more consistent and reliable results can be obtained if one laboratory performs all tests." State law regulates the incidence with which hospitals or physicians must mail tests to the State laboratory. It requires positive results to be reported to State health officials, arranges for further diagnostic tests on "presumptive positives," and offers extensive treatment without charge.

Thus, the differences in state involvement are in some ways very great (see also Appendix C, Table C-2). Yet one apparently illuminating basis for categorizing the programs—between the vast majority of states that have statutory mandated screening and the few that do not—does not provide useful differentiation. Four of the six nonstatutory states (Delaware, North Carolina, Vermont, and Wyoming) have extensive and effective voluntary PKU testing programs, under regulations promulgated by the general authority of their state officials charged with responsibility for public health. The District of Columbia, which dropped its statute because no cases of PKU were being discovered, has only a small program in public health clinics; Mississippi has only cursory regulations, and Arizona has none.

The active nonstatutory programs have heavily involved state boards of health and are generally indistinguishable in form from mandatory programs. In North Carolina, for example, the State Board of Health provides free testing materials; a central, public laboratory undertakes all test analysis; and treatment is provided at no charge to the medically indigent. Aside from being the only state to use the fluorometric technique by itself, North Carolina does not differ significantly in the guidelines it issues from those states whose programs are the result of explicit enabling statutes. Vermont, which offers the services of a state laboratory if desired and which will finance follow-up testing and treatment services, approximates the practices in mandatory states as well. Delaware also offers laboratory services run by a state agency, although it does not appear to have developed any official guidelines on methods of taking tests and dealing with suspected cases of PKU. Screening is not regulated in Wyoming, but follow-up testing is funneled through the University of Colorado Pediatrics Laboratory and is paid for by the State of Wyoming.

Variations in state involvement and methods, as reflected in public health regulations, cannot therefore be predicated entirely on differences among the statutes nor even on whether or not the state has a statute at all. As the Children's Bureau observed early in the initial establishment of PKU screening, very good programs have been established without the enactment of legislation, and a mandatory statute is no guarantee of a successful program.

In analyzing the state regulations, a number of factors stand out; mentioned here are four that seem of special significance.

Test Used The PKU statutes almost universally give the state health departments the authority to regulate screening methods; in the single exception (Nevada) the regulations issued proceed as though such authority had been given. Under such authority, the departments have specified the screening method to be used for PKU detection. In most states the Guthrie inhibition assay is used, alone or in combination with other, unnamed "blood" tests. The District of Columbia uses a urine method (the Phenistix diaper test), and Alabama, Georgia, Louisiana, Missouri, Texas, and Washington permit a urine test in addition to the use of the Guthrie test. North Carolina is alone in relying on the fluorometric test as its sole method, but that test is also included as a method in California, Colorado, Illinois, Louisiana, Minnesota, Missouri, Ohio, Oklahoma, Pennsylvania, West Virginia, and Wisconsin. In addition, Minnesota and Pennsylvania use the La Du method, and Colorado, Minnesota, and Wyoming employ paper chromatography as an alternative method (see Question 1 in Table 3-2).

Testing Auspices Most of the state regulations do not reveal the auspices for the performance of test analysis. In nine cases, however, the regulations make clear that the state is, by rule or practice, the only service in operation, and another five authorize specific laboratories, not operated by the state, to perform the analyses (Question 11 in Table 3-2). This is probably an incomplete listing, because an analysis of other sections of the regulations suggests that in seventeen states screening is provided without charge (Question 3 in Table 3-2). Moreover, in a majority of cases, the state offers to provide test materials, such as filter paper and mailing packages, or test analysis (Question 2 in Table 3-2).

Treatment and Medical Follow-up Twenty-five states provide for treatment and follow-up medical attention in their regulations. Alabama, Colorado, Connecticut, Hawaii, Illinois, Kansas, Kentucky, Louisiana, Missouri, New Hampshire, New Jersey, North Dakota, Ohio, Oregon, Pennsylvania, Texas, Virginia, Washington, West Virginia, and Wisconsin have statutory PKU screening, and Delaware, Mississippi, North Carolina, Vermont, and Wyoming specify by regulation that treatment is part of their voluntary, nonstatutory programs. Seven states give the treatment without charge. In Pennsylvania it is provided free if the physician requests, and in ten other states it is free if the family is "in need." The regulations for seven of the states providing treatment do not specify whether, or when, a charge is made. (See Questions 9 and 10 on Table 3-2.)

Timing and Number of Tests The timing of the initial PKU test is very important for a combination of conflicting reasons. It must accommodate the need to allow enough time to elapse after the initial intake of protein by the baby for an accurately measurable level of phenylalanine to be present, and yet it must be early enough that all, or nearly all, babies are available for screening in a convenient and economical fashion and that they are young enough to be given treatment before significant injury has taken place.

The state regulations show a wide variety of response to these somewhat conflicting demands. Some regulations simply set no time for the blood specimen to be drawn, leaving this to each hospital or physician to determine; the resulting diversity may make it more difficult to attribute significance to any particular level of phenylalanine findings. In ten states, the minimum time for screening is set at 24 hours after the first milk, or other protein, feeding, but still as late as possible prior to discharge. (Most regulations that speak in terms of discharge do not take into account the child whose discharge from the hospital may be delayed for a long period of time for various reasons; apparently, it is assumed that the pediatrician will have the test done without waiting until the time of discharge.) Another ten states set 48 hours as the screening point (with Missouri specifying that this applies to Guthrie and fluorometric samples, but that urine samples should be taken after the child reaches 4 weeks of age). Three other states set the minimum time before testing at 72 hours (including Pennsylvania, which *permits* testing as early as 24 hours but prefers the longer period).

A number of states seem to be concerned that the test might be postponed too long—rather than performed too soon—and these states set outer limits, usually in conjunction with a minimum limit. Nevada sets its outer limit at 5 days; West Virginia at 7 days; Hawaii, Idaho, Maine, Montana, New York, North Carolina, and Virginia at 14 days; California at 20 days; Georgia and Louisiana at 28 days; and the District of Columbia at 6 months (see Question 4 on Table 3-2).

Fewer states have issued regulations covering another important matter—follow-up testing, usually to be performed by the mother in conjunction with the pediatrician or the state health department. Seven states make a second test mandatory, usually 3 to 6 weeks after birth, and another eight recommend that such a test be performed (Question 13 on Table 3-2).

REFERENCES

1. Bessman, S. P., and J. P. Swazey. Phenylketonuria: A study of biomedical legislation, pp. 49–76. In E. Mendelsohn, J. P. Swazey, and I. Taviss, Eds. Human Aspects of Biomedical Innovation. Cambridge, Mass.: Harvard University Press, 1971.
2. Cooper, J. D. Creative pluralism: Medical ombudsman, pp. 46–61. In Research in the Service of Man. Hearings before the Subcommittee on Government Research of the Committee on Government Operations, United States Senate, 90th Congress. First Session on Biomedical Development, Evaluation of Existing Federal Institutions. Feb. 28, March 1, 2, 3, and 16, 1967. Washington, D.C.: U.S. Government Printing Office, 1967.
3. Katz, A. H. Parents of the Handicapped: Self-Organized Parents' and Relatives' Groups for Treatment of Ill and Handicapped Children. Springfield, Ill.: Charles C Thomas, 1961.
4. Mead, M., and M. Brown. The Wagon and the Star. Chicago: Rand McNally, 1967.

TABLE 3-1 State PKU Statutes (As of June 1974)

		(1)	(2)	(3)	(4)	(5)
State	Date of Enactment	Testing Mandatory?	Basis for Avoiding Screening[a]	Population Tested	When Tested	Statute Also Requires[b]
Alabama	1965	Mandated by statute	Religious objection of parents	All children	28 days	Nothing
Alaska	1965; amended 1967	Mandated by statute; testing for other disorders or metabolic errors (that threaten health or intellect) may be made mandatory by Dept. of Health	General parental objection	All children	Newborn (child or infant)	Nothing
Arkansas	1967	Dept. of Health given discretionary power to make PKU (and other) testing mandatory	Religious objection of parents	All children	Newborn (child or infant)	Education
California	1965; amended 1967	Tests for PKU "and other preventable heritable disorders" become mandatory ("shall be administered to each child born in California") once the Dept. of Public Health "has established appropriate regulations and testing methods"	Religious objection of parents	All children	As early as possible	Nothing
Colorado	1965	Mandated by statute; testing for other disorders or metabolic errors (that threaten health or intellect) may be made mandatory by Dept. of Health	Religious objection of parents	All children	Newborn (child or infant)	Education
Connecticut	1965	Mandated by statute; testing for other disorders or metabolic errors (that threaten health or intellect) may be made mandatory by Dept. of Health	Religious objection of parents	Children born in institutions or examined by a physician only	28 days	Nothing

(6) Person Responsible for Reporting Test	(7) Penalty Clause For Not Testing[c]	(8) Provision of Testing Materials and Services by State	(9) Testing Methods Regulated by Dept. of Health	(10) Results to be Reported to State Board of Health or Other Agency	(11) Dept. of Health Must Follow up and Treat
Administrative head of institution (or hospital as corporate entity); physician; person attending neonate not attended by physician	None	No	Yes	"Recording" and "reporting" of results contemplated by statute, but details left to administrators	No
Physician "or nurse who first visits child"	Yes, but does not apply if parents refuse consent	Yes	Yes	All positive results	Yes
No birth certificate issued without proof of test	Health Dept. has injunctive powers to enforce test	Yes	Yes	No requirement	Yes
—	None	No	Yes	No requirement	No
Administrative head of institution (or hospital as a corporate entity); person responsible for registering birth	None	Yes	Yes	"Recording" and "reporting" of results contemplated in statute, but details left to administrators	No
Administrative head of institution (or hospital as corporate entity)	None	No	Yes	"Recording" and "reporting" of results contemplated in statute, but details left to administrators	No

TABLE 3-1 (*Continued*)

State	Date of Enactment	(1) Testing Mandatory?	(2) Basis for Avoiding Screening[a]	(3) Population Tested	(4) When Tested	(5) Statute Also Requires[b]
Florida	1965; amended 1971	Mandated by statute; testing for other disorders or metabolic errors (that threaten health or intellect) may be made mandatory by Dept. of Health	General parental objection	All children	2 weeks	Nothing
Georgia	1966; amended 1972	Mandated by statute	Religious objection of parents	All children	Newborn (child or infant)	Nothing
Hawaii	1965	Mandated by statute	Religious objection of parents	All children	Newborn (child or infant)	Nothing
Idaho	1965	Mandated by statute; testing for other disorders or metabolic errors (that threaten health or intellect) may be made mandatory by Dept. of Health	Religious objection of parents	All children	Newborn (child or infant)	Education
Illinois	1965	Mandated by statute; testing for other disorders or metabolic errors (that threaten health or intellect) may be made mandatory by Dept. of Health	Religious objection of parents	All children	Newborn (child or infant)	Education
Indiana	1965	Statute vests discretionary power in Dept. of Health to make PKU (and other) testing mandatory[d]	Religious objection of parents	All children	Infant	Education
Iowa	1965; amended 1967	Statute vests discretionary power in Dept. of Health to make PKU (and other) testing mandatory[d]	None	All children	Infant	Nothing
Kansas	1965	Mandated by statute	Religious objection of parents	Children born in institutions or examined by physician only	28 days	Education

(6) Person Responsible for Reporting Test	(7) Penalty Clause For Not Testing[c]	(8) Provision of Testing Materials and Services by State	(9) Testing Methods Regulated by Dept. of Health	(10) Results to be Reported to State Board of Health or Other Agency	(11) Dept. of Health Must Follow up and Treat
—	None	Yes, "when not otherwise available"	Yes	All test results	Yes
Physician or Health Dept.	None	Yes	Yes	No requirement	Yes
Physician or person attending neonate not attended by physician	None	No	Yes	"Recording" and "reporting" of results contemplated in statute, but details left to administrators	No
Administrative head of institution (or hospital as corporate entity); person responsible for registering birth	Yes	No	Yes	All positive results	Yes
—	None	Yes	Yes	All test results	Yes
Physician	None	No	Yes	All test results	No
—	None	No	Yes	No requirement	No
Administrative head of institution (or hospital as corporate entity) or physician	None	Yes	Yes	All positive results; "recording" and "reporting" of results contemplated in statute, but details left to administrators	Yes

TABLE 3-1 (*Continued*)

State	Date of Enactment	(1) Testing Mandatory?	(2) Basis for Avoiding Screening[a]	(3) Population Tested	(4) When Tested	(5) Statute Also Requires[b]
Kentucky	1966	Mandated by statute; testing for other disorders (that threaten health or intellect) may be made mandatory by Dept. of Health	Religious objection of parents	All children	28 days	Nothing
Louisiana	1964	Mandated by statute	Religious objection of parents	All children	Newborn (child or infant)	Research
Maine	1965	Mandated by statute; testing for other disorders (that threaten health or intellect) may be made mandatory by Dept. of Health	Religious objection of parents	Children born in institutions or examined by physician only	Newborn (child or infant)	Nothing
Maryland[e]	1965; amended 1967	Mandated by statute	Religious objection of parents	All children	Newborn (child or infant)	Nothing
Massachusetts	1963	Mandated by statute	Religious objection of parents	Children born in institutions or examined by physician only	Newborn (child or infant)	Nothing
Michigan	1965; amended 1967	Mandated by statute	Religious objection of parents	Children born in institutions or examined by physician only	"Before infant is discharged" or according to regulations prescribed by state director of health	Nothing
Minnesota	1965	Mandated by statute; testing for other disorders or metabolic errors (that threaten health or intellect) may be made mandatory by Dept. of Health	Religious objection of parents	All children	28 days	Nothing

(6) Person Responsible for Reporting Test	(7) Penalty Clause For Not Testing[c]	(8) Provision of Testing Materials and Services by State	(9) Testing Methods Regulated by Dept. of Health	(10) Results to be Reported to State Board of Health or Other Agency	(11) Dept. of Health Must Follow up and Treat
Administrative head of institution (or hospital as corporate entity) or person responsible for registering birth	None	No	Yes	"Recording" and "reporting" of results are contemplated in statute, but details left to administrators	No
Physician or person attending neonate not attended by physician	None	No	Yes	All positive results	Yes
Administrative head of institution (or hospital as corporate entity)	None	Yes, on request	Yes	Dept. of Health given power to request records of those making tests, but statute does not require report to Health Dept.	No
Administrative head of institution (or hospital as corporate entity) or person responsible for registering birth	None	—	Yes	"Recording" and "reporting" contemplated in statute, but details left to administrators	No
Physician	None	No	Yes	No requirement	No
Physician	Yes	No	Yes	All test results; also must be reported to parents or guardian	No
Administrative head of institution (or hospital as corporate entity) or person responsible for registering birth	None	No	Yes	"Recording" and "reporting" contemplated in statute, but details left to administrators	No

TABLE 3-1 (*Continued*)

		(1)	(2)	(3)	(4)	(5)
State	Date of Enactment	Testing Mandatory?	Basis for Avoiding Screening[a]	Population Tested	When Tested	Statute Also Requires[b]
Missouri	1965	Mandated by statute; testing for other disorders or metabolic errors (that threaten health or intellect) may be made mandatory by Dept. of Health	Religious objection of parents	All children	10th week	Education
Montana	1965; amended 1973	Statute vests discretionary power in Dept. of Health to make PKU (and other) testing mandatory	No provision	All children	Infant	Nothing
Nebraska	1967; amended 1969	Mandated by statute; testing for other disorders or metabolic errors (that threaten health or intellect) may be made mandatory by Dept. of Health	No provision	All children	Infant	Nothing
Nevada	1967	Mandated by statute	General parental objection	All children	Infant	Nothing
New Hampshire	1965	Mandated by statute	General parental objection	Children born in institutions or attended by physician only	Newborn (child or infant)	Nothing
New Jersey	1964	Statute vests discretionary power in Dept. of Health to make PKU (and other) testing mandatory[d]	Religious objection of parents	All children	Newborn (child or infant)	Educati[illegible]

(6) Person Responsible for Reporting Test	(7) Penalty Clause For Not Testing[c]	(8) Provision of Testing Materials and Services by State	(9) Testing Methods Regulated by Dept. of Health	(10) Results to be Reported to State Board of Health or Other Agency	(11) Dept. of Health Must Follow up and Treat
Administrative head of institution (or hospital as corporate entity), physician, or person attending neonate not attended by physician	Yes	No	Yes	All positive resltsu	No
Administrative head of institution (or hospital as corporate entity) or person responsible for registering birth	None	No	Yes	No requirement	Yes, on request
Administrative head of institution (or hospital as corporate entity)	None	Yes	Yes	All test results	Yes
Administrative head of institution (or hospital as corporate entity), physician, person attending neonate not attended by physician, parent or guardian, "mid-wife, nurse, maternity home . . . attendant on or assisting in any way whatever any infant, or the mother of any infant, at child-birth . . ."	None	No	No	All positive results	Yes
Administrative head of institution (or hospital as corporate entity) or physician	None	No	Yes	No requirement	No
–	None	Yes	Yes	No requirement	No

TABLE 3-1 (*Continued*)

		(1)	(2)	(3)	(4)	(5)
State	Date of Enactment	Testing Mandatory?	Basis for Avoiding Screening[a]	Population Tested	When Tested	Statute Also Requires[b]
New Mexico	1966; amended 1973	Mandated by statute	General parental objection	All children	Newborn (child or infant)	Education
New York	1964	Mandated by statute	No provision	All children	28 days	Nothing
North Dakota	1967	Mandated by statute; testing for other disorders or metabolic errors (that threaten health or intellect) may be made mandatory by Dept. of Health	Religious objection of parents	Children born in institutions or examined by physician only	Newborn (infant or child)	Education
Ohio	1965	Mandated by statute	Religious objection of parents	All children	Newborn (infant or child)	Nothing
Oklahoma	1965	Statute vests discretionary power in Dept. of Health to make PKU (and other) testing mandatory	Religious objection of parents	—	—	Education
Oregon	1963; amended 1965	Mandated by statute[d]	No provision	All children	2 weeks	Education
Pennsylvania	1965	Mandated by statute; testing for other disorders or metabolic errors (that threaten health or intellect) may be made mandatory by Dept. of Health	Religious objection of parents	Children born in institutions or examined by physician only	Newborn (infant or child)	Nothing
Rhode Island	1965	Mandated by statute	Religious objection of parents	Children born in institutions or examined by physician only	Newborn (infant or child)	Nothing
South Carolina	1965	Mandated by statute	Religious objection of parents	Children born in institutions or examined by physician only	—	Nothing

(6) Person Responsible for Reporting Test	(7) Penalty Clause For Not Testing[c]	(8) Provision of Testing Materials and Services by State	(9) Testing Methods Regulated by Dept. of Health	(10) Results to be Reported to State Board of Health or Other Agency	(11) Dept. of Health Must Follow up and Treat
—	None	Yes	Yes	No requirement	No
Administrative head of institution (or hospital as corporate entity) or person responsible for registering birth	None	No	Yes	"Recording" and "reporting" of results contemplated in statute, but details left to administrators	No
Physician	None	Yes	Yes	All positive results	Yes
erson responsible for registering birth	None	No	Yes	No requirement	No
-	None	Yes	Yes	No requirement	No
dministrative head of institution (or hospital as corporate entity), physician, or "public health nurses"	None	Yes	Yes	All positive results	No
lministrative head of institution (or hospital as corporate entity) or physician	None	No	Yes	No requirement	No
sician	None	No	Yes	No requirement	No
	None	No	Yes	"Recording" and "reporting" of results contemplated in statute, but details left to administrators	No

TABLE 3-1 (*Continued*)

State	Date of Enactment	(1) Testing Mandatory?	(2) Basis for Avoiding Screening[a]	(3) Population Tested	(4) When Tested	(5) Statute Also Requires[b]
South Dakota	1973	Mandated by statute; testing for other disorders or metabolic errors (that threaten health or intellect) may be made mandatory by Dept. of Health	Religious objection of parents	All children	Newborn (child or infant)	Education
Tennessee	1968	Mandated by statute; testing for other disorders or metabolic errors (that threaten health or intellect) may be made mandatory by Dept. of Health	Religious objection of parents	All children	Newborn (child or infant)	Education
Texas	1965	Mandated by statute	Religious objection of parents	All children	Newborn (child or infant)	Researc
Utah	1965	Mandated by statute; testing for other disorders or metabolic errors (that threaten health or intellect) may be made mandatory by Dept. of Health	No provision	All children	Newborn (child or infant)	Nothin
Virginia	1966	Mandated by statute	Religious objection of parents	All children	Infant	Educa
Washington	1967	Not mandatory	No provision	All children	Newborn (child or infant)	Nothi
West Virginia	1965; amended 1966	Mandated by statute	No provision	All children	Newborn (child or infant)	Noth

(6) Person Responsible for Reporting Test	(7) Penalty Clause For Not Testing[c]	(8) Provision of Testing Materials and Services by State	(9) Testing Methods Regulated by Dept. of Health	(10) Results to be Reported to State Board of Health or Other Agency	(11) Dept. of Health Must Follow up and Treat
—	None	No	Yes	All test results	No
Person responsible for registering birth, or parent or guardian; at discretion of commission of public health, person charged with seeing that test is conducted "may include" administrative head of institution (or hospital as corporate entity), physician, or "such other person or persons as the commissioner shall deem appropriate"	Yes	Yes	Yes	"Recording" and "reporting" of results contemplated in statute, but details left to administrators	No
hysician or person attending neonate not attended by physician	None	Yes	Yes	All positive test results	Yes
–	None	No	Yes	No requirement	No
dministrative head of institution (or hospital as corporate entity) or physician	None	Yes	Yes	All positive results	Yes
dministrative head of institution (or hospital as corporate entity), physician, or testing lab	None	Yes	Yes	All positive results	Yes
ysician or person attending neonate not attended by physician	Yes	Yes	Yes	All positive results	Yes

TABLE 3-1 (*Continued*)

		(1)	(2)	(3)	(4)	(5)
State	Date of Enactment	Testing Mandatory?	Basis for Avoiding Screening[a]	Population Tested	When Tested	Statute Also Requires[b]
Wisconsin	1965; amended 1969	Mandated by statute; testing for other disorders or metabolic errors (that threaten health or intellect) may be made mandatory by Dept. of Health	Religious objection of parents	Children born in institutions or examined by physician	Infant	Nothing

NOTE: A blank space indicates that the state statute does not contain any information pertinent to the question asked.

[a] "Religious" may refer to a "recognized church" (e.g., in Arkansas) or may have a broader definition, such as "religious beliefs or practices" (e.g., in California).

[b] Some of the statutes go into great detail on the requirement that education about PKU be provided. The following examples suggest the range of concerns in this area.

TENNESSEE—Sec. 53-629. *Information to medical profession—Department to furnish.* The department of public health shall furnish all physicians, public health nurses, hospitals, maternity homes, midwives, and department (sic) of public welfare available medical information concerning the nature and effects of phenylketonuria and other metabolic disorders and defects found likely to cause mental retardation. [Virginia also has a similar provision.]

) erson esponsible for eporting Test	(7) Penalty Clause For Not Testing[c]	(8) Provision of Testing Materials and Services by State	(9) Testing Methods Regulated by Dept. of Health	(10) Results to be Reported to State Board of Health or Other Agency	(11) Dept. of Health Must Follow up and Treat
hysician	None	No	Yes	No requirement	No

REGON—Sec. 433.290. *Board to conduct educational program concerning phenylketonuria.* The State Board Health shall institute and carry on an intensive educational program among physicians, hospitals, public ealth nurses and the public concerning the disease of phenylketonuria. This educational program shall include formation concerning the nature of the disease and examinations for the detection of the disease in infancy order that measures may be taken to prevent the mental retardation resulting from the disease.

Failure to test is usually a misdemeanor.

Rather than making it mandatory for someone (e.g., physician) to test, statute declares it to be "public olicy" that every infant "shall" or "should" be tested.

In 1973, the state established a Commission on Hereditary Disorders with the power to "promulgate rules, gulations, and standards for the detection and management of hereditary disorders." Ann. Code Md., rt. 43, §818. While that law seems to supersede §38A on PKU screening, the latter was not removed from e books.

TABLE 3-2 State PKU Regulations

	(1)	(2)	(3)	(4)	(5)	(6)
State	Test Prescribed	Materials Offered by State	Test Free	When Tested	Presumptive Positive (mg%)	When Test Sen to Lab
Alabama	Guthrie or other unspecified "blood" type test Urine-type test	Yes	—	Just prior to discharge	6	On day sample was collectec or within 24 after sampling
Alaska	Guthrie Inhibition Assay Test	Yes	Yes	Not earlier than 48 hr after milk/protein feeding and as late as possible prior to discharge	—	Specimens to b mailed "immediatel
Arkansas	—	—	—	—	—	—
California	Guthrie Inhibition Assay Test Fluorometric test (McCaman-Robin, etc.)	—	—	Before 20 days: "If born in hospital test before 20 days old; if admitted to a hospital test before 30 days old; if not born or admitted to a hospital between 4–10 days"	—	On day sample was collecte or within 24 hr after sampling
Colorado	Guthrie Inhibition Assay Test Fluorometric test (McCaman-Robin, etc.) Paper chromatography	Yes	Yes	Not earlier than 24 hr after milk/protein feeding and as late as possible prior to discharge	4	Specimens collected fr births in institutions should be mailed in according t the laborat instructions those from noninstitutional births should be mailed with 1 week
Connecticut	Guthrie or other unspecified "blood" type test	Yes	—	Not earlier than 24 hr after milk/protein feeding and as late as possible prior to discharge	4–6	Within 48 hou after sampl was collecte

(7) Person or Organization Receiving Results	(8) Registry of Positives	(9) Treatment Provided by State	(10) Free Treatment	(11) State's Service Only One Legal or Existing	(12) Labs Regulated	(13) 2d Test	(14) Tests Other Than PKU Allowed for
—	—	Yes	If family qualifies under "need test"	—	—	Required	Yes
Physician receives positive reports	—	—	—	Yes	Yes	—	Yes
—	—	—	—	—	—	—	—
A state agency (either local health officer or Dept. of Health) receives all positive reports Physician receives positive reports	—	—	—	—	Yes	—	—
A state agency (either local health officer or Dept. of Health) receives all positive reports Physician receives all reports	—	Yes	Yes	—	Yes	—	—
State agency receives all reports	Yes[a]	Yes[b]	If family qualifies under "need test"[c]	—	Yes	—	Yes

TABLE 3-2 (*Continued*)

State	(1) Test Prescribed	(2) Materials Offered by State	(3) Test Free	(4) When Tested	(5) Presumptive Positive (mg%)	(6) When Test Sent to Lab
Delaware (Regulations cover statewide, nonstatutory program that tests 97% of all neonates)	Guthrie Inhibition Assay Test	Yes	Yes	—	—	—
District of Columbia[d]	Phenistix	—	—	New patients <6 mo old	—	—
Florida	—	—	—	—	—	—
Georgia	Guthrie or other unspecified "blood" type test If parental objection is made to a blood test, urine test is acceptable Urine-type test	—	—	Not earlier than 48 hr after milk/protein feeding and as late as possible prior to discharge Within 28 days of birth or first protein feeding	4	—
Hawaii	Guthrie or other unspecified "blood" type test	Yes	—	Not earlier than 24 hr after milk/protein feeding and as late as possible prior to discharge Within 14 days of birth or first protein feeding	4	—
Idaho	Guthrie Inhibition Assay Test	Yes	—	Just prior to discharge Within 14 days of birth or first protein feeding	4	On day sample was collected or within 24 hr after sampling

(7) Person or Organization Receiving Results	(8) Registry of Positives	(9) Treatment Provided by State	(10) Free Treatment	(11) State's Service Only One Legal or Existing	(12) Labs Regulated	(13) 2d Test	(14) Tests Other Than PKU Allowed for
A state agency (either local health officer or Dept. of Health) receives all positive reports	—	Yes	—	Yes; all testing is done in state labs, but this is not required by statute or regulation	—	—	—
A state agency (either local health officer or Dept. of Health) receives all positive reports	No	—	—	—	—	—	—
—	—	—	—	—	—	—	—
A state agency (either local health officer or Dept. of Health) receives all positive reports Physician receives all reports Hospital receives all tests, including reports designated to be entered into infant's hospital chart	—	—	—	—	Yes	—	—
A state agency (either local health officer or Dept. of Health) receives all positive reports Physician receives positive reports	Yes	Yes	If family qualifies under "need test"	—	Yes	—	Yes
State agency receives all reports	Yes	—	—	No	Yes	—	[e]

TABLE 3-2 (*Continued*)

State	(1) Test Prescribed	(2) Materials Offered by State	(3) Test Free	(4) When Tested	(5) Presumptive Positive (mg%)	(6) When Test Sent to Lab
Illinois	Guthrie or other unspecified "blood" type test	—	—	Not earlier than 24 hr after milk/protein feeding and as late as possible prior to discharge	4	—
Indiana	Guthrie or other unspecified "blood" type test	—	—	Not earlier than 24 hr after milk/protein feeding and as late as possible prior to discharge	—	—
Iowa	Guthrie or other unspecified "blood" type test	—	—	Not earlier than 48 hr after milk/protein feeding and as late as possible prior to discharge	—	—
Kansas	Guthrie Inhibition Assay Test	Yes	Yes	Not earlier than 48 hr after milk/protein feeding and as late as possible prior to discharge	4	Twice weekly
Kentucky	Guthrie Inhibition Assay Test	—	—	—	4	—

(7) Person or Organization Receiving Results	(8) Registry of Positives	(9) Treatment Provided by State	(10) Free Treatment	(11) State's Service Only One Legal or Existing	(12) Labs Regulated	(13) 2d Test	(14) Tests Other Than PKU Allowed for
State agency receives all reports Physician receives all reports	—	Yes	Yes: Not in regulations but treatment is provided at no cost. See Paulissen & Zeldes. "PKU Program in Illinois," Illinois Medical Journal (Dec. 1971)	—	Yes	—	—
A state agency (either local health officer or Dept. of Health) receives all positive reports	—	—	—	—	—	Recommended	—
A state agency (either local health officer or Dept. of Health) receives all positive reports	—	—	—	—	Yes	Recommended	—
State agency receives all reports Physician receives all reports Hospital receives all tests, including reports designated to be entered into infant's hospital chart	Yes	Yes	Yes	Yes	—	Recommended	—
State agency receives all reports Physician receives positive reports Hospital receives all tests, including reports designated to be entered into infant's hospital chart	Yes	Yes	If family qualifies under "need test"	—	—	—	—

TABLE 3-2 (*Continued*)

State	(1) Test Prescribed	(2) Materials Offered by State	(3) Test Free	(4) When Tested	(5) Presumptive Positive (mg%)	(6) When Test Sent to Lab
Louisiana	Guthrie Inhibition Assay Test Urine-type test Fluorometric test (McCaman-Robin, etc.)	Yes	—	Not earlier than 48 hr after milk/protein feeding and as late as possible prior to discharge Within 28 days of birth or first protein feeding	6	—
Maine	Guthrie Inhibition Assay Test	Yes	—	4–6 days postpartum Within 14 days of birth or first protein feeding	4	At least once weekly
Maryland	—	—	—	—	—	—
Massachusetts	Guthrie or other unspecified "blood" type test	—	—	Just prior to discharge	—	—
Michigan	Guthrie Inhibition Assay Test Other tests may be approved on written application to health department	Yes	Yes	Not earlier than 24 hr after milk/protein feeding; not later than 72 hr after milk/protein feeding	—	—
Minnesota	Guthrie Inhibition Assay Test Fluorometric test (McCaman-Robin, etc.) Paper chromatography La Du	Yes	Yes	Just prior to discharge	—	On day sample was collected or within 24 hr after sampling
Mississippi	—	Yes	—	—	—	—

(7) Person or Organization Receiving Results	(8) Registry of Positives	(9) Treatment Provided by State	(10) Free Treatment	(11) State's Service Only One Legal or Existing	(12) Labs Regulated	(13) 2d Test	(14) Tests Other Than PKU Allowed for
State agency receives all reports Physician receives positive reports	Yes	Yes	If family qualifies under "need test"	—	—	Required	—
A state agency (either local health officer or Dept. of Health) receives all positive reports Hospital receives all tests, including reports designated to be entered into infant's hospital chart	—	—	—	Yes	—	Required	—
—	—	—	—	—	—	—	—
—	—	—	—	—	—	Recommended	—
A state agency (either local health officer or Dept. of Health) receives all positive reports Physician receives positive reports	—	—	—	—	Yes	—	—
A state agency (either local health officer or Dept. of Health) receives all positive reports Hospital receives all tests, including reports designated to be entered into infant's hospital chart	—	—	—	—	Yes	Recommended	Yes; statute so provides
—	—	Yes	—	—	—	—	—

TABLE 3-2 (*Continued*)

	(1)	(2)	(3)	(4)	(5)	(6)
State	Test Prescribed	Materials Offered by State	Test Free	When Tested	Pre-sumptive Positive (mg%)	When Test Sent to Lab
Missouri	Guthrie Inhibition Assay Test Urine-type test Fluometric test (McCaman-Robin, etc.)	Yes	Yes (Guthrie)	Guthrie/Fluor: Not earlier than 48 hr after milk/protein feeding and as late as possible prior to discharge Urine: 28 days after birth or later	4	—
Montana	Guthrie Inhibition Assay Test	—	—	Not earlier than 72 hr after milk/protein feeding Within 14 days of birth or first protein feeding	—	On day sample was collected or within 24 hr after sampling
Nebraska	—	—	—	—	—	—
Nevada	Guthrie or other unspecified "blood" type test	—	—	Not earlier than 48 hr after milk/protein feeding and as late as possible prior to discharge Within 5 days	4	—
New Hampshire	Guthrie Inhibition Assay Test	Yes	Yes	Just prior to discharge	4	At least once weekly
New Jersey	Guthrie Inhibition Assay Test	Yes	—	Not earlier than 48 hr after milk/protein feeding and as late as possible prior to discharge	4–8	—
New Mexico	—	—	—	—	—	—

(7) Person or Organization Receiving Results	(8) Registry of Positives	(9) Treatment Provided by State	(10) Free Treatment	(11) State's Service Only One Legal or Existing	(12) Labs Regulated	(13) 2d Test	(14) Tests Other Than PKU Allowed for
A state agency (either local health officer or Dept. of Health) receives all positive reports	—	Yes	—	—	Yes	—	—
A state agency (either local health officer or Dept. of Health) receives all positive reports Hospital receives all tests, including reports designated to be entered into infant's hospital chart	—	—	—	—	Yes	—	—
—	—	—	—	—	—	—	—
A state agency (either local health officer or Dept. of Health) receives all positive reports	—	—	—	—	—	Required	—
Physician receives positive reports Hospital receives all tests, including reports designated to be entered into infant's hospital chart	Yes	Yes	If family qualifies under "need test"	—	—	Recommended	—
A state agency (either local health officer or Dept. of Health) receives all positive reports	—	Yes	If family qualifies under "need test"	Yes	—	—	—
-	—	—	—	—	—	—	—

TABLE 3-2 (*Continued*)

	(1)	(2)	(3)	(4)	(5)	(6)
State	Test Prescribed	Materials Offered by State	Test Free	When Tested	Presumptive Positive (mg%)	When Test Sent to Lab
New York	Guthrie Inhibition Assay Test	—	—	Just prior to discharge Within 14 days of birth or first protein feeding	—	On day sample was collected or within 24 hr after sampling
North Carolina	Fluorometric test (McCaman-Robin, etc.)	Yes	Yes	Just prior to discharge Within 14 days of birth or first protein feeding	3.6	—
North Dakota	Guthrie Inhibition Assay Test	Yes	Yes; state university charges for a second confirmatory test	Just prior to discharge, after 36 hr/milk	4	—
Ohio	Guthrie Inhibition Assay Test Fluorometric test (McCaman-Robin, etc.) Other tests may be approved on written application to Health Department	Yes	Yes	Not earlier than 24 hr after milk/protein feeding and as late as possible prior to discharge	4	Within 48 hr after sample was collected
Oklahoma	Guthrie Inhibition Assay Test Fluorometric test (McCaman-Robin, etc.) Paper chromatography	Yes	Yes (while not in the regulations as of 1966, the State Health Dept. did not charge for test analysis)	Not earlier than 24 hr after milk/protein feeding and as late as possible prior to discharge	4–6	—

(7) Person or Organization Receiving Results	(8) Registry of Positives	(9) Treatment Provided by State	(10) Free Treatment	(11) State's Service Only One Legal or Existing	(12) Labs Regulated	(13) 2d Test	(14) Tests Other Than PKU Allowed for
Hospital receives all test, including reports designated to be entered into infant's hospital chart	—	—	—	—	Yes	—	—
Physician receives all reports Hospital receives all tests, including reports designated to be entered into infant's hospital chart	—	Yes	If family qualifies under "need test"	—	—	—	—
. state agency (either local health officer or Dept. of Health) receives all positive reports hysician receives positive reports ospital receives all tests, including reports designated to be entered into infant's hospital chart	—	Yes	—	Yes	—	Required	—
ysician receives all reports ospital receives ll tests, in- luding reports lesignated to e entered nto infant's ospital chart	—	Yes	—	—	Yes	—	—
tate agency ither local ealth officer or ept. of Health) ceives all ositive reports	Yes	—	—	—	Yes	—	Yes

TABLE 3-2 (*Continued*)

	(1)	(2)	(3)	(4)	(5)	(6)
State	Test Prescribed	Materials Offered by State	Test Free	When Tested	Presumptive Positive (mg%)	When Test Sent to Lab
Oregon	Guthrie Inhibition Assay Test	Yes	—	Just prior to discharge	—	Twice weekly
Pennsylvania	Guthrie Inhibition Assay Test Fluorometric test (McCaman-Robin, etc.) La Du	—	—	Not earlier than 24 hr after milk/protein feeding and as late as possible prior to discharge Prefer not earlier than 72 hr after milk/protein feeding	6[f]	—
Rhode Island	Guthrie or other unspecified "blood" type test	Yes	Yes	—	—	—
South Carolina	Guthrie or other unspecified "blood" type test	Yes	—	Not earlier than 48 hr after milk/protein feeding and as late as possible prior to discharge	4	On day sample was collected or within 24 hr after sampling
South Dakota	—	—	—	—	—	—
Tennessee	Guthrie Inhibition Assay Test	—	—	Not earlier than 72 hr after milk/protein feeding	—	—
Texas	Guthrie Inhibition Assay Test Urine-type test	Yes; urine test not provided, only blood test materials and screening	Yes	Not earlier than 24 hr after milk/protein feeding and as late as possible prior to discharge	4	At least once weekly

(7) Person or Organization Receiving Results	(8) Registry of Positives	(9) Treatment Provided by State	(10) Free Treatment	(11) State's Service Only One Legal or Existing	(12) Labs Regulated	(13) 2d Test	(14) Tests Other Than PKU Allowed for
A state agency (either local health officer or Dept. of Health) receives all positive reports	—	Yes	Yes	Yes	—	Required	Yes
A state agency (either local health officer or Dept. of Health) receives all positive reports	—	Yes	If family qualifies under "need test" Yes, on MD's request	No	—	—	—
state agency (either local health officer or Dept. of Health) receives all positive reports	—	—	—	—	—	—	—
tate agency receives all reports hysician receives all reports ospital receives all tests, including reports designated to be entered into infant's hospital chart	—	—	—	No	—	Recommended	—
	—	—	—	—	—	—	—
	—	—	—	Yes	—	—	No
ysician receives all reports spital receives all tests, including reports designated to be entered into infant's hospital chart	—	Yes	Yes	Yes	—	—	—

TABLE 3-2 (*Continued*)

State	(1) Test Prescribed	(2) Materials Offered by State	(3) Test Free	(4) When Tested	(5) Presumptive Positive (mg%)	(6) When Test Sent to Lab
Utah	Guthrie or other unspecified "blood" type test	—	—	Not earlier than 24 hr after milk/protein feeding and as late as possible prior to discharge	4	—
Vermont (Regulations apply to voluntary program conducted in hospitals)	Guthrie Inhibition Assay Test	—	—	—	—	—
Virginia	Guthrie Inhibition Assay Test	Yes	Yes	Not earlier than 48 hr after milk/protein feeding and as late as possible prior to discharge Within 14 days of birth or first protein feeding	4	On day sample was collected or within 24 hr after sampling
Washington	Guthrie or other unspecified "blood" type test Urine-type test	—	State pays for a confirmatory test after two screening tests	—	—	—

(7) Person or Organization Receiving Results	(8) Registry of Positives	(9) Treatment Provided by State	(10) Free Treatment	(11) State's Service Only One Legal or Existing	(12) Labs Regulated	(13) 2nd Test	(14) Tests Other Than PKU Allowed for
State agency receives all reports Physician receives positive reports Hospital receives all tests, including reports designated to be entered into infant's hospital chart	—	—	—	—	Yes	Required	Yes
A state agency (either local health officer or Dept. of Health) receives all positive reports Physician receives positive reports Hospital receives all tests, including reports designated to be entered into infant's hospital chart	—	Yes	Yes	No	—	—	—
A state agency (either local health officer or Dept. of Health) receives all positive reports Physician receives all reports Hospital receives all tests, including reports designated to be entered into infant's hospital chart	Yes	Yes	If family qualifies under "need test"	—	—	—	—
A state agency (either local health officer or Dept. of Health) receives all positive reports	—	Yes	If family qualifies under "need test"	—	—	—	—

TABLE 3-2 (*Continued*)

State	(1) Test Prescribed	(2) Materials Offered by State	(3) Test Free	(4) When Tested	(5) Presumptive Positive (mg%)	(6) When Test Sent to Lab
West Virginia	Guthrie or other unspecified "blood" type test Fluorometric test (McCaman-Robin, etc.)	Yes	Yes	Within 7 days	4	—
Wisconsin	Guthrie Inhibition Assay Test Fluorometric test (McCaman-Robin, etc.)	—	—	—	6	—
Wyoming	Guthrie or other unspecified "blood" type test Paper chromatography	No	No; state pays for a confirmatory test at the Univ. of Colorado Pediatric Laboratory after two screening tests	—	—	—

NOTE: A blank space indicates that the state statute does not contain any information pertinent to the question.

[a] The "registry" in Connecticut is limited to 5 years; see §19-13-041: "(e) information accompanying each specimen shall be sufficient to identify for future reference the infant from whom taken . . . (g) records of tests shall clearly indicate the tests performed and the results thereof and shall be maintained for a period of 5 years." (There is no discussion of genetic defects in these regulations.)

[b] Program not in formal regulations but provided anyway. See *Metabolic Defects Program and Procedural Manual*, April 1971.

[c] Not in regulations but a need charge imposed; see letter from Sherwin Mellino, Chief, Maternal & Child Health Section, State Department of Health, undated, in *Metabolic Defects Program and Procedural Manual*, April 1971.

(7) Person or Organization Receiving Results	(8) Registry of Positives	(9) Treatment Provided by State	(10) Free Treatment	(11) State's Service Only One Legal or Existing	(12) Labs Regulated	(13) 2nd Test	(14) Tests Other Than PKU Allowed for
A state agency (either local health officer or Dept. of Health) receives all positive reports Physician receives positive reports	—	Yes	Yes; while not specifically stated in regulation, the language strongly suggests that there is no charge for treatment	—	Yes	Recommended	—
A state agency (either local health officer or Dept. of Health) receives all positive reports	Yes	Yes	—	No	Yes	—	Yes; statute so provides
A state agency (either local health officer or Dept. of Health) receives all positive reports	—	Yes	—	No	—	—	—

[d] Regulations apply to public health clinics only. As of early 1973, PKU screening was not being done routinely at D.C. General Hospital.

[e] The Department of Health, Mental Retardation Section is charged with "disseminat[ing] information and advice to the public concerning the dangers and effects of phenylketonuria and other preventable diseases which cause mental retardation," but testing for such other diseases is not made mandatory, although the state board of health has the statutory power to require such additional tests.

[f] 1–3 mg% is defined as the "normal" level, but 6 mg% is regarded as a "presumptive positive" test that should be rechecked.

4 Lessons Learned from the PKU Experience, and Recommendations

Techniques for the mass screening of newborns are currently available for several other inborn errors of metabolism. Some (for galactosemia, histidinemia, and maple syrup urine disease) have been applied to newborn populations; and although the numbers screened and detected are small, problems similar to those for PKU have already been encountered. Variant forms of galactosemia were uncovered in the course of screening, and the question of whether treatment for histidinemia is either effective or necessary is still unanswered. Thus there are lessons to be learned from PKU that will be helpful in considering programs for other disorders.

The objective of PKU screening is the prevention of disability in infants at risk by the institution of effective therapy. To achieve this outcome, three steps are necessary: (a) detection—screening of all newborns; (b) diagnosis—confirmation of a positive screening test; and (c) counseling and treatment—initiation and follow-up with monitoring. The lessons from these three processes in PKU screening will be considered in reverse order.

LESSONS

Treatment and Monitoring

In the early 1960's, when PKU screening became widespread, subjects treated from early infancy had not been followed long enough to predict the extent to which the low-phenylalanine diet would prevent retardation. It was unknown whether specific learning disabilities or behavior problems would develop. Yet most health professionals hailed the diet as highly effective, and there was little organized effort to determine whether, in the long run, screening would meet its objective. Only after a few lonely but loud critical voices were raised, and only after the recognition that optimal phenylalanine levels could not be defined *a priori,* was the Collaborative Project organized in this country to measure the effectiveness of the low-phenylalanine diet and to determine optimal phenylalanine levels. While there was merit in beginning populationwide screening for PKU in order to obtain a sufficient number of infants to test the effectiveness of a rational therapy for a rare disorder in the shortest possible time, procedures should have been developed that could, in a systematic manner, have provided results.

There are different means to this end. A protocol rigidly prescribing management and monitoring procedures (the U.S. Collaborative Project) is one approach, but it may exclude some feasible alternatives as well as missing those in the population who are unable or unwilling to comply. Another approach is the establishment of a Register, as in the United Kingdom (see Appendix H), in which data pertinent to outcome are entered on *all* patients discovered but where management is left to individual physicians, provided they send their data to the Register.

Diagnosis

Most of those involved in the early stages of PKU screening failed to appreciate the extent of variation, including genetic heterogeneity. They assumed that if the blood phenylalanine was persistently above normal, say by a factor of 2 or 3, the risk of retardation was just as great as if it was 20 or 30 times normal. Abundant evidence is now available indicating that persistent but slight elevations are not usually associated with retardation.

The knowledge that variation exists should not be a deterrent to screening, as long as screeners anticipate it. One means of recognition is to have a confirmatory test that provides a more precise indication of the nature of the basic defect than the screening test itself. For PKU this requires liver biopsy, but for other disorders more accessible tissues can frequently be used. (In the few atypical patients in which liver biopsy was performed, residual enzyme activity was found, whereas in classical PKU there was virtually none.) When a more precise diagnostic procedure is not readily available, and when it is difficult to distinguish the biochemical findings associated with the classical condition from those associated with the variants, it is inevitable that some variants will be treated unnecessarily if it is the policy to treat every subject with a persistent biochemical aberration. One way to determine whether a variant is at risk for disability is to withhold treatment from all suspected variants or administer it to half on a random basis.

Such studies are difficult to justify after claims are made that treatment is efficacious and necessary. If the tendency to make unfounded claims continues, perhaps screening programs should begin before any treatment is available. This would permit assessment of the full spectrum of clinical and genetic variation associated with the biomedical aberrations discovered by screening without the intervening effect of therapy.

Both randomized trials and screening before treatment is available are largely research endeavors, and the public—who must consent to be screened and to finance the program—must recognize this. But the practical benefits from this research—screening programs better able to prevent disability without causing harm—are readily recognizable.

Detection

The urine $FeCl_3$ and, subsequently, the tests for blood phenylalanine were used in young infants with inadequate appreciation of the possible ways in which the newborn differs from older subjects. The fact that a screening test is capable of detecting an older individual with a disorder is no guarantee that it will detect the disorder in a newborn. Several solutions are available: (a) Avoid screening during the first few days after birth. (The organization of health services in the United Kingdom facilitated this approach, and the absence of false negatives, as well as the fact that virtually all infants have been screened, justifies it.) (b) If newborns are screened, perform a second test—preferably by an independent method—several weeks later in all infants. This will establish the sensitivity of the test in the newborn period. (c) Establish a central register to which each infant in whom the disorder is discovered clinically (i.e., who was missed by screening) must be reported. This is particularly indicated if routine second testing is not possible. The screening results can be fed back to the screeners so that appropriate modifications can be made. To accomplish this, better record and report systems than are currently used in most states for PKU will be needed.

The objective of screening for inborn errors is the prevention of disability; thus, detection and diagnosis must be completed before irreversible damage occurs. Efficient relations among the source(s) of specimens, the screening laboratory, health professionals responsible for follow-up, and the diagnostic facilities are required. (The shorter time between the first test and follow-up in the United Kingdom than in the United States suggests that the organization of services in Great Britain facilitates coordination.)

Finally, the survey of PKU screening indicates that all laboratories are not equally reliable. Greater centralization of laboratories—provided that their quality is adequately controlled—appears to be a reasonable and economical solution.

Conclusions

In the three areas of treatment, diagnosis, and detection, it is clear that those involved in screening in the early days did not anticipate many problems and failed to see the necessity of documenting their successes. In populationwide programs such as neonatal screening, therefore, general guidelines should be established. They must not be so rigid, however, as to stifle the initiative of those seeking to improve detection, diagnosis, and treatment.

RECOMMENDATIONS

1. All newborns should be screened for PKU by a blood phenylalanine determination. Such screening should be performed at the last possible moment before nursery discharge. This initial screening could be combined with screening for other disorders, such as maple syrup urine disease and galactosemia, in which immediate intervention is imperative.
2. When the initial PKU test is performed on or before the fourth day of life, a second determination of blood phenylalanine should be performed before 4 weeks of age. This test might be combined with others that are more likely to be positive at 4 weeks than earlier (histidinemia and homocystinuria, for instance) and with still others, for which there is no evidence that immediate intervention in the newborn period is necessary.
3. Greater quality control of PKU screening is essential. To accomplish this, screening tests should no longer be carried out in private laboratories or in small states but by regional laboratories. The number of live births necessary for optimal performance of the test should be the prime determinant of the size of each region. Factors such as geographical size and state boundaries would also have to be considered. Regional laboratories could perform other tests as well.
4. A single laboratory—within the Center for Disease Control, for instance—should be responsible for maintaining the proficiency of the regional laboratories.
5. Greater standardization and efficiency of procedures for reporting results to hospitals, health departments, and family physicians are needed, as is a system to monitor test results for statistical purposes. There is too

great a delay, at the present time, between first test and follow-up. Regionalization should facilitate solution of this problem.

6. Infants in whom a diagnosis of PKU is suspected should be referred to a center with experience in diagnosis and management of this disorder before treatment is undertaken. Frequent monitoring of blood phenylalanine is necessary, and this should be accomplished by a laboratory whose proficiency is assured.

The ultimate intellectual and psychiatric results of phenylalanine restriction in PKU are still unknown. Thus, there is a need to combine continued investigation with routine management. This can best be accomplished through centers. Family physicians should be kept fully informed about the patients they refer to the center. This is a key part in the continuing education of physicians in regard to hereditary disorders.

7. If all infants are to be screened, then there is an obligation to ensure that all infants discovered to have PKU receive optimal therapy. Adequate means of financing the costs of special diets and other aspects of care for families not covered by insurance and unable to pay must be a societal responsibility.

8. Continued effort to improve treatment modes is necessary. When private industry cannot pursue this goal, government intervention is needed.

9. In view of the high risk of retardation to the offspring of PKU mothers, screening for PKU should be done as part of early antenatal care because most women currently of reproductive age were not screened for PKU in infancy. Whether a low-phenylalanine diet during pregnancy can prevent retardation in the fetus remains to be established; until its efficacy is proved, termination of pregnancy should be an option.

10. The initial PKU screening trials were undertaken at a time when many questions remained unanswered concerning the detection and treatment of the disease; in a number of localities the initial trials led to very high rates of participation. Nevertheless, despite the unresolved scientific questions, the less than complete coverage of the early screening efforts brought about overwhelming pressure for mandatory PKU screening on the part of local organizations made up mostly of parents of mentally retarded children. Legislators were responsive to such pressure because they saw the proposals as a simple means of eradicating a disease (like any public health measure to stem an epidemic) that was costing the taxpayers money for the care of affected children. There was little recognition of the implications for public policy, or for the impact on individuals who were screened, of the fact that PKU is a *genetic* disease. (The policy, ethical, legal, and cost–benefit implications of this fact are de-

tailed in Part VI, below.) The opposition of physicians to legislation on screening kept them separated from legislative decision-making. (See also Appendix C.)

In order to avoid repetition of this experience of fragmented, uneducated, and hurried decision-making, it is advisable for states, singly or on a regional basis, to establish bodies with ongoing responsibility and competence in the field of genetic screening, including both medical and nonmedical expertise. Such bodies would avoid the dangers of *ad hoc* responses to pleas for state involvement in the increasing number of conditions for which screening will soon become available. Moreover, they could serve a useful review function, making sure that the benefits and costs (direct and indirect, monetary and nonmonetary) are fully accounted for and that the former outweigh the latter.

11. The experience of states with a variety of genetic screening programs indicates that the success of the program, including degree of coverage of newborns, is less dependent on whether it is mandatory than on the way it is organized and operated. A successful program should incorporate, in addition to adequate prescreening professional and public education, (a) properly timed tests, (b) centralized laboratories, (c) careful quality control, (d) rapid follow-up, and (e) state-sponsored medical and nursing consultation for families and free treatment.

12. At the moment, a majority of the PKU statutes provide for parental objections (on religious or other grounds) to screening. If mandatory laws are retained but such provisions are still to be taken seriously, changes will have to be made in the methods of taking specimens, so that parents are made aware of their right to refuse at an early enough time to exercise that right.

IV

SCREENING FOR OTHER DISEASES AND CHARACTERISTICS

To survey currently operating programs of screening for purposes of medical managment, reproductive information, and enumeration and epidemiologic studies, three subcommittees were formed, each to collect information on screening for one of the above aims. Directors and other people involved in projects of all three kinds were interviewed, state health departments were asked to provide information on their programs, and material was collected for an analysis of laws mandating screening for sickle cell anemia. These data, together with other information obtained from the literature, are presented in chapters included in this section. In addition, reviews of the current status of the uses of registers, and of practices and problems raised in screening of relatives of persons detected in population screening programs, are presented. As in the survey of PKU, *genetic screening projects outside the United States were consulted, this time from Canada, and summaries of Canadian experiences are included in Appendix I.*

5 Screening for Medical Intervention

Although screening for early detection of nongenetic disease has been going on for some time, screening for early detection of genetic disease has been conducted for only about 15 years and has been confined, until recently, largely to phenylketonuria. It is now possible to screen for other inborn errors, and since procedures are still not clearly formulated, a survey was undertaken (Table 5-1) of the current state of screening for (a) genetic diseases that are susceptible to treatment or some sort of medical management and (b) genetic characteristics which identify persons as capable of developing a particular disease in the future and for which medical intervention is available. A distinction was drawn in the survey between programs of screening for service to the public with little research content—for example, PKU—and others in which screening was carried out to discover information that may be useful for treatment and management at some future time—for example, alpha-1-antitrypsin deficiency and hyperlipidemia.

SCREENING TO PROVIDE HEALTH SERVICES

Data from a survey of state health departments designed to establish what is currently being done appear in Table 5-1. They represent the health departments' reports of the services now provided in these states; however, it is known that several of the health departments are experimenting with tests they did not mention, or have dropped others that are listed, usually after having discovered that the incidence of the disease in ques-

TABLE 5-1 Survey of State Screening Programs for Inborn Errors of Metabolism (As of January 1974)

State	Type of PKU Law (If Any)[a]	Disorders Screened for and Status of Program[b]		
		PKU	Hemoglobins	Others
Alabama	M	A	Test for abnormal hemoglobins (A)	1. MSUD 2. Tyrosinemia 3. Homocystinuria No positives found after 100,000 tests; discontinued. Will test for other inborn errors as methods are developed
Alaska	M	A	—	No laws, but test for: 1. MSUD (A) 2. Galactosemia (A) since they have specimens and technique fits PKU routine
Arizona	None	—	—	—
Arkansas	V	A	—	—
California	M	A	Sickle cell (limited)	—
Colorado	M	A	—	—
Connecticut	M	A	1. Sickle cell by request (A) 2. Thalassemia by request (A)	1. Galactosemia (A) 2. If galactosemia is positive, test also for G6PD deficiency (A) 3. Tay-Sachs by request (A)
Delaware	None	A	Sickle cell (A)	—
District of Columbia	None	A	—	—
Florida	M	A	—	—
Georgia	M	A	—	—
				—

			—	—
Illinois	M	A	—	—
Indiana	M	A	—	—
Iowa	M	A	—	—
Kansas	M	A	—	—
Kentucky	M	A	Sickle cell: mandatory law; screening required for newborns and to get marriage license	—
Louisiana	M	A	—	—
Maine	M	A	—	—
Maryland	M	A	—	—
Massachusetts	M	A	—	1. Galactosemia (A) 2. MSUD (A) 3. Homocystinuria (A) 4. Tyrosinosis (A) 5. Other metabolic an d renal transport disorders (A) 6. Urine paper chromatography (A)
Michigan	M	A	—	—
Minnesota	M	A	"On a selected basis"—none specified	
Mississippi	None	—	—	Diabetes mellitus (A)
Montana	M	A	—	Mandatory paper chromatography on blood for amino acid screening—as of 7/74
Nebraska	M	A	Sickle cell: supported in part by state, not necessarily ongoing	Tay-Sachs: supported in part by state, not necessarily ongoing
New Hampshire	M	A	—	—
New Jersey	M	A	—	—

TABLE 5-1 *(Continued)*

State	Type of PKU Law (If Any)[a]	Disorders Screened for and Status of Program[b]		
		PKU	Hemoglobins	Others
New Mexico	M	A	Sickle cell: voluntary, aimed at junior high and early high school child	—
New York	M	A	Sickle cell, pending legislation	1. Galactosemia (P) 2. Branched-chain ketonuria (P) 1. Galactosemia 2. Branched-chain ketonuria 3. Homocystinuria 4. Adenosine deaminase deficiency 5. Histidinemia 6. Others may be added Above six may be mandated statewide, pending legislation
North Carolina	None	A	—	1. Blood tyrosine (A) 2. Galactosemia (A) Above two from PKU specimens 1. T-3 (A) 2. T-4 (A) 3. SMA-12 (A) 4. Sugar evaluations (A) Above four by special arrangement —

Ohio	M	A	—	1. Galactosemia (A) 2. Homocystinuria (A)
Oklahoma	M	A	—	Tyrosine planned
Oregon	M	A	—	1. MSUD (A) 2. Galactosemia (A) 3. Tyrosinemia (A) 4. Homocystinuria (A) 1. Hereditary angio-neurotic edema (P) 2. α_1-antitrypsin deficiency (P) (on PKU filter paper)
Pennsylvania	M	A	—	—
Rhode Island	M	A	Sickle cell (A)	1. Homocystinuria (A) 2. Galactosemia (A) 3. MSUD (A) 4. Aminoacidurias (A)
South Carolina	M	A	Sickle cell (A)	—
South Dakota	Just passed PKU law; no funds provided	—	—	—
Tennessee	M	A	—	—
Texas	M	A	—	—
Utah	M	A	—	—
Vermont	None	A (Voluntary; not state-regulated but supported in part by state)	—	—
Virginia	M	A	—	Tyrosine follow-up of Guthrie test (A)
Washington	M	A	—	Others pending legislation. Plan congenital defects and counseling service

TABLE 5-1 *(Continued)*

State	Type of PKU Law (If Any)[a]	Disorders Screened for and Status of Program[b]		
		PKU	Hemoglobins	Others
West Virginia	M	A	—	—
Wisconsin	M	A	—	—
Wyoming	None	A (Hospital-regulated)	—	Paper chromatography in a few PKU screening sites (A)

[a]M = mandatory; V = voluntary.
[b]A = active; P = pilot.

TABLE 5-2 Frequencies of Some Inborn Errors for Which Screening Tests Are Available[a]

Disorder	Number Screened	Affected	Incidence
Phenylketonuria	13,538,912	1,186	1 : 11,500
Maple syrup urine disease	2,972,387	15	1 : 200,000
Homocystinuria	2,654,310	12	1 : 220,000
Histidinemia	1,001,193	41	1 : 24,000
Hartnup disease	554,301	21	1 : 26,000
Cystinuria	554,301	77	1 : 7,000
Galactosemia	3,099,738	41	1 : 75,000

[a] From Levy.[13]

tion did not warrant continued testing. The table, therefore, gives a rough but representative picture of genetic screening now going on in the United States, revealing that some of the states are testing for inborn errors in addition to PKU, most of them even less frequently encountered (Table 5-2 gives the incidence of PKU and other inborn errors in the population).

To obtain some insight into the operation of screening projects other than those for PKU, the Committee obtained detailed information directly from the sponsors of three of the most active ones and additional data on several others—either by interviewing employees of state health departments or as a result of visits by a sociologist employed by the Committee. What follows, therefore, is a composite of data derived from these several sources.

The Tests

Tests for PKU, maple syrup urine disease, homocystinuria, and tyrosinemia are done by modifications of the Guthrie method. Alpha-1-antitrypsin deficiency* and the inhibitor of the first component of complement (a defect in production of this inhibitor produces angioneurotic edema) are tested by fluorescent spot tests devised by Murphy. Others, including argininosuccinicaciduria, are tested by enzyme auxotroph tests, galactosemia by means of an enzyme assay devised by Beutler, and other aminoacidurias by chromatography of urine. Guthrie has contributed largely to this field and is able to test for as many as 11 disorders on a single sample of dried blood.[1] In general, it seems that considerable progress is being made in designing tests that are both sensitive and specific.

* The public health department in Oregon classifies its alpha-1-antitrypsin deficiency screening as a "service" program, but the Committee believes that this screening is still research, and treats it as such in the section on screening for research, below.

In many of the states the assays are done in one or at most a few state laboratories that are easily supervised and in which quality control is readily attained, but in others a great many laboratories may be involved. For example, in California upwards of 150 laboratories test for PKU and under these conditions, as has been described above, quality control is made somewhat more difficult.

Auspices for Screening

As we have seen, responsibility for the supervision of screening for PKU is in the hands of state health departments. Tests for other diseases are tried out from time to time, sometimes becoming a part of the regular procedure but often (after a trial) being discontinued. New tests may be instituted at the urging of an investigator at a nearby medical school, but more often the impulse emanates from the health department itself. Often the test is begun simply because it can be done by a modification of the Guthrie test and uses the sample taken for the PKU screening.

Apart from screening for sickle cell and Tay-Sachs disease, there appears to have been little effort on the part of agencies other than state health departments to promote screening for inborn errors of metabolism except for research purposes. Authorities in state or local medical societies have given the subject little thought or support, and there is little evidence of consultation between them and state health departments about starting new tests. Public participation has been limited to support by disease-related foundations of tests for specific diseases. Evidently, public acceptance of or resistance to screening has seldom been elicited or expressed.

Aims of Screening

As was seen above in the case of PKU, the principal aims of genetic screening are treatment and management. If a disease can be detected early, treatment may be effective in preventing death or developmental retardation; if not, management of some sort may relieve both patient and family of painful and heavy emotional burdens. Since these aims apply to all diseases regardless of frequency, some other reasons must have dictated the selection of the particular conditions listed in Table 5-1. These reasons appear to be (a) the condition is common enough to justify the cost and labor involved; (b) if it is rare, it is possible to add the test to an already existing screening battery with only marginal additional cost, usually by employing a modification of the Guthrie test; (c) all tests can be done on aliquots of the original sample of blood or urine. The last reason may explain why half a dozen states screen for maple syrup urine disease, a condition with a frequency of about 1/250,000 births. The test consists of a microbial assay based on the Guthrie principle that can be done on the same dried blood spot as the PKU test at little added cost.

The validity of this last reason may be questioned, however, in screening for hereditary angioneurotic edema, a consequence of a deficiency of an inhibitor of the first component of complement. Screening newborn infants for this disorder can be accomplished by a fluorescent test using the same blood sample, but the onset is variable and no accepted treatment is available; the wisdom of imparting the information to uncomprehending and anxious families is at least debatable.

Populations and Timing of Screening

In most programs the population screened is unselected. However, not all disorders occur with equal frequency in all populations. For example, tyrosinemia, although very rare in general, is as common as 1/650 in a small Canadian subpopulation, and PKU is less common among blacks than among whites. This probably explains the repeal of the PKU law in the District of Columbia where three quarters of the population is black, although the District health department continues to maintain an active program of screening for that disease.

With few exceptions, the diseases listed in Tables 5-1 and 5-2 have their onset at birth, and for some the urgency of immediate treatment makes immediate screening a necessity. For others, however, specifically α_1-antitrypsin deficiency and hereditary angioneurotic edema, the usefulness of screening newborns is less apparent, since the age of onset of manifestations is variable, some possessors of the genes may escape altogether, and no definitive treatment is presently available for either.

Prescreening Education

A common mechanism for educating parents whose newborn children are to be screened consists of distributing to them a pamphlet containing information about PKU and other diseases for which tests will be carried out. In some hospitals this may be supplemented by teaching sessions for mothers during which the screening is discussed. The purpose of this education is to inform the mother about the impending tests. It is intended to be a part of the consent mechanism, since the consent (or refusal) can be informed only if the parent is aware of the nature of the test to be done.

The effectiveness of these methods is unknown, since it is not clear how much the parents learn, nor what they feel about the test, whether anxieties are aroused, or how intelligible the material is to the general population. In at least one state the pamphlet asks the mother to furnish a urine specimen several weeks after the birth of the child, and since about 75% of the parents do so, it is clear that that part of the material, at least, has been understood.

Informed Consent

Although most states have mandatory statutes for PKU screening, two important questions concerning informed consent were raised in the survey of state practices.

First, in most states, statutes require that parents be given the opportunity to object to the blood sample on religious or other grounds, but it appears that such an opportunity is usually not provided. Rather, the sample is drawn as a routine matter shortly before the infant is discharged from the hospital. Sometimes the information pamphlet, which could alert the mother to the existence of the test and inform her of her right to object, is handed to her as she leaves the hospital—after the blood has been taken.

The second problem of consent arises in those states in which the law mandates only a PKU test but the state health department or other researchers use the blood sample for other metabolic tests. In some programs, almost countless dried blood spots are stored away against the day when additional tests could be done. That such tests might be done would, of course, be unknown to the person from whom the blood was taken. This raises certain legal questions with regard to the ownership of such samples, the consent needed for running tests on them, and the disposition of information. If, for example, it should become possible to do a test for Huntington's chorea on such a sample, what should be done with the information? Should positive results be relayed to the parents or guardians of the person from whom the blood was taken, or, if the individual is old enough, should it be transmitted to him? Little thought has been given to the impact of such tests on the public, and stores of blood, which tend to be regarded as a rich potential source for research purposes, raise important ethical and legal questions that must be faced. (See Part VII, pages 225–271, for more detail.)

In some states blood or urine samples are obtained after hospital discharge, for example, at a month or 6 weeks of age. Since a physician obtains the sample, one may assume that actual or implied consent is obtained, but the Committee's study revealed no information as to how often such consent is actually informed.

The Follow-up

When the result of the screening test is positive, it usually must be followed by a more definitive test. If this is positive, the information is transmitted to the family of the affected child, after which treatment or medical management of some kind is indicated. In most of the programs reviewed, the patient's physician was notified of a definitively positive test, and it was left to him to transmit the information to the family. In one program the physician is bypassed and the family is notified directly. In most instances, the treatment is started and supervised by physicians in teaching hospitals, while counseling and other forms of support may be given by physicians as well as by public health nurses, nutritionists, and others. Assuming that the treatment, which is usually dietary, is being supervised by a specialist, the remainder of the primary care of the baby falls to the family physician or pediatrician.

Although in outline these measures sound simple enough, many problems are encountered. If the diagnosis of a rare inborn error of metabolism with its need for a unique treatment is transmitted to a family through the private physician, difficulties are raised if the physician is himself unfamiliar with the disorder and with the treatment. Genetic counseling appears usually to be left to the physician supervising the treatment and is not generally regarded as a function of the health department. Evaluation of the effectiveness of counseling, of how well information is transmitted to the parents, and of their understanding of the disease is generally wanting, so no one really knows, except in anecdotal ways, what parents think of screening. With these exceptions, most of the programs reviewed run very well. One clinic in which these problems have been examined and carefully evaluated is that of the Children's Hospital of Montreal; this program could serve as a model for others[2] (see Appendix I for a full discussion of screening practices in Canada).

Involvement of Patients' Physicians

Patients' physicians often know little about the disorders for which screening is being done, and this condition is not effectively ameliorated by sending them pamphlets and fliers prior to instituting a new test. A common pattern is for the physician to announce his ignorance when informed that he has a patient in his practice with a rare inborn error and to ask the clinic director or state health department to assume responsibility for the treatment of the disease. On the other hand, in those programs that deal directly with the family and bypass the physician, the physician is often angered at what seems to be tampering with his patients.

Tests of Relatives

In general, screening programs assume no responsibility for tests for the carrier state in relatives of persons discovered to have inborn errors of metabolism. These relatives may themselves be at risk or may wish to know their genotypes. As far as the screening authority is concerned, this is left either to the families themselves, who may discuss the matter with their own doctor, or to the physician supervising the treatment.

Costs

Costs are generally calculated in oversimplified ways (see Chapter 12 for more detail). Many states simply divide the total funds allocated by the legislature by the number of tests. Others divide the amount of state money that must be added to other screening costs by the number of times the new test is carried out. In one state that has an elaborate screening program, the cost is calculated by dividing the total amount of money provided by the state for screening by the number of babies multiplied by the number of metabolic errors tested for to give an average cost per test. In all such instances, funds provided by sources other than the state, as well as nonmonetized costs, tend to be overlooked. It is evident that standard methods for cost accounting must be applied.

Regionalization

The possibility of regional centers is the object of considerable interest. Already, some of the less populous Western states send their PKU samples to another state for assay. Negotiations are going forward in both the Northwest and the Northeast for regional centers, each embracing several states. It has been suggested that such regionalization would reduce the number of laboratories carrying out tests and would facilitate quality control and reduce costs. In addition, by concentrating experience with screening in a small number of people, standardization would be accomplished and the institution of new tests would be simplified.

SCREENING FOR RESEARCH

Alpha-1-Antitrypsin Deficiency

Alpha-1-antitrypsin is a proteolytic enzyme inhibitor found among the human serum proteins.[3-5] Its electrophoretic mobility and other properties have been characterized, but its function is not clearly understood. A deficiency of this inhibitor was discovered in Sweden a number of years ago and was seen from the beginning to be associated with obstructive pulmonary disease. Family studies using a quantitative assay of inhibitor as the phenotype reveal that the deficiency is genetically determined. The homozygote shows very low activity, while the heterozygotes show around 60% activity.

Since these original studies were undertaken, many varieties of alpha-1-antitrypsin have been discovered, and they are classified under the heading of the Pi (protease inhibitor) system. More than 20 alleles are now known. The most frequent of them is Pi^M; two others, Pi^S and Pi^Z (both occurring in most populations with frequencies of greater than 1%) produce deficiency, Pi^Z more than Pi^S. Pregnancy, inflammatory disease, oral contraceptives, and some vaccines elevate the level of alpha-1-antitrypsin in the blood. The ZZ phenotype, with very low levels of inhibitor, is associated in perhaps 80% of its possessors with severe emphysema with onset at 20 to 30 years of age. In other persons, the same phenotype is associated with infantile cirrhosis. Occasionally an individual may have both these diseases.

In the United States, the study of the alpha-1-antitrypsin system and the relationship of its alleles to disease has been carried out by a number of investigators, all working together with the support of interrelated grants and contracts awarded by the National Institutes of Health. Two reference laboratories were established for the standardization of techniques, a newsletter is published, and all the investigators meet from time to time to compare results. Several of these investigators reviewed their work with the Committee.

Measurement Several methods of measurement of phenotype are available, including assays of serum trypsin inhibition, radioimmunodiffusion, and electroimmunoassay. These quantitative methods will detect the *ZZ* phenotype with certainty, but the heterozygous states *MZ, MS,* and *SZ* can be established with certainty only by means of electrophoretic typing methods, which are still rather complex and laborious. Automated systems for quantitative measurement have been developed, so that hundreds of serum samples could be screened for Pi type *ZZ* in a single day. Thus, if screening for the *ZZ* type should be considered beneficial, methods exist for processing large numbers of samples. All samples detected by screening would then need to be definitively typed.

Relation to Disease Most screening programs are concerned with the frequency of the various alleles, with the discovery of new alleles, or with efforts to determine whether the various heterozygous states are associated with disease.

The *MS* phenotype is found in 5–7% of most populations studied, while the *MZ* is found in 3–5%. Of all of the phenotypes, only *ZZ* and *SZ* have regularly been associated with disease, but some investigators believe that the *MZ* and possibly *MS* phenotypes are also associated with pulmonary disease. The latter possibility has been tested both retrospectively and prospectively: Some studies of the incidence of the various phenotypes in clinics treating emphysematous patients have shown excesses of the *MZ* phenotype among these patients, but the status of *MS* is less clear. In Rochester, a prospective study is being carried out with the double objective of determining the prevalence of the Pi types in an adult childbearing population and of discovering a pool of second-generation heterozygotes for long-term prospective pulmonary studies in an effort to determine the relationship of the various phenotypes to chronic respiratory disease. In all these studies the relationship of smoking to obstructive pulmonary disease and the α_1-antitrypsin phenotypes has been examined. A connection has been established with the *ZZ* phenotype, but although the results of some of the retrospective studies are suggestive, an unequivocal connection with the heterozygous states cannot yet be made. In the prospective study, no association has yet been discovered.

All these projects have brought out a number of problems inherent in research screening programs: (a) Many, if not most, of the studies already in the literature cannot be evaluated because of lack of standardization of the techniques for assay of inhibitor levels and determination of Pi type. (b) Many of the studies were not carried out according to good epidemiologic design. The numbers were often inadequate and controls were often insufficient. (c) There may be a "survivor effect." That is to say, assuming the *MS* and *MZ* heterozygotes are more prone to pulmonary disease than *MM*, the older the subjects screened, the less likely such heterozygotes will be represented. (d) Emphysema itself is very difficult to diagnose, so that the base-line frequency of emphysema in the population at any given age is not determined.

Other problems relating to the social impact of these screening programs are also apparent. In all the studies reviewed, little was offered the participants in the way of preliminary education, there was not much evaluation of the impact of a positive test result, and little follow-up was reported. In general, persons discovered to be either homozygous or heterozygous were told they ought to stop smoking, but in few instances was it determined whether such persons did stop or how they felt about being told to stop. It was also sometimes suggested to heterozygotes that they "choose their occupations wisely," that they seek early treatment for respiratory infections, and that they be certain to have immunization against influenza at times when that virus is epidemic. It was not known whether any of the subjects carried out these suggestions.

Persons with *ZZ* phenotype are definitely known to be at risk. So far, no evaluations have been reported of the effect of discovering that one has genes capable of ending one's life in an especially unpleasant way, perhaps in early middle age. Neither is it known what people do with the knowledge or how they feel about it, especially people who have never heard of alpha-1-antitrypsin and are unable to grasp its meaning with any precision. Neither is anything known of attitudes of insurance companies toward persons with the *ZZ* or any other phenotype.

Costs Costs for determination of phenotypes varied from $1.50 to $30.00. It is difficult in this case to reckon a cost–benefit relationship since the benefits of screening are so uncertain.

Summary In summary, although it seems clear that the *ZZ* phenotype is deleterious, and that the *SZ* phenotype is probably harmful, the hazards of the other heterozygous states remain to be described. Until this question is cleared up and since so little evaluation has been made of the social impact of screening for this characteristic, it seems likely that screening for α_1-antitrypsin variants will remain, for the time being, a research activity.

Familial Hyperlipidemia and Premature Atherosclerosis

Epidemiologic studies have distinguished several causative factors of coronary artery disease: hyperlipidemia, hypertension, cigarette smoking, and diabetes. Hyperlipidemia is defined as an increase in the concentration in circulating blood plasma or serum of cholesterol or triglycerides or both. For clincial purposes, hyperlipidemia has been translated into hyperlipoproteinemia; of this there are at least five types, based on variations in lipid levels in the blood and on the qualities and quantities of the lipoproteins. These types are descriptively useful, but probably none is due to a single genotype.

There are now several effective and practical means of reducing hyperlipidemia, including diet and some drugs, but it has not so far been demonstrated unequivocally that lowering the blood lipids will reduce the risk of premature vascular disease. Most atherosclerosis is believed to be less influenced by genetic than by cultural factors, including particularly the diet, and when mass prophylaxis has been recommended, it is mainly to alter these cultural factors.

Studies of genetic causes of hyperlipidemia carried out by Goldstein and others[6,7] and by Kwiterovich and others reveal three main patterns of distribution of hyperlipidemia in families[8]: In one pattern, all affected persons have hypercholesterolemia alone; in the second, all affected persons in families have hypertriglyceridemia alone; and in the third, some of the affected persons have hypercholesterolemia, some hypertriglyceridemia, and some both. The pedigrees of these families suggest single-gene inheritance, but one cannot rule out more complex modes of transmission. About 1% of the population has one or another of these forms of hyperlipidemia.

In addition to these three apparently mendelian forms of hyperlipidemia, there are others, also familial, whose distribution suggests some multigenic origin. Goldstein showed that of 500 patients with myocardial infarction under 60 years of age, about one third had hyperlipidemia. Of these, a third had disease of polygenic or possibly nongenetic origin, a third had combined hypercholesterolemia and hypertriglyceridemia, and approximately one sixth had familial hypertriglyceridemia alone and another sixth had hypercholesterolemia alone.

The relationship of genetic hyperlipidemia to heart disease was studied by Goldstein by comparing the incidence of myocardial infarction among the members of the families with hyperlipidemia with those of control families. His index cases were individuals under 60 who had had myocardial infarction. When the records of relatives of individuals who had had myocardial infarction and hyperlipidemia were scrutinized, there were twice as many persons who had suffered myocardial infarctions among these relatives as among relatives of a control group (ascertained through a patient with myocardial infarction whose serum lipids were normal).

Screening for Hyperlipidemia It is a matter of consequence to screening programs that among hyperlipidemic families the lipid patterns in children are not the same as those of the adults. Hypercholesterolemia appears at birth, but hypertriglyceridemia does not, reaching its full expression only in adults. For the combined type, neither hypercholesterolemia nor hypertriglyceridemia appears in children. Thus, screening at birth or in childhood would be feasible only for hypercholesterolemia.

Screening for hypercholesterolemia at birth has been carried out in several large studies.[9,10] In four of these, cord blood was collected from 7,200 newborn babies. Three to five percent of these had cholesterol values above the 95th percentile, but it cannot be ascertained how many of these babies have familial hypercholesterolemia. Neither is it known how many infants with normal cord blood levels may manifest familial hypercholesterolemia later in life. If these two questions are to be answered, family studies must be done for each kind of infant and the babies must be re-evaluated later, at least after their first birthday. Even this latter evaluation is complicated by the marked effect of diet on plasma lipids during the first year of life. Results of studies to answer the first question are beginning to be reported, and the incidence of familial hypercholesterolemia ascertained at birth varies from .0025 to .005. These individuals are designated as suffering from familial hypercholesterolemia not only because of continued hypercholesterolemia a year after birth but also because of the presence of affected persons in their families. Most infants with elevated cord blood cholesterol levels are found a year later to have normal levels. The answer to the second question—how many infants with normal cord blood cholesterol levels develop hypercholesterolemia at one year of age—is less clear. Apparently, it does occur, but no one knows with what frequency.

Agreement has not been reached on the best test to use in screening for hypercholesterolemia in the newborn period. Measurements both of cholesterol and of low-density lipoproteins appear to be important, but more information is required before it can be said whether one or both of these measurements are necessary.

As to treatment, dietary restrictions instituted as early as possible should be the best form of treatment; but side effects, if any, are still unknown, and it cannot be said unequivocally that such early treatment is effective in the prevention of premature atherosclerosis.

Thus the question of how to screen for genetic hyperlipidemias remains unresolved. To be truly efficient, it might have to be done three times: A first screen at birth might detect familial hypercholesterolemia, provided family studies were done on infants with high cord blood cholesterol levels and the cholesterol level were checked again at 1 year of age. If a second screen were done at age 5 or 6 years, hypertriglyceridemia would begin to be discovered; and if it were done in high school, the rest of the familial hyperlipidemias would make themselves known. It is also possible that almost as much information might be learned if adults were screened at 25 or 30 years of age and then the children of affected persons studied. Another way of approaching the problem might be for pediatricians to inquire about the incidence of myocardial infarction in the previous two generations on both sides of the family. Infants with a positive family history could then be screened.

Here again, as in screening for other characteristics, little is known about the impact of the news of a genetic predisposition to disaster on individuals who must live with the information. In addition, since it is not yet certain that dietary or drug intervention in fact prevents vascular damage (even though that seems reasonable), it is possible that even if screening techniques were simple, accurate, cheap, and capable of giving maximum information at any time of life, one could not be sure that one had not discovered something about which nothing could be done. Studies also need to be done to discover the effectiveness of attempts to modify dietary habits. Modification of smoking habits, also a risk factor for myocardial infarction, has been only partially successful.

It is likely that screening for hyperlipidemias in children will remain, therefore, in the research area for some time to come.[11]

Hypertension

Widespread population screening for hypertension is now being advocated. Although there is a large body of literature on the influence of the genes on blood pressure, nothing is known about these genetic influences to suggest that a screening test would be capable of predicting future elevations of blood pressure. On the basis of blood pressures taken very carefully in small children, Kass has shown that, although the pressures rise with age, they tend to remain in a fixed position relative to others.[12] That is, apart from a few specific types of hypertension, persons whose blood pressures were found to be high in middle life had pressures on the high side in young adulthood, teenage, childhood, and infancy; if the pressure in middle years is low, so was it low earlier. It is not known to what degree such blood pressure differences may be the result of the genotype or of special dietary or even intrauterine experiences, so that it is premature to think of screening for any genetic factors now.[13]

REFERENCES

1. Guthrie, R. Mass screening for genetic disease. Hosp. Pract. 7(6):93–100, 1972.
2. Clow, C. L., F. C. Fraser, C. Laberge, and C. R. Scriver. On the application of knowledge to the patient with genetic disease. Prog. Med. Genet. 9:159–213, 1973.
3. Sharp, H. L. Alpha-1-antitrypsin deficiency. Hosp. Pract. 6(5):83–96, 1971.
4. Mittman, C., T. Barbela, and J. Lieberman. Antitrypsin deficiency and abnormal protease inhibitor phenotypes. Arch. Environ. Health 27:201–206, 1973
5. Mittman, C., and J. Lieberman. Screening for alpha-1-antitrypsin deficiency. Israel J. Med. Sci. 9:1311–1318, 1973.
6. Goldstein, J. L., W. R. Hazzard, H. G. Schrott, E. L. Bierman, and A. G. Motulsky. Hyperlipidemia in coronary heart disease. I. Lipid levels in 500 survivors of myocardial infarction. J. Clin. Invest. 52:1533–1534, 1973.
7. Goldstein, J. L., H. G. Schrott, W. R. Hazzard, E. L. Bierman, and A. G. Motulsky. Hyperlipidemia in coronary heart disease. II. Genetic analysis of lipid levels in 176 families and delineation of a new inherited disorder, combined hyperlipidemia. J. Clin. Invest. 52:1544–1568, 1973.

8. Kwiterovich, P. O., Jr., D. S. Fredrickson, and R. I. Levy. Familial hypercholesterolemia (one form of familial type II hyperlipoproteinemia). A study of its biochemical, genetic, and clinical presentation in childhood. J. Clin. Invest. 53:1237–1249, 1974.
9. Kwiterovich, P. O., Jr. Neonatal screening for hyperlipidemia. Pediatrics 53:445–457, 1974.
10. Goldstein, J. L., J. J. Albers, H. G. Schrott, W. R. Hazzard, E. L. Bierman, and A. G. Motulsky. Plasma lipid levels and coronary heart disease in adult relatives of newborns with normal and elevated cord blood lipids. Amer. J. Hum. Genet. (In press)
11. Zinner, S. H., P. S. Levy, and E. H. Kass. Familial aggregation of blood pressure in childhood. N. Engl. J. Med. 284:401–404, 1971.
12. Kass, E. Personal communication to the Committee.
13. Levy, H. L. Genetic screening. Adv. Hum. Genet. 4:1–104, 1973.

6 Screening to Provide Reproductive Information

One objective of genetic screening is the discovery of persons possessing particular genotypes in order to provide them with information that may be relevant to their reproductive decisions. Such persons may be the carriers of genes for sex-linked or autosomal recessive traits, or of autosomal dominants that are latent during reproductive years or only minimally expressed. The assumption behind such screening is that awareness of such genes is an important ingredient in decisions about reproduction. To have the knowledge is to enhance freedom of choice.

Screening of this kind is already being done in the United States, both for health service and for research. For example, carriers for hemoglobinopathies and Tay-Sachs disease are the objects of some programs, while in others amniocentesis is being used to discover fetuses with Down's syndrome. A representative view of the accomplishments and unresolved issues of these and other programs was an object of the Committee's inquiry. Persons actively involved in many such projects were interviewed; their observations and data from the recent literature are included in this chapter.

SCREENING FOR HEMOGLOBINOPATHIES

Screening for sickle cell anemia and sickle cell trait is being conducted as a public service in many places, while the search for thalassemia trait remains largely in the area of research.

Sickle Cell Anemia and Sickle Cell Trait

It has been recognized only recently that sickle cell anemia is a disorder in which there is a wide variation in severity, time of onset, frequency of crises, length of life, and functional status of affected individuals. Although many patients die before adulthood, those who do survive past adolescence often find gainful employment, have families, and function as useful citizens. The cost of care for sickle cell anemia is high because of frequent episodes of pain and thrombotic crises that require repeated and sometimes prolonged hospitalization. There is still no effective treatment for the disorder.

Classical sickle cell anemia is the most common of the various sickle cell diseases and results when a child inherits the gene for hemoglobin S from each of his parents. Other sickle cell diseases are the result of combinations of the gene for hemoglobin S with such other alleles as those specifying hemoglobin C, hemoglobin D, β-thalassemia, and persistent fetal hemoglobin. Clinical disease in these disorders is usually less severe than in classical sickle cell anemia. The carrier state for hemoglobin S occurs in 8–10% of the American black population; that for hemoglobin C in 2–3%; and that for β-thalassemia and persistent fetal hemoglobin in 1–2% and 0.1%, respectively.[1]

Screening programs for sickle cell disease and trait have evolved in a rapid, haphazard, often poorly planned fashion, generated in large measure by public clamor and political pressure. Six programs were reviewed by the Committee (Appendix A, p. 275). The general characteristics of these programs are described below.

Objectives Some of the programs are well planned with clearly thought out and stated objectives; others were initiated simply because it was fashionable to do so. Some of the programs are mainly investigative, studying, among other things, the effectiveness of educational and counseling techniques. The objective of some is simply to discover persons with sickle cell anemia without particular concern for the trait. Others offer to test everyone who wants to be tested and to provide education and information about sickle cell disease and trait; most offer reproductive advice, particularly for couples who both have sickle cell trait.

This last objective exposes an important inconsistency in screening for sickle cell trait. There is now no prenatal test available for sickle cell disease, with the choice of a therapeutic abortion if indicated; thus the current alternatives to taking a rather high risk with each pregnancy are limited to artificial insemination or adoption. How to decide in advance which individuals will find such information helpful and which will be merely threatened is an unresolved question.

Tests There is general agreement that electrophoresis is the best test and that Sickledex or slide tests alone are inadequate. The latter distinguish only Hg S and give no information about other hemoglobin abnormalities.

Auspices and Settings Projects have been carried out under a great variety of auspices. Some have been sponsored by local Sickle Cell Foundations, some are under the direction of state health departments, and others are directed by city health departments. Some projects are offered as a service in hospital clinics, others partly as a service, partly as research, by individual investigators. Sickle cell testing has also been carried out by the Black Panthers and other "black awareness" groups, without medical supervision. In some instances, programs have been unwittingly in competition with one another, and in big cities it is possible that individuals have been tested more than once. Since 1971, sickle cell disease centers intended to promote screening, management, counseling, and research, have been supported by the National Institutes of Health and the Health Services Administration.[2]

A wide range of settings have been used, including hospital clinics, health centers for adults, prenatal clinics, well-baby clinics, schools, public health clinics, private practitioners' offices, and churches.

Populations Some of the programs test all who present themselves, regardless of age or condition. Others are aimed at unmarried adolescents and young married people. Newborn babies, schoolchildren, both primary and secondary, young people in the Job Corps, infants in well-baby clinics, and mothers at prenatal clinics have all been mentioned as target populations.

Educational Programs Most projects make some attempt to educate the population to be screened, using television, radio, newspaper articles, pamphlets, and other literature. In addition, visual aids are used and lectures are given, often just before the screening is to be done. Physicians, nurses, teachers, public health department personnel, and technicians have all been employed in providing the education. The educational material generally consists of information about the nature of the disease, its genetic origin, the segregation of genes, the odds for the disorder, gene frequency, and the nature of sickle cell trait, with emphasis on its distinction from the disease. In most programs, little attempt is made to determine whether the educational efforts have been successful. Those studies that have been made reveal that while retention of the information offered is directly correlated with educational attainment, it is especially difficult to transmit the abstract ideas of probability, and the results of such efforts vary widely.

Too little attention has been paid to the reasons some persons participate in these screening programs and others do not. One cause for noncompliance must be that despite the educational programs, many people remain ignorant of the disease; this, too, appears to be related to educational and social status.[3] Nor are ignorance and misinformation about sickle cell disease confined to the lay public. One study revealed that of 160 physicians polled, 1 in 7 believed that sickle cell trait is a disease, 1 in 5 thought it was difficult to distinguish trait from disease, and 1 in 2 was unaware of the existence of the SC and S-thal phenotypes.[4]

Legislation In the period from 1971 to 1973, pressures from health, community, and political groups combined to spur a number of states to adopt laws promoting or mandating sickle cell screening. Again, Massachusetts led the way with the adoption in mid-1971 of a statute "requiring the testing of blood for sickle trait or anemia as a prerequisite to school attendance." To date, 16 other states and the District of Columbia have enacted statutes on sickle cell testing, although amendments to the legislation establishing some of these programs have by now, in effect, abolished them.

Seven of the programs were mandatory as of June 1974 (Question 1 in Table 6-1), but the mandatory nature of the programs was undercut by provisions for objection by the screenee on general grounds in three states and on religious grounds in a fourth (Question 2 in Table 6-1). Moreover, the requirement in the National Sickle Cell Anemia Control Act that state programs be run on a voluntary basis to qualify for federal support has continued to cause states to change mandatory programs into voluntary ones. In the voluntary programs studied by the Committee, consent is asked but the amount of information given the screenee or presented in the consent form varies. In some hospitals where hemoglobin electrophoresis is routinely performed as part of the diagnostic workup on patients at risk for hemoglobinopathies, consent is not asked, which violates the patient's right to have the test omitted.

As mentioned above, some of the statutory sickle cell screening programs are directed at schoolchildren, others at marriage license applicants (under a strained analogy to the serologic test for syphilis usually required for a marriage license), and a few at pregnant women or newborn babies (Question 3 in Table 6-1). Only Kentucky's statute now actually makes reference to a single racial group (blacks) being singled out for screening; but a majority of the other statutes are drawn, with varying degrees of candor or obfuscation, so as to achieve similar results (Question 16, and accompanying notes, in Table 6-1). Most states do not attach any penalty to violation of the statute, but four states provide for fine or imprisonment (Georgia, Indiana, Kansas, and Kentucky) and five withhold marriage licenses or school attendance from those not complying with the statute (Illinois, Indiana, Massachusetts, Mississippi, and New York). (See Question 9 in Table 6-1.)

Given the great concern over the potential abuse of data on a person's sickle cell status, it is somewhat surprising that only four states (Kansas, Maryland, Massachusetts, and Virginia) make the results of screening confidential by statute (Question 15 in Table 6-1). All these provisions were enacted in 1973, after a great deal of criticism had been leveled at the initial effort at legislation. In the projects studied by the Committee, confidentiality had generally been maintained, although the great variety in auspices under which the testing was done meant varying degrees of formality of record-keeping. Two of the Committee's informants revealed that a city school system had asked for the results of tests but were refused this information. It was not clear why the schools wanted the results.

Most of the statutes do not require that any state agency be informed of screening results (Question 7 in Table 6-1), and more remarkably, only six of the statutes specify at all who should receive test results (Question 8 in Table 6-1). The Illinois and Indiana statutes provide that positive results of sickle cell screening will be funneled back through the physician conducting the test; in Georgia, Maryland, Massachusetts, and New York test results go to the person screened or to a parent of that person.

The fact that sickle cell screening legislation was enacted on a less carefully thought-out basis than PKU screening laws, and as a result of different and more diverse pressures, is also shown by the fact that there are requirements for research in only three states (Louisiana, North Carolina, and Ohio) and for educational activities in only another five (Maryland, Massachusetts, Mississippi, New Mexico, and Virginia), all states with statutes enacted or modified late in 1972 or in 1973 (see Question 5 in Table 6-1).

To some extent, however, sickle cell legislation initially followed the same pattern as PKU—sudden public awareness of the availability of simple testing methods that could "prevent" a serious disease, leading to organized pressure to make all susceptible individuals undergo the test. But the central difference in the means of prevention between PKU and

TABLE 6-1 State Sickle Cell Statutes (As of June 1964)

Key

Numbers in parentheses refer to column heads.

(1) Is sickle cell testing mandatory?
 a) test for sickle cell is mandated by statute
 b) statute vests discretionary power in the department of health to make sickle cell testing mandatory if the department deems it necessary
 c) test for sickle cell is nonmandatory

(2) Is there a provision for avoiding screening on the basis of:
 a) religious objections of parents
 b) general objections of parents
 c) objection of (adult) person to be tested
 d) no provision

(3) Who is to be tested?
 a) all schoolchildren
 b) all newborns
 c) pregnant women
 d) applicants for a marriage license

(4) When should the child be tested?
 a) newborn
 b) entering school

(5) In addition to testing, does the statute require:
 a) research
 b) education
 c) no other requirements

(6) Who is responsible for reporting the test?
 a) physician
 b) parent

(7) Must the results of the test be reported to the state board of health or other state agency?
 a) all results
 b) all positive results
 c) "recording"/"reporting" contemplated by statute but details left to administrators
 d) no requirement

(8) Who, in addition to state officials, receives results of testing?
 a) physician receives all positive results
 b) person tested
 c) parents of person tested

(9) What penalty attaches to violation of the statute?
 a) fine or imprisonment
 b) exclusion from school
 c) withholding of marriage license
 d) no penalty clause

(10) Must the state provide testing materials and/or services?

(11) What test is prescribed for initial sickle cell screening?
 a) electrophoresis or other standard test

b) test to be designated by state board of health or other state agency
c) no test prescribed by statute

(12) Is the department of health responsible for follow-up activity including treatment?

a) yes
b) counseling only
c) no provision

(13) By statute, must all testing be performed in a state-run laboratory?

(14) If tests are conducted in other laboratories, are the laboratories regulated by the state?

a) regulated by another statute
b) regulated by sickle cell statute

State	Date of Enactment	(1)	(2)	(3)	(4)	(5)
Arizona	1972, amended 1973	c[2]	b,c	a,c,d	b	c
California	1973	—	d	a[11]	—	c
Georgia	1972	a[3]	a,c	b,d	a	c
Illinois	1971, amended 1973	a[4]	b[9]	a,d[4]	b	c
Indiana	1972,[1] 1973	a[4]	a	a,d[4]	—	c
Kansas	1973	—	d	—	—	c
Kentucky	1972	a	d	b,d[12]	a	c
Louisiana	1972	c	b	a,b	a,b	a,b
Maryland	1972, amended 1973	c	b, c	—	—	b
Massachusetts	1971, amended 1973	a[5]	d	a[5]	b	b
Mississippi	1972	b[6]	d	a[6]	b	b
New Jersey	1972	—	d	[13]	—	c
New Mexico	1973	a[7]	d	a[7]	—	b
New York	1971, amended 1972	a[8]	c[10]	a,d[8]	b	c
North Carolina	1973	c	c	[14]	—	a,b
Ohio	1972	—	d	—	—	a,b
Virginia	1972, amended 1973	c	c	—	—	b

NOTE: A blank space indicates that the state statute does not contain any information pertinent to the question.

Notes

Numbers here refer to those in the body of the table.

[1] INDIANA—The provision mandating the testing of marriage license applicants was enacted in 1972; the provision mandating the testing of schoolchildren was enacted in 1973.

[2] ARIZONA—The Department of Health Services "may require that a test be given" to "any identifiable segment of the population" determined to be "susceptible" at a "disproportionately higher ratio" than the rest of the population, but consent of the person to be tested or his parent (if such person is a minor) must be obtained.

[3] GEORGIA—§53-216 mandates that each marriage license applicant be *offered* a sickle cell anemia test "as well as counselling . . . that a carrier of the inheritable hemoglobin type of sickle cell anemia may convey to his or her offspring the sickle cell anemia trait or the disease sickle anemia." §88-1201.1 provides that all newborn infants "who are susceptible or likely to have . . . sickle cell anemia or sickle cell trait" shall be tested.

[4] ILLINOIS; INDIANA—As physician determines.

[5] MASSACHUSETTS—As commissioner of public health determines to be susceptible to sickle cell anemia.

c) no regulation

(15) Are the results of the test required by statute to be kept confidential?

(16) Is there a provision for screening on a racial basis?

a) specific reference to blacks or Negro race

b) statute contemplates that only *some* children need to be tested

c) no differentiation made or contemplated

(17) How does the statute describe what is being tested for?

a) meniscocytosis

b) sickle cell anemia

c) sickle cell disease

d) sickle cell syndrome

e) sickle cell trait

(6)	(7)	(8)	(9)	(10)	(11)	(12)	(13)	(14)	(15)	(16)	(17)
—	d	—	d	no	b	c	no	a	no	b[2]	b
—	c	—	d	[22]	c	c	no	a	no	b[11]	e
—	d	c[18]	a	yes[23]	c	b[23]	no	a	no	b[3]	b,e
—	b	a	b,c	yes[24]	c	c	no	a	no	b[4]	b
[15]	a[16]	a[16]	a,b,c	no	a,b	c	no	b	no	b[4]	b
—	d	—	a	no	c	b[28]	no	a	yes	c	b,e
—	d	—	a	no	c	b	no	a,b	no	a	c,e
a	b[17]	—	d	yes[25]	c	a	no	c	no	c	a
—	c	b,c[19]	d	no	c	c	no	a	yes	c	—
—	c	b,c[19]	b	yes[26]	b	a[29]	no	c	yes	b[5]	b,e
—	d	—	b	no	c	c	no	c	no	b[6]	b,e
—	d	—	d	no	c	c	no	a	no	c	b
—	d	—	d	yes[27]	c	c	no	c	no	b[7]	b,e
—	d	b,c[20]	b,c[21]	yes[21]	c	a[30]	no	a	no	b[8]	b
—	d	—	d	yes[14]	c	b	no	c	no	c	d
—	d	—	d	no	c	a[31]	no	a	no	c	c
—	c	—	d	no	b	b	no	c	yes	c	b

[6] MISSISSIPPI—As Board of Health determines to be particularly susceptible to sickle cel anemia.

[7] NEW MEXICO—For "all school-age children who may be susceptible" to sickle cell anemia.

[8] NEW YORK—Mandatory for city schoolchildren only; as physician determines necessary for other schoolchildren. Mandatory for each marriage license applicant not of Caucasian, Indian, or Oriental race.

[9] ILLINOIS—Tests for schoolchildren but not marriage license applicants may be avoided on "constitutional" grounds.

[10] NEW YORK—Test may be avoided by religious objection of *child*, or of marriage license applicant.

[11] CALIFORNIA—§307 mandates that the health screening and evaluation aspect of each county's "child health and disability prevention program" include for each child a test for sickle cell anemia, "where appropriate."

[12] KENTUCKY—Only members of the "Negro race" are tested.

[13] NEW JERSEY—Children under 21 years.

[14] NORTH CAROLINA—The Department of Human Resources shall make available testing and counseling services for any persons so requesting, without cost to such persons.

[15] INDIANA—The governing body of each school corporation must file a report with the state board of health.
[16] INDIANA—For results of schoolchildren's tests only.
[17] LOUISIANA—Positive results on newborn children must be sent to the Department of Public Health; positive results on schoolchildren must be sent to the parish or city school board of the area in which the child resides.
[18] GEORGIA—Provides for reporting only in cases of positive results on newborn children.
[19] MARYLAND; MASSACHUSETTS—Results shall be made available to the person tested, or if the person tested is under 18 years, to his parent or guardian.
[20] NEW YORK—Parents of schoolchildren shall be notified of positive results; marriage license applicants shall be notified of all results.
[21] NEW YORK—Rather than excluding child who does not furnish certificate of testing, the school gives parents 15 days notice that child will be tested mandatorily; parents could choose to remove child from school and place him in school not requiring test (e.g., private school; out-of-state school, etc.).
[22] CALIFORNIA—Statute is unclear whether county, in establishing a child health and disability prevention program, has the obligation of providing testing materials or services.
[23] GEORGIA—Counseling for children free, but statute does not specify charges for testing; adults must pay for both counseling and testing (absent "adequate state appropriations or Federal aid") but price charged cannot exceed one dollar.
[24] ILLINOIS—If parent is unable to obtain sickle cell test for his child, the test will be provided by the local health department or the school district under an agreement with either licensed physicians or a voluntary agency.
[25] LOUISIANA—Each child entering school must have a test for meniscocytosis administered by his or her family physician *or by the parish health unit* in the parish where the school is located; the attending physician of a newborn child shall cause said child to be subject to a test for meniscocytosis.
[26] MASSACHUSETTS—The 1973 amendment provides that the state shall furnish facilities for a *voluntary* screening program; this appears to supplement the mandatory school testing program enacted in 1971.
[27] NEW MEXICO—For "any person unable to afford the services of a physician."
[28] KANSAS—Counseling must be provided without charge to anyone requesting counseling relative to sickle cell anemia.
[29] MASSACHUSETTS—Any screening program that may be established "shall include provisions for a complete health education and post-screening counseling service and for such treatment of those affected by any blood abnormality as the commissioner by regulation may determine to be appropriate or practical."
[30] NEW YORK—If parent or guardian is unable or unwilling to provide treatment for afflicted pupil.
[31] OHIO—The director of health shall "provide for rehabilitation and counseling of persons possessing the trait of or afflicted with this disease."

sickle cell (treating homozygotes versus counseling heterozygotes on reproduction), the consequent problems in finding an ideal age for screening, and the racial nature of the condition led to much more criticism of sickle cell screening. Moreover, legislation tended to be drafted by legislators rather than by interest groups; it was often done hurriedly, for political reasons, and without the coordinated effort that had occurred in the case of PKU. As a result, when strong opposition developed and the federal statute somewhat pre-empted the field, the flood tide of sickle cell screening statutes rapidly ebbed.

Transmission of Results and Counseling The methods of communicating the results of screening are as variable as other aspects of these projects. It is sometimes done by telephone or by letter and occasionally by a home visit from a public health nurse or by a communication from a physician. In some programs, which screen only for sickle cell disease, information about trait is not transmitted at all.

Most programs include counseling, not only to discuss reproductive odds, but also to clear up any misapprehensions about the test and the meaning of the result. The counseling is done by physicians, nurses, students, and technicians, as well as by other members of the community especially trained for the purpose. Generally, the counseling is given sometime after the subject has been informed that he is a carrier. Sessions vary in length and in content and are carried out in clinics, community centers, schools, well-baby clinics, or wherever the screening was done. The choice of a location for counseling may inadvertently lead to a breach of confidentiality, because persons seen entering a room known to have been set aside for counseling of carriers may become labeled as carriers whether they are or not.

Large numbers, perhaps a majority, of individuals found to be carriers for hemoglobin S do not return for counseling, so their response to the discovery of their genotype is unknown. How effective the counseling has been for those who do return is also unclear, although a few studies reveal that significant numbers of people fail to remember what they have been told, or have misapprehensions about the information. For example, it is difficult to teach some carriers that they do not have a disease. It is especially important that this be understood, not only by the carriers themselves, but also by the general public; misunderstanding by either group may lead to carriers being—or feeling that they are—stigmatized by the test results. In one study in which infants and children were tested, the knowledge of parents of carriers was shown to be better than those of noncarriers. That is, the latter were more likely to believe erroneously that being a carrier was an illness that required additional food and extra rest and that might impair the development of the child.[5]

Hazards of Screening In addition to the stigma resulting from general misunderstanding about sickle cell trait, discrimination of other sorts is also a hazard of screening. Since the emphasis in sickle cell programs is on the effects of being a carrier on reproduction, it is not surprising that a major effect of screening results is on the marriageability of those found to be positive. This type of stigmatization was poignantly demonstrated in a screening program in a community in Greece conducted for the express purpose of discovering carriers so as to eliminate the disease.[6] Marriages there are generally arranged by the parents, so it was thought that matings between carriers should easily be avoided if the hemoglobin status of all marriageable persons was known. At the end of the study, the frequency of sickle cell disease had not diminished, but young women known to be carriers were no longer regarded as desirable objects for matrimony in that village and went elsewhere. Although young women in North America may not experience this hazard, sufficient attitudinal studies have not yet been carried out to eliminate it altogether.

Evidence of stigmatization in the United States is seen in job discrimination, in proposals to limit admission to the armed forces to noncarriers, and in increases in insurance premiums.[7] Nine of twelve insurance companies in one sample charged higher rates for individuals with sickle trait even though mortality curves for such individuals do not differ significantly from blacks without the trait.[8] The screening of school-age children for sickle cell trait is subject to particular hazards, since the natural caution and fears of parents and teachers may lead to unnecessary but unavoidable restriction on activities and unconscious but irreversible curtailment of expectations for performance and achievement. All of these results of "labeling" therefore reflect misunderstanding about the significance of being a carrier.

Even when the information is correctly understood, harm can be done by screening. The discovery of nonpaternity is such a hazard. Testing has been known to result in marital rifts and divorce when a child is discovered whose genotype cannot be accounted for. Some counselors attempt to explain the child's genotype as a new mutation, but parents are often not persuaded. This outcome could be guarded against by indicating in the educational materials, and when obtaining informed consent, that the test can uncover nonpaternity.

Family Testing When an individual is discovered to be a carrier, it is a general rule to suggest that other members of the family be tested, particularly to discover matings in which both partners are heterozygous. How frequently the screenees comply with this recommendation is not known. How far it should be pushed is in any case debatable: It is in family testing that nonpaternity is discovered, and there is so little constructive to offer the carriers who might be discovered by vigorous pursuit of the relatives.

The Present State of Sickle Cell Screening Although there have been many mistakes and some controversy, sickle cell screening is continuing in a more certain and businesslike atmosphere.[2,9-11] The establishment of sickle cell centers for testing, counseling, and research has helped in promoting education and understanding, and community organizations have helped in setting priorities and working toward unified aims. Misconceptions about sickle cell trait are being dispelled, and there are fewer allegations of job discrimination. Further, some of the mandatory state laws have been repealed or modified. Some of the early practices of sickle cell screening programs are lessons in what not to do; we may look forward to the useful employment of the wisdom of the veterans of these projects to provide guidance to initiators of future screening programs for other conditions.[12-13]

Thalassemia

Thalassemia major is a severe disease with less variability than sickle cell anemia. Homozygotes for severe α-thalassemia are usually spontaneously aborted or stillborn; β-thalassemia, or Cooley's anemia, is a severe, crippling disease that often results in early death. The β-thalassemia gene exists with greatest frequency in Mediterranean populations, but a variant is found also in perhaps 1–2% of U.S. blacks. Occasionally individuals are found with the $\beta^{S/Thal}$ genotype.

A few screening projects currently in operation aim to detect thalassemia carriers. One representative program, carried out in Connecticut, studied populations of Greek and Italian descent, including some high school students. Red cell size, measured in a Coulter counter, was the test selected after other tests were found wanting. Positive results were checked with assays for serum iron and A_2 hemoglobin, which is usually elevated in this condition.

A communitywide educational campaign was carried out in which Cooley's anemia and thalassemia trait were clearly differentiated. Persons with positive results were offered counseling in which the relevant genetics was discussed. Most persons found to have the trait were said to have availed themselves of this service, but since neither the success of the educational program nor the effectiveness of the counseling was evaluated, what the screenees actually learned is unknown.

The need for or usefulness of screening for thalassemia trait is not yet settled. In the first place, there is little point in screening for the disease, which will in any case announce itself. In the second place, screening for thalassemia trait in order to provide reproductive information is of doubtful value on two counts. The methods, while reliable in competent hands, are not simple and cheap and are easily abused; and the potential for causing anxiety is as great as in the sickle cell program without, once again, any reproductive alternative other than to avoid having children. Furthermore, people of Greek and Italian ancestry are outbreeding with such frequency as to reduce the incidence of thalassemia major so that we no longer know what that incidence is, although it is known to be considerably less than that of sickle cell disease. Perhaps for the moment the availability of a test for thalassemia should be made known and provided for those who feel a strong need to have it done.

Antenatal Diagnosis

Antenatal diagnosis of sickle cell disease and thalassemia might provide some forward impetus to screening for these conditions because it would offer a worthwhile reproductive alternative to taking the risk, remaining childless, or adoption. Progress has been made toward this end in two ways: by the invention of methods to measure β-chain synthesis in fetal blood and to sample blood from the placental circulation.

There is little adult hemoglobin in fetal erythrocytes at times favorable for antenatal diagnosis; therefore it has been necessary to devise a method to test for the synthesis of β chains.[14,15] Such a method has been reported, and β chains have been observed to be produced in the red cells as early as the second month of gestation. Futhermore, the method allows the distinctions of all the various hemoglobin chains, including β^S, and by comparing the amounts of one to others, it is possible to diagnose the thalassemia states. Until very recently, all this work was done, perforce, on erythrocytes obtained from dead fetuses, and although the AS and S-thal phenotypes have been detected, none has been found to have either sickle cell disease or thalassemia major. More recently, however, erythrocytes have been obtained from the placental circulation of living fetuses with results that substantiate previous observations, and although heterozygotes for Hb S have been detected, no homozygotes have yet been detected.[16,17]

The discovery of a method to detect the abnormal hemoglobin states antedated the capability to make the prenatal diagnosis of disease because of the difficulty in obtaining fetal blood. Unfortunately, amniotic fluid contains too few fetal erythrocytes to study by biochemical techniques, so if a diagnosis of these conditions is to be made *in utero,* it must be done on red cells obtained from the living fetus, or the fetal aspect of the placenta. Progress is being made in the uses of a fetoscope for this and other purposes, and no doubt such diagnosis will soon be possible.[18]

It is unlikely, however, that fetoscopy will soon become widely employed or that antenatal diagnosis for any hemoglobinopathy is about to become a routine test. Both procedures are and must remain for some time in the domain of research. For example, many technical details must be worked out before settling on the best fetoscope and the best way to obtain placental blood; and since so few experiments have been done, no one knows how great, or even what, the risks are. As for the hemoglobin analyses, these have been carried out so far by a few experienced investigators; in addition to their costliness, they are by no means ready for routine use. For the time being, then, antenatal diagnosis of the hemoglobin diseases must remain under investigation.

The question of whether antenatal diagnosis and abortion of SS fetuses *should* be done is in any case moot, because it raises a dilemma raised by all disorders of variable expression. While severe cases of sickle cell disease make a misery of an abbreviated life, milder ones are compatible with a long and satisfying existence. Since the prenatal diagnosis cannot predict which path the individual will take, the decision to continue or to terminate a pregnancy may be clouded for those parents to whom the idea of abortion is at best an unattractive one.

TAY-SACHS DISEASE

Tay-Sachs disease is a lipid storage disorder characterized by neurologic deterioration beginning 3 to 6 months after birth and progressing to death by 4 to 6 years of age. Most patients must eventually be institutionalized, and all die in early childhood. Biochemically the condition is characterized by an abnormality of the enzyme hexosaminidase A (Hex A), a lysosomal enzyme present in both serum and tissues. The disorder occurs rarely in all populations, but among Ashkenazi Jews it appears with a frequency of about 1 in 3,600 births. It is inherited as an autosomal recessive, and 3–4% of Ashkenazi Jews are carriers. It can be diagnosed prenatally from cultured amniotic fluid cells taken early in the second trimester of gestation.

Tay-Sachs disease is an ideal disorder for screening for reproductive counseling for the following reasons: (a) It is mainly confined to a defined population. (b) There is a simple, reliable, automated, and relatively inexpensive test for detecting the carrier state. (c) There is a positive reproductive alternative for couples, both of whom are carriers, because the disorder can be diagnosed prenatally at a time when induced abortion can be carried out safely. This allows such couples to plan for unaffected children while avoiding having children with the disease.

Screening Programs

Tay-Sachs screening was begun by Kaback in the Baltimore–Washington area in 1971; other projects are currently under way in many communities, having spread very rapidly.[19] Table 6-2 summarizes Dr. Kaback's

TABLE 6-2 Spread of Tay-Sachs Screening Programs in the United States and Abroad

		Initiator of Program			Type of Testing			
			Professional					
Year	Number of Programs	Lay	Geneticist	Other	Mass Only	Hospital Only	Both	Undecided
1971 (7 mo)	10	3	2	5	0	0	9	1
1972	17	4	9	4	4	1	8	4
1973	7	1	4	2	1	1	2	3
Total	34	8	15	11	5	2	19	8

experiences as a consultant in helping to organize new programs in the United States and abroad. Most of these (19 out of 30) were in the Northeast or North Central states, one was in the Northwest, and ten were in Southern states. Two programs were begun in Canada, one in England, and one in South Africa. In addition to these, screening for Tay-Sachs is known to be going on in many other places, all programs having been started less than 3 years ago. The Committee sampled the experiences, presumably representative, of three of the U.S. programs.

Objectives

The aim of Tay-Sachs screening is to discover couples, both of whom are carriers of the Tay-Sachs gene and who therefore have a risk of 0.25 for a defective child. A reasonable alternative to reproductive curtailment may be offered such couples in the form of antenatal diagnosis and abortion of affected fetuses. This approach has the double virtue of brightening the reproductive outlook of potentially afflicted families and of reducing the incidence of Tay-Sachs disease in the community at large. It is worth noting that, in contrast to screening for other conditions (for example, sickle cell anemia), Tay-Sachs projects can afford the limited objective of discovering couples only, since the genetic aim is tied to the positive option of antenatal diagnosis. Thus there may be no particular incentive for a single person to know his genotype prior to marriage; indeed in some programs unmarried people are discouraged from being tested.

Auspices and Settings

The first Tay-Sachs screening project was undertaken as a research enterprise.[20] The plan was to do the testing in large groups using facilities made available principally by synogogues. Table 6-2 reveals that mass screening is still in vogue, but that opportunities are also available at hospitals where couples may present themselves at appointed times. The table also reveals the mixture of lay and medical people involved in starting new programs. The laymen are representatives of the Tay-Sachs Foundation or other community leaders; the professionals are medical geneticists, laboratory directors, or interested physicians. Financial support at first was derived principally from Tay-Sachs Foundation chapters and other donors, as well as from contributions from the screenees themselves; but recently some states have made funds available, and state health departments are taking an interest.

Prescreening Education

This has been accomplished by enlisting the help of volunteers to develop community support, by articles in both parochial and secular newspapers, through the social functions of the synagogue and in premarital counseling by rabbis, by television and radio programs, as well as by spot advertisements, and by pamphlets and other written materials. Efforts are usually also made to alert physicians, who will presumably recommend screening for their patients. The material presented consists of the characteristics of the disease, including its genetic origin, its incidence and the frequency of the carrier state, the odds for having an affected child given the genotypes of the potential parents, and the nature and risks of amniocentesis, antenatal diagnosis, and abortion of affected fetuses. Emphasis is laid upon the opportunity screening may provide for couples at risk to have babies free of this dreadful disease.

It is not yet clear how successful each of these educational methods is. There is some evidence that the mass media and word-of-mouth are most successful.[21] Physicians and rabbis, although both are given high marks as potential advocates, do not fulfill this expectation, since neither group is the source of any significant number of referrals.[22] What causes some persons to submit to the screening test while others do not has been studied.[23] Those who do avail themselves of the service know more about the disease and have greater educational experience. They are younger than the noncompliers, plan to have more children, and are more sensitive to their susceptibility to the disorder, although less concerned with the seriousness of being discovered to be a carrier. These differences may be evidence of the effectiveness of the prescreening education, since if one knows the probability of being a carrier and also knows that, although the disease is disastrous, one can be assured of a nonaffected baby by antenatal diagnosis, then one's sense of susceptibility is heightened while the seriousness of being found to be a carrier is diminished. The noncompliers were found characteristically not to know either the carrier rate or much about antenatal diagnosis.

Populations

So far, Tay-Sachs screening has been promoted only among Ashkenazi Jews. In general, young couples are the principal object, but some programs test anyone who presents himself and others screen high school or college populations specifically. Married women tend to predominate (their husbands are frequently "too busy"), and if they are found not to be carriers, there is no need to screen their husbands. When a woman is pregnant, she must have the more definitive leukocyte test. Pregnant women already in the late second or third trimester are best left untested.

The Test and Results

The test for carriers consists of measuring the resistance of serum hexosaminidase A to heat inactivation. Occasionally the result is inconclusive, particularly during pregnancy or if a woman is using birth control pills. If so, the test must be repeated using leukocytes rather than serum—a more discriminating, but technically more demanding, procedure. If the result of this test is positive, it should be further supported by evidence that at least one parent is also a carrier of the mutation. False positive and false negative results due to simple classification error can be reduced by subjecting the results of enzyme assays to appropriate statistical procedures.[24] Such false results may also be obtained by mishandling the specimen. Errors may also be produced in assays of amniotic cells. For example, enzyme from maternal blood in the fluid or maternal cells as passengers in the fluid give a false negative result on assay of uncultured fluid. Contamination of cultures by bacteria that contribute their own Hex A activity may do the same. While genetic heterogeneity may contribute unexpected results, it is rare.

In Kaback's experience of 17,000 people screened, 17 couples were found to be at risk. Of these, eight have had pregnancies, and one affected fetus has so far been discovered and aborted.

Consent and Counseling

Signed consent is not always obtained in mass screening programs. Since the screening is voluntary, some program directors have assumed that proffering oneself for the test is evidence of consent, although the extent of the screenee's information is seldom asked. On the other hand, some projects take pains to provide information at the time of the screening; in these, at least, it may be presumed that no one is tested without at least an opportunity for as full an explanation as he might wish.

The results of the test are usually transmitted by letter, or for those demonstrated to be carriers, by telephone or by interview with a physician. When both parents are shown to be carriers, an interview is the rule. The impact of discovery that one is a carrier has not been studied systematically. Anecdotal evidence suggests that most people are not overwhelmed, but detailed knowledge of their feelings and thoughts is wanting. Counseling is likely to be, at best, informal, unless the screenee shows overt evidence of needing more attention.

Costs

Cost accounting, while generally informal and incomplete, suggests that screening pays for itself in that if it were carried out in the target population, the costs of prevention of Tay-Sachs disease would be considerably less than the outlay for the treatment of the predicted cases.

In general, screening for Tay-Sachs disease has been well received and has been useful to those who have availed themselves of the service. Many pregnancies of carrier couples have now been monitored with minimal error or confusion. Many questions, however, remain unanswered. For example, it is not yet clear whether the mass screening approach is the most economical and effective method. Among other things, the attendant fanfare may arouse an unreasonable amount of anxiety about a disease with an incidence of only 1/3,600 even in the highest-risk group. Mass screening seems to attract mainly the more educated who are attuned to health-related matters and fails to attract some significant number of others. This leads one to wonder if the same, or even better, results might be achieved if it were possible to teach physicians (perhaps especially obstetricians) to make the test a routine part of their patient care. Possibly the health maintenance organization (HMO) will become the ideal setting for this and other kinds of screening. But if this is what the future brings, it will be in part because mass screening has raised the interest of the public and physicians alike.

SCREENING BY AMNIOCENTESIS

The ability to make an antenatal diagnosis is an outcome of the newly developed techniques for growing human cells *in vitro,* for analyzing their chromosome composition, and for assaying the activities of many of their enzymes.[25] The method involves transabdominal removal of a sample of amniotic fluid early in the second trimester of pregnancy, followed by culture of amniotic cells. At an appropriate time the cultivated cells are analyzed for evidence of the disorder that constituted the reason for doing the amniocentesis. It is to be emphasized that the procedure is never done as a fishing expedition, but only upon indication, and with a specific disorder in mind. Although an unanticipated condition is sometimes discovered, the aim of the procedure is to determine whether the fetus has a particular disease, not to assure the prospective parents of a normal, healthy baby. It is done regularly now in a few places, but is still far from routine. Indeed it must be considered as experimental, since the extent of the risk is not yet fully known even when performed by highly skilled obstetricians.

Amniocentesis is used for screening in two ways: in the narrow sense of examining a fetus whose probability of being diseased is signaled by the known genotypes of parents or other relatives; and in the more conventional sense of screening for reproductive information by offering a defined population the choice of whether to allow a diseased fetus to go to term. The latter is the more frequent use of amniocentesis, but in contrast to other screening tests, both are rare.

Screening for Down's Syndrome

It is well known that the incidence of Down's syndrome rises with maternal age, taking a particularly rapid upturn after age 30. The risk for mothers of 35–39 years of age is of the order of 1/60, and this rises to 1/40 for mothers over 40 years of age. Perhaps 10% of all pregnant women are over 35, of whom about one third (or 3% of all pregnant women) are over 40. This means that about 60% of all mongoloid babies are born to mothers above 35 years of age, and if these women were to choose amniocentesis and antenatal diagnosis followed by termination of affected fetuses, the incidence of Down's syndrome would be reduced by more than half.

In addition to the rising incidence of the disease with maternal age, other reasons for limitation of the procedure to this age group are the uncertain risks of abortion or damage to the fetus due to the amniocentesis itself, the cost of at least $150 for the procedure, and the present lack of facilities, competence, and experience required for both obstetric and laboratory aspects. The justification for doing it at all is the burden on both the parents and the state of a child who can never become self-sufficient. Many calculations have been made of the costs of the care of such patients; while they vary as to accuracy, all expose the immense disparity between the cost of the amniocentesis and a lifetime of demanding and expensive care.

Although screening for Down's syndrome by amniocentesis is still experimental in the sense that the risks have not been precisely defined, they are sufficiently low that the procedure is being offered in a few centers as a "service" whose feasibility is still being studied. Some of the questions and problems that are the objects of continuing investigation are discussed in the following sections.

Technique Misdiagnosis appears to be less troublesome than might have been anticipated, although it is occasionally reported, sometimes as a result of contamination of the culture with maternal cells. Multiple pregnancies may pose difficulties since one fetus may be diseased and the other normal. In good hands the cell culture, karyotyping, and biochemical analyses give reliable results, but none of these techniques should be attempted in any but well-equipped laboratories with experienced personnel. The expense, complexity, and variety of these procedures strongly urge the institution of regional facilities that, while narrowing the experience of each laboratory, would deepen it. Direct analyses of amniotic cells and fluid, although appealing because they could give early answers, have not proven reliable.

Maternal Age Some clinics use 35 years as the lower limit of age for screening for Down's syndrome by amniocentesis; some set it at 40, a few somewhere above 30 but less than 35. But since only half or a little more of all babies with Down's syndrome are born to mothers over 30, leaving a sizable number who would be undetected by current screening practices, why should not screening by amniocentesis be extended to all pregnant women? The reasons are practical and compelling. The facilities and manpower are lacking, and it is still not known that the risks do not outweigh the benefits. The probability of a fetus with Down's syndrome is about .0017 for all ages, while that for any chromosome abnormality is about .005. Thus, even if the risk were less than the benefit, the probability of adventitious findings is greater than that of the discovery of the characteristic for which the screening is to be undertaken.

Sociologic Problems The first problem in this area is the abortion decision. Most investigators take the view that amniocentesis and abortion are to be considered separately; that is, a woman should not be asked for a conditional agreement to an abortion before the amniocentesis is done. Parents cannot be sure in advance how they will greet the news of a defective fetus, and the record shows cases of pregnancies brought to term despite this knowledge. The impact of this and other aspects of the procedure on prospective parents requires study. It is a further example of a new technologic advance that, in its advocacy of abortion, does violence to what was once thought to be an inviolable moral principle, a principle that, it should be added, is still so regarded by some. There has been too little attention paid so far to detailed examination of the thoughts, feelings, and attitudes of women who have undergone amniocentesis, or of those of their husbands.

A second important problem is the promotion of screening. When, if ever, should screening by amniocentesis for Down's syndrome be publicly advanced like other screening tests? There is a difference between public promotion and a recommendation made in the privacy and traditional atmosphere of the doctor's office. The question is, should amniocentesis for pregnant women over 30 years of age be pressed publicly and with vigor, or should the educational efforts be limited to notifying the public of its availability and to instructing physicians in their duty to make it available to their parents?

The third problem is what should be done about adventitious findings. The incidences of chromosomal abnormalities other than trisomy 21 also rise with maternal age, so that unexpected aberrations are occasionally discovered. This occurs also when the amniocentesis is done for biochemical indications when a karyotype is made to diagnose the sex of the fetus. A lethal or severe disease poses no problem of what to say, but sex chromosome aneuploidy does. There appears to be no alternative to telling the parents. But to convey the clinical nuances and variable expectations for persons with the XXY or XYY chromosome constitution to parents to whom the event is entirely unexpected and who may know nothing at all of the condition—or worse, who may believe that such people must inevitably end up at variance with society—is a job to tax the skill of the most experienced counselor.

Finally, the future will surely bring certain legal questions. For example, when will it become malpractice to fail to recommend amniocentesis to women over 35 years of age? There may be also questions of insurability. Will insurance companies ever have the right to refuse to insure a woman who refuses amniocentesis and to pay costs if she has a baby with Down's syndrome?

Amniocentesis for Sex Determination Fetal sex is easily determined by chromosome analysis, so it is perfectly possible to carry a fetus of one sex to term while aborting a fetus of the other sex. Since most parents are unlikely to be casual or frivolous about making such a request, an obstetrician must consider what answer he can give when a serious question is asked. Abortion of all male fetuses of women known to be heterozygous for hemophilia is sometimes done, and there are other sex-linked lethal or severe disorders that might reasonably be given the same consideration.

It is the idea of screening with fetal sex as the only indication that must be examined. There is no estimate of prevailing attitudes, but it is likely that most parents and obstetricians would draw back from such a procedure. Perhaps it is the ethical reservation about this indication for abortion that accounts for the lack of enthusiasm for this procedure as a public screening service.

ALPHA-FETOPROTEINS IN SCREENING FOR NEURAL TUBE DEFECTS

Neural tube defects, including anencephaly and meningomyelocele, occur with an average frequency of 1 or 2 per 1,000 live births, though in some populations the frequency approaches 1 per 100 live births. When one such child has been born in a family, the probability for another in subsequent pregnancies rises to around 5%.[26] These figures make desirable a simple and economical screening test that could make an accurate diagnosis early enough in pregnancy to make the option of abortion feasible.

We do not now have such a test, but a beginning has been made.[27] Alpha-fetoprotein (AFP) is an α-1-globulin synthesized by embryonal liver cells, the yolk sac, and the fetal gastrointestinal tract. Its functions are unknown. The fetal serum concentration of this protein rises from the 6th week of embryonic life, reaching a peak at the 12th to 14th week and then declines constantly, synthesis ceasing with birth. It is found in amniotic fluid at much lower concentrations than in serum, and Brock and Sutcliffe have demonstrated an excess of it in the fluid of women carrying fetuses with neural tube defects.[28] Since then others have confirmed this discovery, and a screening test of sorts, applicable only to pregnancies of women with previously affected babies, or possibly to women who themselves have spina bifida, is in the process of being worked out. Milunsky has, however, reported assays of AFP in the amniotic fluid of both normal and abnormal pregnancies.[27] So, while it is clear that neural tube defects, especially anencephaly, are often associated with elevated amniotic AFP, so are such other conditions as fetal death, Rh immunization, twins, and threatened abortion. When the results of amniotic AFP levels, sonography, and x-ray are combined, about 85% of open neural tube defects can be diagnosed prenatally.

Even if this test can be made reliable, specific, and adequate in every way, it could still be applied only to those few women who had some reason to fear the outcome of their pregnancy. Facilities for amniocentesis for all pregnant women are not now available. But if a good serum test for AFP could be contrived, all pregnancies could be screened. This condition seemed to be fulfilled when one case of anencephaly was diagnosed *in utero*—accurately, as it turned out, since after confirmation by analysis of amniotic AFP, as well as by sonography and x-ray, an anencephalic fetus was aborted.[29] Subsequent studies have dimmed this prospect, however, and the serum test is not yet regarded as a reliable diagnostic indication.[30,31]

The advent of an effective test poses the same dilemma raised by sickle cell disease. Anencephaly is uniformly lethal, but meningomyelocele varies in its manifestations. While the severe cases of the latter raise the question only of whether to try some treatment, milder ones are not incompatible with a life which, if not normal, can be satisfying.[32] Some estimate of future function, or at least whether treatment is likely to help, can be made postnatally; but if the prenatal test cannot make the same distinctions, then the parents will have to confront a difficult decision.

REFERENCES

1. Motulsky, A. G. Frequency of sickling disorders in U.S. blacks. N. Engl. J. Med. 288:31–33, 1973.
2. Jackson, R. E. A perspective of the national sickle cell disease program. Arch. Intern. Med. 133:533, 1974.
3. Young, W. I., J. Peters, H. B. Houser, and E. B. Jackson. Awareness of sickle cell abnormalities. A medical and lay community problem. Ohio Med. J. 70:27–30, 1974.
4. Kellon, D. B., and E. Beutler. Physician attitudes about sickle cell disease and sickle cell trait. (Editorial) JAMA 227:71–72, 1974.
5. Hampton, M. L., J. Anderson, B. S. Lavizzo, and A. B. Bergman. Sickle cell "nondisease." A potentially serious public health problem. Amer. J. Dis. Child. 128:58–61, 1974.
6. Stamatoyannopoulos, G. Problems of screening and counseling in the hemoglobinopathies, pp. 14–15. In A. G. Motulsky and F. J. G. Ebling, eds. Fourth International Conference on Birth Defects, Vienna, Austria, Sept. 2–8, 1973. Abstracts of Papers. International Congress Series No. 297. Amsterdam: Excerpta Medica Foundation, 1973.
7. Whitten, C. F. Sickle-cell programming—an imperiled promise. N. Engl. J. Med. 288:318–319, 1973.
8. Bowman, J. E. Personal communication.
9. Rutkow, I. M., and J. M. Lipton. Some negative aspects of state health departments' policies related to screening for sickle cell anemia. Amer. J. Publ. Health 64:217–221, 1974.
10. Fielding, J., P. Batalden, G. Tolbert, R. Bennett, and S. H. Nelson. A coordinated sickle cell program for economically disadvantaged adolescents. Amer. J. Publ. Health 64:427–432, 1974.
11. Gaston, M. Screening for sickle cell disease. So. Med. J. 67:257–258, 1974.
12. Whitten, C. F., and J. Fischoff. Psychosocial effects of sickle cell disease. Arch. Intern. Med. 133:681–689, 1974.

13. Motulsky, A. G. Screening for sickle cell hemoglobinopathy and thalassemia. Israel J. Med. Sci. 9:1341–1349, 1973.
14. Kazazian, H. H., Jr., and A. P. Woodhead. Adult hemoglobin synthesis in the human fetus. Ann. N.Y. Acad. Sci. (In press)
15. Kan, Y. W., A. M. Dozy, B. P. Alter, F. D. Frigoletto, and D. G. Nathan. Detection of the sickle gene in the human fetus. Potential for intrauterine diagnosis of sickle-cell anemia. N. Engl. J. Med. 287:1–5, 1972.
16. Hobbins, J. C., and M. J. Mahoney. In utero diagnosis of hemoglobinopathies. N. Engl. J. Med. 290:1065–1067, 1974.
17. Chang, H., J. C. Hobbins, G. Cividalli, F. D. Frigoletto, M. J. Mahoney, Y. W. Kan, and D. G. Nathan. In utero diagnosis of hemoglobinopathies. Hemoglobin synthesis in fetal red cells. N. Engl. J. Med. 290:1067–1068, 1974.
18. Scrimgeour, J. B. Fetoscopy, pp. 12–13. In A. G. Motulsky and F. J. G. Ebling, eds. Fourth International Conference on Birth Defects, Vienna, Austria, Sept. 2–8, 1973. Abstracts of Papers. International Congress Series No. 297. Amsterdam: Excerpta Medica Foundation, 1973.
19. Kaback, M. M., R. S. Zeiger, L. W. Reynolds, and M. Sonneborn. Approaches to the prevention and control of Tay-Sachs disease. Prog. Med. Genet. (In press)
20. Kaback, M. M., and R. S. Zeiger. The John F. Kennedy Institute Tay-Sachs Program: Practical and ethical issues in an adult genetic screening program, pp. 131–145. In B. Hilton, D. Callahan, M. Harris, P. Condliffe, and B. Berkley, eds. Ethical Issues in Human Genetics. Genetic Counseling and the Use of Genetic Knowledge. New York: Plenum Press, 1973.
21. Ivker, F., H. Rothschild, W. Van Vean, W. Danos, N. Manowitz, and M. Miller. Characterization and motivational factors influencing participants and non-participants in a voluntary community screening program. Amer. J. Hum. Genet. 25(6):35A, 1973.
22. Beck, E., S. Blaichman, C. R. Scriver, and C. Clow. Advocacy and compliance in genetic screening. Behaviour of physicians and clients in a Tay-Sachs program. N. Engl. J. Med. (In press)
23. Becker, M. H., M. M. Kaback, I. M. Rosenstock, and M. V. Ruth. Some influences on public participation in a genetic screening program. J. Commun. Health (In press).
24. Gold, R. J. M., U. R. Maag, J. L. Neal, and C. R. Scriver. The use of biochemical data in screening for mutant alleles and in genetic counselling. Ann. Hum. Genet. 37:315–326, 1974.
25. Milunsky, A. The Prenatal Diagnosis of Hereditary Disorders. Springfield, Ill.: Charles C Thomas, 1973.
26. Carter, C. O. Spina bifida and anencephaly: A problem in genetic–environmental interaction. J. Biosoc. Sci. 1:71–83, 1969.
27. Milunsky, A., and E. Alpert. The value of alpha-fetoprotein in the prenatal diagnosis of neural tube defects. J. Pediat. 84:889–893, 1974.
28. Brock, D. J., and R. G. Sutcliffe. Alpha-fetoprotein in the antenatal diagnosis of anencephaly and spina bifida. Lancet 2:197–199, 1972.
29. Brock, D. J., A. E. Bolton, and J. M. Monaghan. Prenatal diagnosis of anencephaly through maternal serum—alpha-fetoprotein measurement. Lancet 2: 923–924, 1973.

30. Seller, M. J., J. D. Singer, T. M. Coltart, and S. Campbell. Maternal serum—alpha-fetoprotein levels and prenatal diagnosis of neural-tube defects. Lancet 1:428–429, 1974.
31. Harris, R., R. F. Jennison, A. J. Barson, K. M. Laurence, E. Ruoslahti, and M. Seppälä. Comparison of amniotic-fluid and maternal serum alpha-fetoprotein levels in the early antenatal diagnosis of spina bifida and anencephaly. Lancet 1:429–433, 1974.
32. Lorber, J. Selective treatment of myelomeningocele: To treat or not to treat? Pediatrics 53:307–308, 1974.

7 Screening for Enumeration, Monitoring, and Surveillance

We commonly think of epidemiologic studies as including three sequential levels of research. *Descriptive epidemiology,* the first and lowest level, is confined to studies of the distribution of disease, traits, risk factors, or other health-relevant data in a population, cross-tabulated by various population characteristics. *Analytic epidemiology* builds on prior descriptive work in an effort to explain why disease states, traits, risk factors, and the like are distributed in a particular way; in other words, it represents an effort to identify the causes of the disease or other variable being studied. *Experimental epidemiology* builds on knowledge obtained at the first two levels and represents attempts to intervene in disease or disease-related processes. At the moment, genetic screening for enumeration would appear to be geared primarily toward the descriptive level of epidemiology and secondarily toward the analytic.

The Committee reviewed the activities of several projects screening for chromosome abnormalities, of others involved with monitoring the incidence of congenital malformations, and of still others whose primary purpose was the gathering and storage of data in registries.

SCREENING FOR CHROMOSOME ABNORMALITIES

Seven studies, covering some 67,000 individuals, were examined in some detail. (Much of the data from these studies appears in references 1–5.) Five of the studies dealt with newborn populations at various hospitals in the United States and Canada. The newborn studies continued for periods ranging from 1 to 9 years, with 1,000–34,000 individuals surveyed in each. A recent report indicated that in a sample of 344 cases of early neonatal death, 6% were associated with a chromosome abnormality.[6] One study involved 7-year-olds enrolled in a collaborative study in six cities, and one involved institutionalized juvenile delinquent or emotionally disturbed males of less than 18 years of age. The primary objective in all these surveys was research, but in some, follow-up and genetic counseling were available. The service element was large or small, depending on the philosophy of the investigator. At one extreme was the viewpoint that every newborn should be screened, at least to the extent of having placental cells examined for Barr bodies, because individuals with sex chromosome abnormalities are at increased risk. An abnormal Barr body count or a discrepancy between the apparent sex of the newborn and the Barr body analysis is associated with an elevated mortality, indicating the need for early diagnosis of sex chromosome abnormalities, if we are to learn to cope with their higher than average perinatal risk.

Some studies provided no information to the families about the screening. In others, questionnaires or booklets given at the time of hospital admission or birth of the baby provided a certain amount of information. But even in these cases consent forms were rarely used, refusals were also rare, and it is uncertain whether the mother always knew her baby was having a chromosome study.

Usually, two karyotypes were prepared on each individual. In one study, placental amnion was examined for Barr bodies or Y bodies to evaluate the sex chromosome constitution, and karyotypes were performed on the aberrant cases, as well as on patients with a clinical diagnosis of Down's syndrome.

The choice of controls for studies of the clinical effects of some of the chromosome variants was solved in various ways: selecting the next baby of the same race, sex, and birth weight; using the sib nearest in age; and so on. In the study of institutionalized XYY males, four controls per case were included, matched for age, weight, and institution.

The results of all these studies were somewhat variable, in keeping with the relatively small sample size of some of the studies. The incidence of sex chromosome variations ranged from 1 to 3.3 per 1,000 and that of autosomes from 1 to 4 per 1,000, with overall values ranging from 3 to 5.8 per 1,000. In two studies, involving 14,000 and 34,000 individuals respectively, seasonal variations in incidence of both sex chromosome abnormalities and Down's syndrome were noted. In contrast, their incidence in 6,000 7-year-olds of both sexes from the collaborative study was 3.2 per 1,000. The incidence of XYY males ranged from 0 to 0.3 per 1,000 in the newborn surveys, with a mean value of about .2 per 1,000 males. An incidence of 4 per 100 was noted among a small sample of mentally disturbed, institutionalized juvenile delinquent males.

What information on the results of the screening was given to families? This varied from none at all, to a general statement that a chromosome variant of unknown significance has been found, to a specific statement that a chromosome abnormality was present. The information given to the parents of controls also varied from study to study. Some were told their baby had normal chromosomes; others were asked to join the study as normal controls.

The response of parents to the information given was assessed in some of the studies. Anger and anxiety were noted, and evaluation at a later date in one study showed that without follow-up the parents usually forgot details but remembered that there was something wrong with their child's chromosomes. In addition, some persons telephoned months or years later to report that their child was *not* retarded, although the possibility of developmental retardation had never been raised.

Follow-up was carried out in several of the studies, evaluating both the individuals noted to have a chromosome variant and the controls. The primary purpose of the follow-up was to detect and study any behavioral or clinical effects associated with particular chromosome variants. Little or no attention was paid to determining the retention of information given to parents at the time of initial screening, although in one such study it was noted that most of it was not remembered. However, the information was imparted in a rather general, noncommittal way in order to avoid frightening parents unnecessarily, and it is possible that the failure to remember may have been related to the ambiguous message delivered.

The importance of the educational aspects of screening was brought out in all the studies. Screening programs have great potential for education, not only of the screenees, but also of the physicians, public health personnel, and other persons involved in their organization. The need for safeguards to assure the confidentiality of information was also made evident, along with the possible stigmatization of individuals found to have any kind of an aberration, whether clinically significant or not.

Screening programs for chromosome variants, as mentioned above, are carried out primarily for research purposes. Even so, the liaison among screening authority, the screenee's physician, and the screenee should be kept at an optimum. This is not always done. In one study, the family did not know a screening program was in progress, no informed consent was obtained, and no follow-up was carried out. In another center, however, sex chromosome constitution was determined on umbilical or placental tissue and patients with sex chromosome abnormalities or clinical features of Down's syndrome were karyotyped as part of the medical service accorded the newborn infant. That is, both analyses are regarded as a natural part of the proper management of the obstetric patient and the delivery. This view places the screening in a medical context, which carries certain implications for the kind of informed consent that is sought and the kind of follow-up that is indicated. In particular, certain individuals can be placed in what could be called an undefined high-risk category. If this approach were also to be used with individuals who are found to have a variant of one of the autosomes, at least one in 200 newborns would be involved—and perhaps more as new chromosome banding techniques are used to pinpoint chromosomal changes, and more minor variants are consequently picked up. When, on the other hand, screening is defined as research requiring selection and examination of controls, follow-up of the controls may represent a threat, since the continuing interest in such children might suggest to their parents that there was a medical reason for it.

One view holds that chromosome screening of newborns should no longer be regarded as primarily a research tool but that it should be seen as an important medical service. This appears to have only limited justification. While some of the individuals with chromosome variants might benefit from more intensive medical supervision than that offered other children, the absence of specific therapies sets a limit on the potential value of such a course of action. Although learning disabilities and speech problems do appear to be common in some of the sex chromosome aneuploidies and might be helped to some extent by treatment, it is possible that harm could be done by the adverse effect that information about karyotype abnormalities might have on the individual and the family.[7-9] Hard data on this question are still limited, although in one study children with chromosomal mosaicism did not show the behavioral abnormalities seen in children with the chromosome change in all their cells. The parents of both groups received the same information, so the noted difference is not attributable to parental expectation.

Little attention was given to cost in the presentations of chromosome screening before the Committee. A rough estimate of $20–30 for a karyotype study limited to two cells, and $5 for X and Y body screening of amnions, may not be out of line. It is possible that fully automated methods suitable for wide-scale screening will lower costs to as little as $3–5 per individual analysis if, say, all the newborns in a city of the size of Denver are screened, but this cost is not all-inclusive.

Mistakes in diagnosis did not receive much attention, either because they rarely occur or because they are rarely detected.

MONITORING AND SURVEILLANCE

The Committee looked at various programs for monitoring and surveillance for congenital malformations or genetic disorders, registries for storage and recovery of such information, and the uses to which such registries are put. Five such programs are reviewed below.

The Center for Disease Control

Three studies from the Center for Disease Control (CDC) were reviewed. The purpose of these studies was to devise monitoring systems that would permit review of the incidence of particular malformations from time to time, in order to recognize sudden increases so that steps could be initiated to determine the cause of the increase and control it.

The first of these studies covered 28,000 births in 20 hospitals in Atlanta, Georgia. All newborns, and any infant with a chromosomal or structural or biochemical abnormality diagnosed under the age of 1 year and admitted to one of the hospitals, entered the study. Center physicians abstracted information from the medical records library, newborn nursery, and obstetric service of each hospital, accepting the diagnoses recorded there. It was presumed that diagnostic deficiencies would remain fairly constant, so that real fluctuations in the incidence of congenital abnormalities could be recognized from the records used. The average incidence of these abnormalities was about 2.5% per year. All the material was transferred into a registry and the incidence of many malformations was tabulated and compared, monthly, semimonthly, bimonthly, and annually, with baseline figures gathered during previous years.

Socioeconomic data, evidence of environmental exposures, and family history information were obtained by interviewing the parents of affected children 1 or 2 months after the birth of the infant. The interview was arranged through the pediatrician and obstetrician in charge of the patient. About 5% of the physicians declined to cooperate, about 5% of the parents failed to cooperate, and 5% more were lost in some way, giving about 85% compliance. Two full-time nurses, a full-time interviewer, and a half-time statistical clerk were required to carry out this study, in addition to CDC physicians.

The second study involved a surveillance of malformations in northern Florida. A surveillance form was filled out by medical records librarians on all births in the area and sent to the CDC for processing. Some 12,000 births were monitored, giving a rate of malformations of 1.5%. One of the aims of this study was to discover the needs of the families of the babies with malformations. Accordingly, each family so diagnosed was visited by an emissary from the Child Health Section of the State Department of Health. This study revealed many unmet needs, and the Health Department in Florida feels that the surveillance program can help identify families early who need the services of a variety of state agencies.

The third study took place in Nebraska, where the legislature passed a law in July 1972 setting up a birth defects program that includes genetic counseling, a registry, and money for medical education. The role of the CDC was to help in surveillance. As in the second study, the information sent in was abstracted from records by medical records librarians, and again an incidence of about 1.3% was found. Despite inaccuracies in physicians' diagnoses, errors in transcribing records, and deficiencies in birth certificates, therefore, it is unlikely that surveillance and monitoring can be much improved unless new, and far more expensive, methods for discovery of cases are used.

Questions were left unanswered concerning the interviews with the parents of malformed children. There was little or no provision for genetic or other counseling, and anxieties and needless misapprehension may have been engendered. There were other questions as to who controls the data and the registry, who gets access to it, and whether or not the families had consented to have their names in such a registry. In a number of on-going programs there has been little or no consultation with the public in advance. That is, these studies are done without any representation for the people who are being studied.

The Fetal Life Study of Columbia University

The Fetal Life Study of Columbia University in the City of New York was reviewed briefly. This study, which collected data from 1946 until 1970, was designed as a prospective epidemiologic survey of pregnancies and pregnancy outcomes. Large amounts of data on a relatively small number of patients were collected, tabulated and stored, first on punch cards and later on magnetic tape, for computer retrieval and analysis. The study illustrated the immense technical complexity of collection, storage, and retrieval of information.

The British Columbia Registry

The British Columbia Registry was instituted over 20 years ago as a registry of handicapped persons that was operated by the Division of Vital Statistics of the Health Branch of the Province of British Columbia. Like others, this registry is both a research instrument and a source of important services. The registry collects the names and diagnoses of children with malformations or genetic diseases and continually updates and amends the information.

The functions of the registry now include providing incidence and prevalence figures (monitoring), prevention, genetic counseling, and follow-up of special cases. It can be used for long-term follow-up studies and to predict what the needs of the handicapped children might be in adolescence, for example. It also acts as a coordinating center to facilitate referral of cases by family physicians to agencies that can provide the appropriate help. It is in direct telephone contact with all the public health units in the province and has been helpful in providing all kinds of health services. Within 48 hours of the birth of a child, a public health nurse fills in a card, which is then picked up by the local health unit. The health nurse then visits the home to get further information. The British Columbia Registry now contains about 50,000 names.

Among the capabilities of a registry is the ability to identify persons who are at risk for genetic diseases but who don't know it. It is uncertain whether it is either ethical or legal to bring this risk to the individual's attention. This is usually done only if the individual through whom the original information was obtained will allow it.

The British Columbia Registry feeds information into a federal registry in Ottawa, which will eventually cover all the provinces of Canada. Since the registry is part of the vital statistics function of the provincial health department, the issue of confidentiality is built into the training of personnel and the registry is thus as confidential as a death record, birth record, or marriage record. More important, the registry personnel never contact the patient. If someone wishes to do a study, it must be approved by the Public Health Service. Registry records in Canada can never be brought into court or subpoenaed. Registration is entirely voluntary and consent must be given for a name to be included. These safeguards are difficult to observe in practice, so it is possible that names may be included without the person's permission, or without truly informed consent about the potential hazards of being included in a registry.

It may be that at least part of the success of the British Columbia Registry is due to the fact that it can operate in an environment where there is a National Health Service. Such an environment allows relationships between physicians and public health personnel to be well structured and well developed.

Kaiser-Permanente of California

The Kaiser-Permanente program in California provides an example of the development of registries within a health care delivery system. The population sample covers 10 hospitals, 1.2 million people, and 14,000 deliveries a year.

There are three registries. The chromosome abnormality registry is run by the physician who does 95% of the karyotyping and follow-up. Hand punchcards are adequate for keeping track of the 250 patients currently registered and the 50 new cases each year from 175 that are karyotyped. The cardiac abnormality registry is maintained by the pediatric cardiologist who takes care of all the children with congenital heart disease in this northern California catchment area. It too is a hand punch system. The third registry is a newborn surveillance system to keep track of prenatal and perinatal problems. It is maintained by the doctors in charge of the eight newborn nurseries. At present, autopsy findings are not recorded on the punchcards completed in the nurseries.

This program was of exceptional interest because large group practices and health maintenance systems are expected to become even more important in the future, and their involvement in monitoring and surveillance might minimize problems of confidentiality, misunderstanding, or lack of needed counseling. Interviewing would presumably be done by trusted health personnel rather than by potentially threatening strangers.

The Commission on Professional and Hospital Activities

Some of the activities of the Commission on Professional and Hospital Activities (CPHA) were reviewed. The CPHA was started in 1953 to see whether data could be gathered from many different hospitals in a uniform manner and displayed in such a way that patterns of patient care could be analyzed by diagnosis and operation, with the objective of improving the quality of in-patient care. Today, 1,860 hospitals participate in this program. They discharge 15 million patients per year, 40% of the U.S. total. A program is currently being worked out with the Center for Disease Control (described above) to use these data to monitor the rates of occurrence of congenital malformations in the United States. A baseline will be constructed using data for the four years 1970–1973, and monitoring will start with 1974 data. Changes, particularly unusual increases, will be quickly spotted using this magnetic-tape-computerized system and the projected input from 1.2 million births a year. Confidentiality is maintained because data are filed by hospital numbers without the names of the patients. The disadvantages of the system are that it depends on medical records librarians to abstract the cards onto a one-page data sheet; there are inadequate data about certain items such as the family, maternal age, and details of pregnancy; and there is a deficiency in the coverage of lower socioeconomic groups and university hospitals.

REFERENCES

1. Lubs, H. A., and F. H. Ruddle. Applications of quantitative karyotypy to chromosome variation in 4400 consecutive newborns, pp. 119–142. In P. A. Jacobs, W. H. Price, and P. Law, eds. Human Population Cytogenetics. (Medical Monographs 5.) Baltimore: Williams & Wilkins, 1970.
2. Hamerton, J. L., M. Ray, J. Abbott, C. Williamson, and G. C. Ducasse. Chromosome studies in a neonatal population. Can. Med. Assoc. J. 106:776–779, 1972.
3. Gerald, P. S., and S. Walzer. Chromosome studies of normal newborn infants, pp. 143–151. In P. A. Jacobs, W. H. Price, and P. Law, eds. Human Population Cytogenetics. (Medical Monographs 5.) Baltimore: Williams & Wilkins, 1970.
4. Borgaonkar, D. S., and S. Shah. The XYY chromosome male—or syndrome. Prog. Med. Genet. (In press)
5. Jacobs, P. A., M. Melville, S. Ratcliffe, A. J. Keay, and J. Syme. A cytogenetic survey of 11,680 newborn infants. Ann. Hum. Genet. 37:359–376, 1974.
6. Machin, G. A. Chromosome abnormality and perinatal death. Lancet 1:549–551, 1974.
7. Robinson, A., M. Puck, and K. Tennes. The 47,XXY karyotype. Lancet 1:1343, 1974.
8. Leonard, M. F., G. Landy, F. H. Ruddle, and H. A. Lubs. Early development of children with abnormalities of the sex chromosomes: A prospective study. Pediatrics 54:208–212, 1974.
9. Garvey, M., and D. E. Mutton. Sex chromosome aberrations and speech development. Arch. Dis. Child. 48:937–941, 1973.

8 Registries of Genetic Disease and Disability, and Family Screening

The previous chapter described various programs that, among other things, store information on genetic disease and disability. Some of these were registries. This chapter reviews the stated objectives of health registries, discusses certain problems regarding their current status, makes suggestions for their improvement, and discusses the problems of extending screening, either through a physician or through enumeration of some sort, to family members known as being possible carriers of or at risk from genetic disease.

DEVELOPMENT OF HEALTH REGISTRIES

In simplest form, a registry is merely a list of individuals (or objects) that have in common one or more attributes deemed of interest. These persons may, for example, belong to a single age set, possess a specific disease or tumor, or own a particular make of automobile. Registries can be further characterized in terms of some of their properties.

The unit of registration may be an individual in one instance, or a group, such as a nuclear or extended family, in another. The registry may be supported primarily by private funds and depend upon voluntary cooperation, or it may have some form of governmental financing, and possibly legislation to compel individual, group, or population involvement. Its activities may be limited or undefined in time. Registries may or may not be population based; that is, they may or may not relate to a definable population—most extant registries probably do not. Efforts to enroll persons in a given registry may be on a casual basis, or on a systematic, actively pursued one, and enrollees may or may not be directly contacted by the individuals who maintain the registry. Finally, responsibility for the registry may be vested in one institution or agency, or it may be shared. There are clearly other ways in which registries may be characterized, but these are the most relevant for our purposes.

The registration of individuals for medical or public health objectives is largely a development of the twentieth century. The most conspicuous use of registration for public health purposes is in the numerous local and regional tumor registries. Some of these, the Connecticut Tumor Registry, for instance, have been in existence for four decades or more.

Chief among the stated objectives of most health registries are the following:

- To prevent disease, either through preventing the birth of an individual who might be affected, as in the case of a genetic registry, or through assurance of proper prophylactic practices where such exist
- To ensure prompt and correct diagnosis
- To provide, through referral, proper treatment for a rare disorder, when few physicians will know the current status of therapy for the disease
- To detect and eradicate life-threatening complications when they arise
- To evaluate prevalence and incidence and thereby identify possible high-risk populations whose health care requirements might differ from those of other groups
- To afford better evaluation of the natural history of the disease
- To appraise the impact of a given disease on a population and to evaluate changes in that impact resulting from exposure to environmental changes, for example, chemical mutagens
- To evaluate health care needs and the distribution and adequacy of health care facilities with reference to a particular set of diseases—in this instance those with an inherited basis.

Few, if any, of the current registries of inherited disease or congenital defects address themselves to all these objectives. Most have more limited interests, largely ascribable to the sequence of events that prompted the development of the registry. Thus, for example, the National Center for Disease Control's Congenital Malformations Surveillance System emphasizes a continuing monitoring of the prevalence and incidence of certain malformations with a view to early recognition of significant changes in those frequencies.[1] The Maryland Psychiatric Case Registry, on the other hand, stresses among its objectives provision of a laboratory for solving the methodologic, legal, financial, and administrative problems in the establishment and maintenance of psychiatric registries and their use in training and guidance of medical and paramedical personnel.[2]

PROBLEMS WITH REGISTRIES

A variety of problems, some technical and some not, have combined to compromise achievement of the general aims listed above. One such problem is the unambiguous and accurate identification of the unit of registration (the person, for example, or a family). It is generally assumed that if a sufficiently large number of items of information can be recorded on a group of individuals, each array will be unique and thus will establish the identity of the individual. As the number of items increase, however, manipulation of the information becomes more difficult and the likelihood of error in one or more items of information increases. This has prompted some individuals to urge the wider use of unique identifiers, such as social security numbers, but these alternatives have their own problems. Accuracy of identification, thus, becomes a matter of cost.

The advent of large-scale, fast digital computers has made possible achievement of objectives or registries that were previously unattainable or prohibitively costly. For example, the linking of multiple sources of information on a given person or event by machine, a task that would be impracticable by hand, is not only possible but potentially inexpensive. Conceivably, many such data might be of a demographic nature routinely collected by various governmental agencies, e.g., birth, death, and marriage records. The computer also promises more effective utilization of the data that are collected.

Data management and file structure are other areas where further advances would be welcomed. Much more is known about the logic of data files than was known a decade or two ago, and it is now possible to move within the structure of a file more rapidly. This diminishes the expense of data retrieval, an important consideration because the cost of data management and processing can escalate rapidly. As file size and number of accessions to the file increase, methods of file record management become extremely critical. Tiny inefficiencies become costly. Random-access storage devices have materially reduced data retrieval costs, and new technologic developments have contributed to a substantial lowering of the expense of data storage.

Quality control is another matter of moment, particularly to those individuals who propose to use registries as aids to research. While the requisite verification of information is not formidable as long as a register or file remains small, as a registry grows large and accessions occur more frequently, quality control can become difficult and expensive.

The use of data from registries (particularly detailed ones maintained in computers) poses numerous unresolved legal and ethical issues, however.[3] Among these issues are the specificity and reliability of the data, the confidentiality of the information, the centralization of registries with overlapping interests into a single registry (avoiding duplication but perhaps heightening the possibility of invasion of privacy), and the security of provisions that govern the private segments of the data file. In the Maryland Psychiatric Case Registry, the confidential nature of the data is protected from court subpoena, and the reporting physician or agency is not legally liable for damages resulting from the submission of these data to the registry. All forms that contain identifying information are kept locked up at all times except when in active use by authorized personnel, and tapes containing identifying information can be referenced only by specific computer programs. Whether these precautions are adequate to ensure confidentiality of the individual record and the anonymity of the person is moot, but they evince a general concern.

It may also be anticipated that registries of disease, particularly those that are family oriented, will frequently identify individuals with disease who may be unaware of that fact. Not all will view this new-found information as a blessing (as has been mentioned in earlier sections of this report); when to divulge such information and to whom remains unclear. Other troublesome issues involve the determination of who is to have access to the registry, under what circumstances, and to what part of the accumulated file. How are such decisions to be reached in a manner equitable to the person registered, to others, and to society, and what mechanisms of appeal are to exist?

Ultimately, the value of registries will presumably be determined not only by their potential and actual contributions to treatment, research and training in the health sciences, but also by their impact upon issues of public policy, ethics, and morals.

FAMILY SCREENING

When a patient is discovered to have a genetic disease, his relatives are immediately marked with some calculable probability of having at least one copy of the gene (or, less commonly, the chromosome) that caused it. The patient with the disease thus becomes the point of departure for a search for others who might also have the disease or the genes as yet unexpressed, or who are carriers for a gene that could be the source of disease in offspring. This is screening, but not quite the same as population screening, since here the population is defined by kinship and would, therefore, be limited in number, although not necessarily in geographic distribution. Earlier sections of the report have referred fleetingly to the opportunities and problems associated with collecting and disseminating genetic information on relatives. This section discusses the issues systematically.

Overt or Latent Disease

It is common practice when, for example, a patient with Wilson's disease is discovered, to test the sibs for latent evidences of the disease. This is simply good medicine, since early treatment may prevent the onset of irreversible manifestations. Because Wilson's disease is a recessive characteristic and a rare one, it is unlikely that collateral relatives will have it too; but for some dominant diseases the picture is different. Intestinal polyposis is one such disorder, and it has a fatal outcome due to malignant degeneration of the polyps. This disaster can be prevented by a timely resection of affected bowel, so it ought to be someone's responsibility to communicate the discovery of the disease in one person to his relatives.

There are also other conditions, perhaps of less urgency, the news of which might be passed on to relatives. Some, such as the various hyperlipidemias, represent indicators of future disease that might be controlled by dietary discipline; others, such as glucose-6-phosphate dehydrogenase deficiency, are not diseases at all, except under rather specific and usually avoidable conditions. Here the transmitted information may permit a relative to escape a disease that he was unaware was in store for him by avoiding those drugs and medications that promote hemolysis.

Reproductive Information

A second aim of family screening is to apprise relatives of probabilities for carrying genes that may be associated with disease in their offspring. While this issue may not be a pressing one if the disease in question is a rare recessive, it becomes urgent when it is sex-linked, regardless of rarity. That is, the female relatives of the mother of a child with hemophilia, for example, are themselves at risk for affected boys. If a hemophilic child is the first and only affected boy in an extended family, it is, of course, possible that he represents a new mutation; but if his mother can be shown to be heterozygous, then all her female relatives are at risk and ought, perhaps, to know it.

Unresolved Questions

Whose Responsibility? Physicians are accustomed to dealing directly only with patients encompassed by their "practice," that is, those persons who have asked them to see to their medical problems. For this reason, doctors are unlikely to see family screening as their duty; indeed, they are unlikely to think of it at all. Furthermore, they may even be made uneasy by the idea of proposing health measures, unasked, to persons who may be someone else's patients. On the other hand, the issue may be managed by the family of the affected patient. That is, the family may assume the responsibility of transmitting information provided by their own doctor to such relatives as they may decide should have it. Thus the question becomes a part of genetic counseling, in which the uses of genetic information are always left to the discretion of the recipients. Unfortunately, the literature is generally silent on this important issue, so that we do not know in any detail how often or in what ways physicians and genetic counselors deal with it, nor what the outcomes are.

If genetic screening becomes an important function of state health departments, the dissemination of information to relatives might become a part of their mission. There is an analogy with the search for contacts of patients with infections, which is a common health department occupation. But this analogy is incomplete, because the search for contacts is carried out to protect society, while genetic screening is done only in the interest of each particular individual. On the other hand, assuming confidentiality could be maintained, and with the voluntary collaboration of affected patients or their parents, there seems no particular reason why, *under conditions that remain to be defined,* screening carried out under the auspices of health departments could not be extended to sibs and collateral relatives. The legal aspects of the question are discussed in Part VI, Chapter 10.

It has been suggested that genetic registries could be useful in identifying relatives at risk for genetic disease.[4-6] This could be accomplished by entering each family ascertained through, for example, a screenee found to have a specific gene or disease. If extended pedigree information were entered, the computer could calculate the risk for each person and the registry officials could notify such persons, perhaps through their family physicians. A few such registries are now in existence, as described above, but little is known of the details of their operation as detectors of persons at risk. Such uses of registries should be the subject of research for some time to come, since there are many problems of confidentiality, invasion of privacy, even of misidentification, to surmount before they are ready to become an ordinary part of public service offered by health departments.

Counseling in Family Screening To be told the diagnosis of a disease when one is sick, while sometimes shocking, has at least the logic of fitting a name and prognosis to the ills one feels; but to learn that one is doomed to a disease of late onset, or that one possesses the genetic capacity to harm one's offspring, is a new and unexpected experience to all but a few. It is not surprising, therefore, that some families may hesitate to pass on risk probabilities to their relatives, or to be the instrument through which they may be subjected to test. And, indeed, the issue of whether they should, and if they should, what the circumstances should be, are not yet settled.

There is no question that the potential for anxiety and emotional damage is great. The polar positions are represented by the following examples. The most favorable situation occurs when a gene is discovered whose effects can be definitively detected in those at risk, and something can be done about preventing the disease or treating it. An example of this might be a sex-linked recessive disease in which the mother of an affected boy can be shown definitely to be a carrier, and in which the affected fetuses of known heterozygous maternal relatives can be diagnosed. The least favorable example is that of a lethal or seriously debilitating autosomal dominant disease of late onset that can be neither prevented nor treated. For everything in between the duty of the physician or counselor is not clear, although he must surely discuss the matter thoroughly, advising the family of the risks for their relatives and of the availability and reliability of appropriate tests to resolve those risks for some and to make them a certainty for others.

Summary

Testing sibs of a child who has a genetic disease is simply good medicine and is only technically to be regarded as screening, but the pursuit of collateral relatives with the intention of providing risk probabilities or screening tests is not envisioned in ordinary practice and lacks precedent. Without the empirical data that normally provide his direction and inform his decisions, the physician is left to proceed according to his own social and ethical imperatives, and these may often dictate that he do nothing. Before family screening can become an accepted medical or health measure, a great deal of investigation is necessary into the feelings and attitudes of parents who are to be asked to share information with their sibs and other relatives, into the mechanisms by which that information can be transmitted, and into the feelings and attitudes of the recipients. We need some actual evidence of the cost-to-benefit ratios of informing relatives for many different diseases. Perhaps the anticipation of undue anxiety will be discovered to have been exaggerated. Perhaps sibs, uncles, aunts, and cousins will be found to be generally grateful for having been warned.

REFERENCES

1. U.S. Department of Health, Education, and Welfare, Public Health Service, Center for Disease Control. Congenital Malformations Surveillance. November–December 1973. Atlanta, Ga.: U.S. Department of Health, Education, and Welfare, March 1974.
2. Maryland Department of Mental Hygiene and the National Institute of Mental Health. Maryland Psychiatric Case Register. Description—History, Current Status, and Future Uses. Washington, D.C.: U.S. Department of Health, Education, and Welfare, 1967.
3. U.S. Department of Health, Education, and Welfare. Records, Computers, and the Rights of Citizens. Report of the Secretary's Advisory Committee on Automated Personal Data Systems. HEW Publ. No. (OS) 73-94. Washington, D.C.: U.S. Department of Health, Education, and Welfare, 1973.
4. Smith, C., S. Holloway, and A. E. H. Emery. Individuals at risk in families with genetic disease. J. Med. Genet. 8:453–459, 1971.
5. Emery, A. E. H. The prevention of genetic disease in the population. Internat. J. Environ. Studies 3:37–41, 1972.
6. Miller, J. R., Personal communication.

V

CURRENT STATE OF READINESS TO PROMOTE AND ACCEPT GENETIC SCREENING

9 Knowledge, Attitudes, and Behavior

The success of a screening program depends upon public acceptance, and informed consent depends on adequate knowledge and understanding. If genetic screening is to play any significant part in preventive medicine, it will be because the public knows and understands its aims and impact and because physicians approve of it and advocate it. Accordingly, the Committee devoted some time to a discussion by experts in health education and the means of influencing health behavior. In addition, a national study of physicians' attitudes toward screening and genetics was commissioned (Appendix G). This chapter contains an analysis of data concerning the knowledge and attitudes of physicians; a discussion of public knowledge and attitudes, and of the principles governing health behavior; and a review of genetic counseling as it might apply to genetic screening.

PHYSICIAN KNOWLEDGE OF AND ATTITUDES TOWARD GENETIC SCREENING

A survey was undertaken during late winter and spring of 1974 to identify potential barriers to physicians' screening for genetic disease.*

* The survey was accomplished by means of a mail questionnaire sent to a probability sample of board-certified pediatricians, obstetricians/gynecologists, and family physicians. Appendix G contains an explanation of how the sample was selected, what the response and nonresponse rates were, and a copy of the questionnaire. It also contains detailed tables of the summary findings presented in this section.

Particular attention was devoted to ascertaining the views of practicing physicians about the risk of genetic health problems; the consequences of genetic problems for the affected child, family, and society; and whether they believe that there currently exist effective preventives, treatments, or cures for various conditions, including counseling, abortions, and medical treatment and management. Also studied were physicians' attitudes toward genetic screening in general, and, for those who favor screening, their views about whether responsibility for screening should be a public or private matter, and how costs of screening should be met. Finally, opinions were solicited on such related matters as genetic counseling, abortion, the role of law in screening, and the usefulness and propriety of genetic registers.

Findings

Education On the subject of education, it was found that nearly three quarters of the group reported that no courses in genetics had been available during their medical training. Even among those in practice less than 6 years, only half reported that such courses had been available to them. Concerning the education of the public, most physicians believed that there should be more emphasis on genetics in primary medical education, as well as continuing education at higher levels.

Knowledge Regarding physicians' knowledge about genetics, it was found that there are substantial differences among specialties in the perceived frequency of genetic defects, with pediatricians and obstetricians believing them to be more frequent than family practitioners did (see Table G-3 of Appendix G). They also differ widely within and among specialty groups in their perception of the subjective risks of genetic disease associated with stated mathematical probabilities of occurrence of hemophilia, Tay-Sachs disease, Down's syndrome, and cleft lip/palate (see Appendix G, Tables G-5 through G-8). Pediatricians, again, attribute the highest risks to these conditions, with obstetricians next, and family practitioners attributing lowest risks. Interestingly, more than half the sample (it should be remembered that the sample is composed of physicians) believed that sickle cell trait causes occasional or frequent medical problems.

A majority agreed with the statement that many metabolic errors are inborn and further that such errors will be shown to have genetic determinants (Appendix G, Table G-10). As with other responses, however, the family practitioners and obstetricians were much less sure about the latter than pediatricians.

Slightly less than half the sample believed that cessation of all treatment for genetic disorders would have an extremely serious impact on affected children and their families (see Table G-11, Appendix G), but once again there was substantial disagreement among specialists, with a majority (56%) of pediatricians believing the impact would be extremely serious, compared to 45% of the obstetricians and only 29% of the family practitioners. The same pattern of response occurred, but at a lower general level, when the question was directed at the impact on society as a whole of ceasing all treatment.

Experience More than a third of the sample reported that they have had very little or no contact with potential or actual genetic disease. In addition, of the conditions reported as "genetic," up to 10% could not be confirmed as such by the survey analysts because they were too vaguely described to be identified or were incorrectly classified as genetic. Here again pediatricians were the most accurate, followed by obstetricians and then by family practitioners. Referrals of patients for determination of genetic diseases within the last 5 years have also been made primarily by pediatricians and obstetricians. A majority of pediatricians and obstetricians reported that they used general criteria for such referral, but only just over 20% of family practitioners did so.

Attitudes toward Management of Genetic Problems Counseling, therapy, and abortion were all considered appropriate and generally effective measures for various conditions by significant numbers of the physicians questioned. Further questions were asked concerning counseling, and the answers betray a certain ambivalence. Although most of the sample (family practitioners less than the others) believed that their own genetic counseling of patients has been partially or highly effective, less than 2% believed that physicians in general are currently competent to provide such counseling, and only 13% believed additional training would make them competent. On the other hand, less than half of the obstetricians thought trained genetic counselors were needed, and even fewer of the other two specialties thought so.

Attitudes toward Screening Wide variation among specialties was observed in perceived importance of detecting potential or actual genetic disorders, with pediatricians most frequently believing in the importance of detection and family practitioners least often agreeing with that position. Nearly three quarters of the respondents believed that screening for particular traits or conditions should be encouraged, but over half, with little variation by specialty, are opposed to mandatory screening.

Concerning attitudes toward genetic screening *per se,* about half of each specialty group preferred that such tests be offered only as part of regular medical practice, with most of the rest expressing a preference for community-organized campaigns. There was general agreement among respondents that if such programs were organized, it should be done by health departments or by medical societies. With regard to financing, 40% thought the individual screened should pay for the service, with another 25% favoring payment by state or local government.

More than 80% of the respondents favored screening to increase scientific knowledge, but only about a quarter of the physicians believed that the benefits of PKU and sickle cell screening have outweighed the costs. Finally, more than 40% of the physicians were opposed to a regional or national genetic registry.

Interpretation of Results

The survey showed that less than half the physicians surveyed believe it is extremely important to detect potential or actual genetic disorders, while nearly all of the remaining physicians believe such detection is "important" rather than "unimportant." Those who (a) know more about genetics, (b) believe risks of contracting specified genetic disease are relatively high, (c) have had direct experience with genetic disease, (d) believe the impact of untreated genetic disease to be extremely serious, and (e) believe that PKU and sickle cell screening have been beneficial are the most likely to believe the detection of genetic defects is extremely important. The same pattern is seen among those favoring community-wide screening for particular traits, favoring prenatal screening for inborn errors for which no postnatal therapies are available, believing that genetic counseling clinics and trained counselors are desirable, believing that screening for at least some conditions should be required by law, and believing that the incidence of genetic disease is relatively high.

These findings suggest that the medical profession as represented by the three specialties studied is not as a whole ready to accept the importance of genetic disease and of screening for it at the present time. But the findings do suggest that such readiness could be increased if the physicians had greater knowledge of genetics, deeper appreciation of the impact of untreated genetic disease on affected families, and more direct experience with genetic disease.

PUBLIC KNOWLEDGE, ATTITUDES, AND BEHAVIOR

As the previous section showed, physician knowledge of and experience with genetic disease are not by any means perfect. It is clear, however, that the more physicians know, the more likely they are to appreciate the impact of genetic disease and to favor the detection and treatment of it. The same is very likely to be true of the public, who can be expected to have a lower level of knowledge than practicing physicians. This section of the report is devoted to a discussion of the knowledge and attitudes of the public and how they might be influenced to increase the likelihood of public acceptance of screening and preventive measures.

The Health Belief Model

In recent years a theory has been developed to explain the conditions under which people take action to prevent, detect, and diagnose disease. In addition, much knowledge has been acquired from studies of persuasion that seems relevant to the problems of public programs for genetic screening. These topics will be discussed in general terms here (specific suggestions can be found in Part VII in the section on public education, p. 244).

It should be made clear at the outset that most of the relevant research has been done in connection with health conditions other than the inborn errors of metabolism,[1-4] although there has been one study on factors influencing the decision to participate in screening for the Tay-Sachs trait. Therefore, the applicability of this research to the public's future response to genetic screening programs cannot be taken for granted.

The major variables in the model are drawn and adapted from general social-psychological theory; the variables deal with the subjective world of the behaving individual and not with the objective world as described by others. The focus in the application of the model is to link current subjective states of the individual with current health behavior. As will be seen, it has been shown to have utility in explaining behavior even in the presence of symptoms of illness.[5-7]

A truism in social psychology is that motivation is required for perception and action. Thus, people who are unconcerned with a particular aspect of their health are not likely to perceive any material that bears on that aspect of their health. Even if, through accidental circumstances, they do perceive such material, they will fail to learn, accept, or use the information.

Such concern or motivation is not only a necessary condition for action; motives also determine the particular ways in which the environment will be perceived. That a motivated person perceives selectively in accordance with his motives has been verified in many laboratory studies[8] as well as in field settings.[3]

The explanation of health behavior grows out of such evidence. Specifically, it includes three classes of variables: (a) the general level of health motive or health concern exhibited by the individual, (b) the psychological state of readiness to take specific action, and (c) the extent of the belief that a particular course will be beneficial in relation to the psychological costs of taking that action.

Health Motivation Motivation may be defined as differential emotional arousal in individuals caused by some given class of stimuli, in this case health matters. Health motivation may be conceived as including negative components—avoidance of ill health or conditions that might put one at risk of suffering illness—and it may include positive components—striving for a sense of good health and well-being.

Readiness to Act Two principal dimensions define whether a state of readiness to act exists: (a) the degree to which an individual feels vulnerable or susceptible to a particular health condition and (b) the extent to which he feels that suffering that condition would have serious consequences in his case. As indicated, readiness to act is defined in terms of the individual's point of view about his susceptibility to and the seriousness of various health conditions, rather than objectively.

Perceived Susceptibility Perceived susceptibility refers to the subjective risks of contracting a condition or of possessing a particular trait. Individuals vary widely in the acceptance of personal susceptibility to a condition. At one extreme is the individual who denies any possibility of his contracting or transmitting a given condition or possessing a particular trait. A more moderate case is the person who may admit to the "statistical" possibility of its occurrence but to whom this possibility has little personal reality. At the other extreme is a person who says he feels in real danger of contracting or transmitting a given condition or of possessing a particular trait.

Perceived Seriousness Convictions concerning the seriousness of a given health problem may also vary from person to person. The degree of seriousness may be judged both by the degree of emotional arousal created by the thought of a disease and also by the kinds of difficulties the individual believes a given health condition will create for him.

A person may, of course, see a health problem in terms of its medical or clinical consequence. But the perceived seriousness of a condition may, for a given individual, include such broader and more complex implications as the effects of the disease or trait on his self-image, his job, his family life, and his social relations. Thus a person may not believe that tuberculosis or the sickle cell trait are medically serious but may nevertheless believe that either condition would be serious if it created important psychological or other tensions within himself or his family. There is probably some "optimal" level of perceived seriousness in producing a favorable readiness to act. Too little or too much perceived seriousness can produce a response that is not well adapted to the objective situation.

Perceived Benefits of Taking Action and Barriers to Taking Action The acceptance of one's susceptibility to a disease or trait that one believes to have serious implications provides a force leading to action, but it does not define the particular course of action that is likely to be taken. The direction the action will take is also influenced by beliefs regarding the relative effectiveness of known, available courses of action in reducing the health threat to which the individual feels subject. An action is likely to be seen as beneficial if it relates to the reduction of one's perceived susceptibility to or seriousness of an illness or trait. Again, the person's belief about the availability and effectiveness of various courses of action, and not the objective facts about the effectiveness of action, determines what course he will take. And his beliefs in this area are undoubtedly influenced by the norms and pressures of his social group.

An individual may believe that a given action will be effective in reducing the threat of disease but may also see the action as having high psychological costs, including inconvenience, expense, unpleasantness, pain, or embarrassment. These negative aspects of health action arouse conflicting motives. Several resolutions of the conflict are possible. If the perceived benefits of action are great and the costs or negative aspects are seen as relatively weak, the action in question is likely to be taken. Action is less likely the more the reverse is true. Where the potential benefits of action are seen as great and the barriers to action are also great, the conflict may be more difficult to resolve.

What does the individual do if the situation does not provide acceptable alternatives to resolve his conflicts? Experimental evidence obtained outside the health area suggests that one of two reactions occurs. First, the person may attempt to remove himself psychologically from the conflict situation by engaging in activities that do not really reduce the threat. Vacillating between choices may be an example. A second possible reaction is a marked increase in fear or anxiety.[9] If the anxiety or fear becomes strong enough, the individual may be rendered incapable of thinking objectively and behaving rationally about the problem. Even if he is subsequently offered a more effective means of handling the situation, he may not accept it, simply because he can no longer think constructively about it.

Cues to Action The variables that measure perceived susceptibility and severity, as well as the variables that define perceived benefits and costs of taking action, have all been subjected to and generally validated by research. However, one additional variable, which has not been subjected to careful study, is necessary to complete the model.

A cue or a trigger to trip off appropriate action is also necessary. The level of motivation provides the energy or force to act; the perception of relative benefits provides a preferred path of action. However, the combination of these can reach considerable levels of intensity without resulting in overt action unless some instigating event occurs to set the process in motion. In the health area, such events or cues may be internal (e.g., perception of bodily states) or external (e.g., interpersonal interactions, the impact of communication media, knowledge that someone else has become affected, or receiving a postcard from the dentist).

The required intensity of a cue sufficient to trigger behavior presumably varies with differences in the level of readiness. With relatively low psychological readiness (i.e., low motivation, little acceptance of the susceptibility or severity), intense stimuli will be needed to trigger a response. On the other hand, with relatively high levels of readiness, even slight stimuli may be adequate.

Evidence

A large number of major investigations whose design was largely or entirely determined by this model of health belief have been undertaken. For the most part, they have provided support for its usefulness in helping to explain individuals' responses to preventive and screening programs and the degree of compliance with medical regimens.

The pertinence of the model to genetic screening is illustrated by a recent study that analyzed factors influencing members of an identified Jewish population in the Baltimore–Washington area to participate in screening for the Tay-Sachs trait.[10] The education of the target community began 6–8 weeks before initiation of mass screening. Multiple educational approaches were used to saturate the communities with accurate and clear information. These included the press, TV, radio, letters from rabbis, fliers from community organizations, medical presentations to the community, telephone calls from trained volunteers, brochures from physicians, and other special mailings. Lists of the target population were available, so it could be ascertained that all members of the target group—couples of childbearing age—were exposed to at least some of these educational activities.

As applied to the Tay-Sachs situation, the explanatory variables were defined as follows: *Health motivation* included two components: (a) a positive response indicating a desire to have (additional) children and (b) a set of generalized items about typical health behavior, such as the frequency with which the person thinks about his own health and whether he generally goes to the physician if he feels sick. *Perceived susceptibility* included the person's belief that he could carry the Tay-Sachs gene and transmit it to his progeny. *Severity* was interpreted as the individual's views of the potential impact of learning that he was a carrier, especially with regard to future family planning. *Perceived benefits* were defined in terms of a personal evaluation of how much good it would do the potential carrier to be screened for the trait. Did he really need to know or want to know his carrier status? *Barriers to action (costs)* were not measured in this study. They might include, however, the usual monetary or convenience factors, as well as threats we currently know very little about, for example, the impact on an individual of learning that he is a carrier of some recessive trait. How does it affect his self-image, his perception of his health and of his well-being? Does it affect his marriage? How does it influence future family planning?

In all, nearly 7,000 adults, estimated as 10% of the total eligible population of childbearing age, were screened during the first year of the study, all drawn from lists of synagogue membership and names in predominantly Jewish neighborhoods. All adults who appeared for screening were asked to complete a brief questionnaire just before going through the screening process; 500 of these were selected as the participant sample. In addition, 500 questionnaires were mailed to a random sample of nonparticipants who had been invited in for screening; here the response rate was 82%. It should be noted that both respondents and nonrespondents had received informational material on Tay-Sachs disease and screening. Comparisons were made between 500 randomly selected participants and 412 randomly selected nonparticipants who responded to the mailed questionnaire.

The participants were significantly younger than the nonparticipants, had fewer children, were less likely to have completed their families, and were slightly better educated. Turning to the health belief variables, the participants differed sharply in the first component of health motivation (desire to have children)—82% of those who expressed the desire to have more children participated in the screening program, while less than 19% who did not desire future children participated. There was no significant difference in participation according to the second motivational measure used (typical health behavior). The perceived susceptibility measure was significant, being highly correlated with participation in the screening program. Perceived severity was also significant, but this time it was negatively associated with participation.

When the three foregoing variables were combined, it became apparent that while each of the three is associated with participation, perceived susceptibility and the desire to have more children were connected, while perceived severity played an independent, explanatory role. For persons who desire additional children, moderate perceived susceptibility and low perceived severity best explain participation in the program. Among those who are not motivated to have additional children, high perceived susceptibility and low perceived severity best explain participation. Irrespective of motivation, the combination of high perceived susceptibility and low perceived severity best accounts for participation.

Benefits-to-Barriers Ratios Among those individuals who indicated that they planned to have more children, more nonparticipants than participants indicated that the discovery that either or both husband and wife were carriers would change their future child-planning behavior; frequently they reported that they would have no additional children. One possible interpretation of this finding is related to beliefs exhibited by participants and nonparticipants about the transmission and detection of Tay-Sachs disease and about reproductive alternatives.

The impact of learning that one member of a married couple was a carrier had a very different effect on participants and nonparticipants. Participants were much less likely than nonparticipants to alter their plans. More of the participants had apparently learned that carrier status in only one member of the couple poses no dangers. However, in response to the question on the impact if *both* parents were found to be carriers, while participants were again less likely to change their reproductive plans than nonparticipants, they did indicate they would reduce the number of children they would have or that they would use "other" approaches. In nearly every case where the "other" category was used, participants went on to explain that they would elect to use amniocentesis (fetal diagnostic test) in order to continue to have children. Very few of the nonparticipants displayed knowledge of the availability of amniocentesis; rather, they tended to indicate that, in the event either member or both members of a couple were found to be carriers, they would not have further children.

Since more participants than nonparticipants learned about the fetal diagnostic test, it may be inferred that screening conferred considerable benefits on participants: (a) They could rule out the possibility that both parents carried the recessive gene, or (b) if both proved to be carriers, amniocentesis could rule out the possibility that the fetus had the disease, or (c) if the fetus were diseased, they could elect to abort it. While nearly all the study respondents (participants and nonparticipants) held attitudes favoring abortion in the event that a fetus had Tay-Sachs disease, the nonparticipants could not have seen as much benefit in screening, since they did not give evidence of having learned about amniocentesis.

Barriers to screening were minimized in the described study by offering the test at low cost to a relatively affluent group and at convenient times and locations. Such financial and situational factors could, however, prove to be important for other target groups.

One final consideration should be emphasized. It is believed that in this case perceived severity associated with the Tay-Sachs trait reached such high levels that it caused persons to avoid participation in the program. It has always been believed that what is needed for appropriate behavior is an "optimal" balance of perception of health motive, vulnerability, severity, and the psychological benefit–cost ratio; where the balance among these is either quite "low" or quite "high," professionally recommended behavior is not to be expected. The truth of this assertion, however, can come out only in studies that use measures sensitive to variations in the degree to which each variable is present.

The Relationship between the Health Belief Model and Demographic Factors Questions have been raised about the relationship between the health belief model and demographic factors because research on utilization of health services shows that demographic factors distinguish high from low utilizers. Generally speaking, scores on the variables in the health belief model are distributed unevenly in the population, high scores tending to be more prevalent among whites, among females, among persons of relatively high socioeconomic status, and among the relatively young. One might conclude that it is not the person's socioeconomic status, race, sex and age that determine action but his motives and beliefs. However, research that controls for variation in health beliefs shows that the seeking of Papanicolaou screening is more probable among whites, among persons of higher socioeconomic status, and among the relatively young. Apparently, both the beliefs and the sociologic characteristics, while closely related, make independent contributions to behavior.*

* It may be pointed out that the model described may also have usefulness in explaining behavior of providers of health care as described in the previous section. In a case study of responses to the Asian influenza epidemic of 1957, physician behavior was attributed to the same kinds of variables that appeared to explain consumer behavior.[3] Private practitioners, compared to public health physicians, exhibited low perceived importance of influenza, did not expect a dangerously high prevalence of the disease, and did not expect serious impact on their clientele. They also voiced greater doubts about the efficacy of the influenza vaccine. And, in general, they showed much less interest than public health physicians in planning and participating in immunization programs.

Table 9-1 summarizes the nature of the variables that have been shown to be useful in explaining and predicting health behavior as they might apply to attitudes and behavior of providers and clients of genetic screening. It would seem well worthwhile to test the total model in the context of a number of developing genetic screening programs.

Persuasion

The foregoing material suggests that if providers and consumers possessed an optimal balance of the several motives and beliefs described, they would support and participate in genetic screening programs. Even in the absence of good data concerning client attitudes toward genetic screening, it is nearly self-evident, given the widespread public ignorance and misunderstanding of biology and genetics, that very few persons possess the combination of motives and beliefs that would stimulate them to seek out genetic screening on their own. The problem that arises is how to persuade those without the requisite degree of motivation and beliefs to behave in the recommended ways. Here one must deal with two separate questions: (a) Can behavior be modified without first modifying the

TABLE 9-1 Variables Affecting Provider and Consumer Acceptance of Genetic Screening

Variable	Provider Attitudes	Client Attitudes
Health motive	General salience and perceived importance of genetic risks and disease	Overall concern with health and illness and with health of unborn or living children
Perceived vulnerability to serious disease	Conditions to be screened for would have serious enough impact to justify genetic screening	Feelings of susceptibility of self or children to particular conditions and moderate degree of severity of such conditions
Perceived efficacy of intervention	Reliable methods exist for diagnosing and successfully "treating" or managing genetic diseases	Early detection of traits or disease is possible and beneficial
Perceived barriers to screening	Financial and psychological costs to patient as well as professional time are not excessive relative to expected benefits; negative side effects such as possible damage to fetus or to parents are outweighed by benefits	Financial and other (e.g., religious) barriers to obtaining benefits are outweighted by potential benefits; negligible negative side effects to self or child; low impact of learning about genetic "defects" on self-image

underlying motives and beliefs? (b) Can such motives and beliefs themselves be modified through persuasion?

The first question will be dealt with here. The second will be reserved for consideration in the section on public education in Part VII (p. 244).

Can Behavior Be Modified without a Direct Attack on Motives and Beliefs? Individuals can sometimes be persuaded to behave in particular ways, rather independently of their belief systems. Structuring of the environment in particular ways will increase the probability of certain behavior. The use of law is a prime example of such a structuring of the environment. In the area of health care the individual who finds himself (through whatever processes) in the health care system is likely to submit to the variety of tests and procedures that his physician recommends. Thus, most Papanicolaou screening is done in the context of regular medical care and is accepted by many women who are not particularly motivated to seek such a test on its own merits. Most adult immunizations are also received in this manner.

Insofar as genetic screening or any other health procedure can be made part of the ordinary process of delivering care, it is likely to be accepted by a large proportion of individuals submitting to such care. Before this can happen, however, professional associations and practicing physicians will need to perceive genetic screening as a useful preventive procedure.

In another sphere, we know from studies in group dynamics that groups have power to influence the behavior of their members even without direct attempts to modify pertinent motives and beliefs.[11] If a majority of members of any group are persuaded to adopt a particular action, such as screening for disease, they will exert pressure on the remaining members of the group to adopt the majority position. (It is an interesting and encouraging fact, however, that such behavioral changes frequently lead to subsequent modifications in associated beliefs to bring the individual's beliefs into consonance with his behavior.[12])

But in at least some cases it is clear that direct influence on the motive and belief system is not necessary in order to accomplish behavioral change. Nevertheless, there are a number of reasons for trying to modify the psychological underpinnings of behavior.

- It should be recognized that the establishment of a norm (whether through law or social agreement) will ultimately result in behavioral patterns in which the norm becomes the model behavior exhibited by the group; substantial numbers will nevertheless not conform to the established norm. Despite speed limits, for instance, there remain many drivers who typically exceed them. Despite current norms in medical practice, to cite a more relevant example, there are many clients who do not conform in that they do not see a physician until symptoms render them incapable of normal functioning.

• There are large groups in the population who are not in any organized health care system and who consequently do not seek health services at all, except in emergencies. Such persons clearly cannot be reached by a reorganization of the current health care system if that reorganization is independent of changes in motivation.

• The argument is sometimes made that, if economic barriers to receipt of health care were removed, most persons would obtain regular health care. Available research evidence shows that when economic barriers to care are reduced or eliminated, utilization of services increases somewhat among poorer persons but does not attain the level of care received by the more affluent. Furthermore, even among the more affluent, there are obvious failures to seek needed health care.

• Many of the practices associated with good health entail personal living habits undertaken without professional health care. Dietary practices, physical exercise, smoking, and the like all reflect patterns of behavior that are not very much influenced by professional contact.

• Finally, the ethical principle of self-determination, which most professionals espouse, may not be consistent with a direct attack on behavior. Insofar as possible, individual action should result from informed self-interest. Use of the hidden persuaders of social engineering—behavior modification and artificially created group pressures—without concomitant education would be inconsistent with this philosophical tenet.

For these five reasons, therefore, we must conclude that direct efforts to modify behavior without simultaneously modifying its psychological underpinnings can be only partially effective and may not always be ethical. Efforts should thus be made to work more directly with motives and beliefs themselves, as well as with behavior. Recommendations based upon research and experience are offered to those responsible for planning educational programs in Part VII (p. 244).

GENETIC COUNSELING

Earlier sections of the report have dealt with physicians' knowledge of and familiarity with screening. The perceptions and awareness of potential screenees that are the prelude to acceptance of preventive measures, together with some barriers to understanding that may preclude that action, have also been discussed. There is one more element in this transaction because, even when the physician is persuasive and the subject proffers himself readily, if the results and implications of the test are not effectively transmitted, then the process will have failed in its purpose. This section is concerned, therefore, with the means by which the result of the screening test may be transmitted to and comprehended by the screenee.

Physicians are accustomed to informing and counseling their patients with the intention of making management a collaborative process to which both parties make appropriate contributions. But they have too seldom asked whether the collaboration works, or how frequently their instructions and advice are misunderstood or ignored. Nor does the literature reveal much systematic study of the requirements for fulfillment of the aims of such counseling. Genetic counseling is simply a special case of this aspect of the physician's work, adding information about the odds and discussions of the options for reproductive outcomes to the more conventional content of counseling.[13-17]

Requirements and Content

Successful genetic counseling requires an accurate diagnosis, a complete family history, and a knowledgeable and well-trained counselor. The counseling session includes a description of the disease or trait under consideration, with prognosis; attention to the social and psychological impact of the disease upon the patient and his relatives; probabilities for future reproductive outcomes, together with some discussion of such possible reproductive alternatives as antenatal diagnosis and adoption, or simply control of reproduction by contraception or sterilization; and finally, some consideration of the odds for possession of specific genotypes by sibs and collateral relatives, including whether (and under what conditions) they should be informed.[18-22]

The Counselor

The role of the primary physician makes him the ideal counselor. Unfortunately, many doctors are unacquainted with the often rare disorders and are uneasy discussing genetic odds, so counseling is frequently carried out in genetics clinics, where diagnoses can be confirmed and counselors with knowledge of and experience in both medicine and genetics are to be found.[10] Counselors are not invariably physicians, however, and recently some schools have begun to train college graduates to fill a growing need for which the supply of physician–geneticists is inadequate. These nonmedical counselors function best in specialty clinics where the counselee perceives them to be one among others, all moving under the direction of the patient's own doctor toward a solution to his problem.

Counseling Evaluation

No one can doubt that experienced and sensitive counselors are usually effective in transmitting their message.[23,24] They know a good deal of genetics, are attuned to the emotional and educational status of their clients, and recognize the value of reinforcement in making a lesson memorable.

Barriers to Comprehension of Counseling All counseling is not so effectively done, however, as is suggested by reports that the message is not equally well understood by all counselees.[25-30] This lack of success is due in part to a want of knowledge, experience, and ability to communicate of some counselors, and in part to the presence of factors that impair the receptivity of the counselees (as has been discussed in the previous section). Some of the latter factors are discussed in the following paragraphs.

Denial A few parents or patients simply deny the seriousness of the disease at hand, or their own part in its genesis. For example, it may be difficult, or impossible, for a parent to accept that he has contributed a gene that has harmed his child.

Comprehension of Probability There is much variation in ability to grasp the abstraction of odds, which may account for the frequency with which counselees forget them or misapply them. And it has been observed that even those who memorize the odds may not appreciate their meaning, or may fail to realize that they apply independently to each pregnancy.

Knowledge and Intelligence Clearly the educational status, life experiences, and intellectual capacities of the recipients of counseling are important in determining how much they can absorb and how they will use the information. For example, many counselees are seriously handicapped by a lack of even the simplest knowledge of medicine or human biology, or worse, by misinformation that must somehow be eradicated before useful information can be discussed with profit.

Evaluation of Success of Counseling Counseling may be said to have been successful if, in possession of the facts, a counselee makes a reproductive decision that in his judgment is appropriate for him and his family. Thus subsequent reproductive curtailment cannot be regarded as evidence of success of counseling in general, although it may be an appropriate sign in particular cases. It is very difficult to assess, however, whether the counselee is truly in possession of the facts, how he has interpreted them, and whether his subsequent reproductive behavior has been appropriate.

The counselee's information might be assessed with accuracy by asking pointed questions, although that is seldom done; but his synthesis of the information and how he is likely to use it is less easily appraised. Indeed the relationship of knowledge to attitudes toward reproduction has not been demonstrated; that is, attitudes toward further childbearing and actual reproductive performances after counseling were found in one study to be uncorrelated with socioeconomic level, educational attainment, knowledge of the genetic aspects of the disease in question, general knowledge of biology, and ease in handling probabilities.[25] Thus, knowledge of genetic facts and odds, while necessary, is not all that goes into decisions made after genetic counseling.

It is generally agreed that reproductive decisions are strongly influenced by the parents' sense of the burden imposed by the disease upon an affected child and upon themselves. Indeed, the burden may be the paramount consideration, since parents are known to accept high risks where the disease is mild or its duration brief; but they may be unwilling to run low risks when the disease is disabling or chronic.[23] It has also been observed, however, that the opposite behavior sometimes prevails; that is, some persons take chances with severe, chronic disorders, while others forego reproduction rather than take even small chances.[23]

These attitudes have not been well studied, but several suggestions have been made to account for them.[31] For example, there are differences of temperament that may be reflected in caution or daring in the face of risks. This may be expressed as a sense, on the one hand, of having bad luck, of being especially vulnerable, or, in contrast, of being especially fortunate. Further, apparently there are differences in the interpretation of "high" or "low" risk, so that what seems a sure thing to one person may be an unacceptable gamble to another; and finally, behavior that may seem irrational may represent the triumph of motives that overwhelm both risk and burden—for example, religious beliefs or a consuming desire for a child.

These are properties of the personality and beliefs of the counselee, characteristics that the counselor is not likely to be able to change and to which he must, therefore, adapt himself. But in accepting them he must be sure that unrealistic views of odds are not due to ignorance of those empiric risks that represent the chances we all take in many aspects of our lives. For example, a probability of 0.1 or 0.01 for a specific adverse reproductive outcome should be seen against the observed and known probability of disaster for any pregnancy.

Counseling and Genetic Screening

Counseling of persons identified in screening projects should not differ in principle from advice and information given to persons discovered through more conventional medical channels. The job will still entail description of the disorder, a discussion of reproductive odds and options, and psychological and emotional support. But there are important practical differences.

- The most frequent questions confronting the genetic counselor are those posed by the parents of a genetically afflicted child who initiate discussion of the chance that a subsequent pregnancy will result in another affected baby. Here, the questions revolve around a patient with a disease whose impact the family has experienced. But the object of screening is to identify persons who may have a predisposing genotype but who are not yet ill, or persons who are carriers for genes that are associated with disease only in homozygotes. Although these persons will have given the possibility of disease some thought, or they would not have come forward to be tested, they are unlikely to have experienced the disease and may be unprepared for it—both in their ignorance of its characteristics and prognosis and in their ability to withstand its emotional impact. Most persons can accept discovery of disease or trait with moderate but bearable strain, but for some it will be a stunning blow. For these latter persons, the problems of counseling will be intensified.
- When a disease is discovered through the usual medical channels, the mechanisms for moving the patient on to management and treatment are usually well worked out; and as one aspect of management, counseling has its times, places, and methods. But the role of genetic counseling in genetic screening programs is only now being clarified; and while it is clear that the service is essential, the exact procedures governing where and how it is best done, and how often and by whom, are not yet worked out.
- The authors of papers on genetic counseling (who tend to be physicians) reveal a distinct preference for physicians as counselors in genetics clinics, and it is in such clinics that counseling is said to be most effectively administered.[22] Such clinics are most likely to be found in teaching hospitals, where they serve as a consultation center for a wide area.

Unfortunately, these resources as they are presently constituted will be of only peripheral value to large screening programs, since they cannot accommodate the number of persons who will need counseling or may wish to have it. Even current screening projects, which include sickle cell trait and Tay-Sachs disease, turn up numbers of potential counselees sufficient to overwhelm presently available facilities. This means that new sources of counselors must be developed, which in turn requires new teaching programs to produce nonmedical persons of high qualifications who not only are capable of dealing with questions raised by current screening but also are easily adaptable to new projects. Such training should be designed and supervised by medical geneticists in conjunction with teachers of public health and preventive medicine. It might be that the new schools of allied health sciences will see this curriculum as a logical extension of their work.

In summary, if the participants in genetic screening are to have the benefits the projects are designed to provide, counseling must be made available to all who require it. Failure to provide it breaks the continuity of the flow of information that begins with the prescreening education and imperils fulfillment of the intent of the screening because, if the result of failure to counsel is unwarranted anxiety or inappropriate indifference, the purpose of the program will have been compromised.

REFERENCES

1. Gochman, D. S. Children's perceptions of vulnerability to illness and accidents. Publ. Health Rep. 85:69–73, 1970.
2. Hochbaum, G. M. Public Participation in Medical Screening Programs: A Socio-psychological Study. U.S. Dept. of Health, Education, and Welfare, Public Health Service Publ. No. 572. Washington, D.C.: U.S. Government Printing Office, 1958.
3. Rosenstock, I. M., G. M. Hochbaum, H. Leventhal, *et al.* The Impact of Asian Influenza on Community Life: A Study in Five Cities. U.S. Dept. of Health, Education, and Welfare, Public Health Service Publ. No. 766. Washington, D.C.: U.S. Government Printing Office, 1960.
4. Rosenstock, I. M. Why people use health services: Milbank Mem. Fund Quart. 44 (Suppl.):94–127, 1966.
5. Becker, M. H., R. H. Drachman, and J. P. Kirscht. A new approach to explaining sick-role behavior in low-income populations. Amer. J. Publ. Health. 64:205–216, 1974.
6. Kasl, S. V., and S. Cobb. Health behavior, illness behavior, and sick-role behavior. I. Health and illness behavior. Arch. Environ. Health 12:246–266, 1966.
7. Kasl, S. V., and S. Cobb. Health behavior, illness behavior, and sick-role behavior. II. Sick-role behavior. Arch. Environ. Health 12:531–541, 1966.
8. Bruner, J. S., and C. C. Goodman. Value and need as organizing factors in perception. J. Abnorm. Soc. Psychol. 42:33–44, 1947.
9. Miller, N. E. Experimental studies of conflict, pp. 431–465. In J. McV. Hunt. Personality and the Behavior Disorders. Vol. 1. New York: The Ronald Press Co., 1944.

10. Becker, M. H., M. M. Kaback, I. M. Rosenstock, and M. V. Ruth. Some influences on public participation in a genetic screening program. J. Commun. Health (In press).
11. Cartwright, D., and A. Zander, eds. Group Dynamics: Research and Theory. 2nd ed. New York: Harper & Row, 1960.
12. Festinger, L. A Theory of Cognitive Dissonance. Evanston, Ill.: Row, Peterson and Co., 1957.
13. Childs, B. Genetic counseling: A review of the literature. In B. H. Cohen and P. C. Huang, eds. Genetic Issues in Public Health. Springfield, Ill.: Charles C Thomas (In press).
14. World Health Organization. Genetic Counselling. WHO Tech. Rep. Ser. No. 416. Geneva: World Health Organization, 1969.
15. Fraser, F. C. Genetic counseling. Hosp. Pract. 6(1):49–56, 1971.
16. Sly, W. S. What is genetic counseling? Birth Defects Series 9(4):5–18, 1973.
17. Stevenson, A. C., and B. C. C. Davidson. Genetic Counselling. Philadelphia: Lippincott, 1970.
18. Murphy, E. A. The rationale of genetic counseling. J. Pediat. 72:121–130, 1968.
19. Murphy, E. A., and G. S. Mutalik. The application of Bayesian methods in genetic counselling. Hum. Hered. 19:126–151, 1969.
20. Epstein, C. J. Social aspects of medical genetics. Med. Ann. D.C. 36:224–227, 1967.
21. Motulsky, A. G., and F. Hecht. Genetic prognosis and counseling. Amer. J. Obstet. Gynecol. 90:1227–1241, 1964.
22. Epstein, C. J. Who should do genetic counseling, and under what circumstances? Birth Defects Series 9(4):39–48, 1973.
23. Carter, C. O., J. A. F. Roberts, K. A. Evans, and A. R. Buck. Genetic clinic. A follow-up. Lancet 1:281–285, 1971.
24. Emery, A. E. H., M. S. Watt, and E. Clack. Social effects of genetic counselling. Brit. Med. J. 1:724–726, 1973.
25. Leonard, C. O., G. A. Chase, and B. Childs. Genetic counseling: A consumers' view. N. Engl. J. Med. 287:433–439, 1972.
26. Sibinga, M. S., and C. J. Friedman. Complexities of parental understanding of phenylketonuria. Pediatrics 48:216–224, 1971.
27. Reiss, J. A., and V. D. Menashe. Genetic counseling and congenital heart disease. J. Pediat. 80:655–656, 1972.
28. McCrae, W. M., A. M. Cull, L. Burton, and J. Dodge. Cystic fibrosis: Parents' response to the genetic basis of the disease. Lancet 2:141–143, 1973.
29. Taylor, K., and R. E. Merrill. Progress in the delivery of health care. Genetic counseling. Amer. J. Dis. Child. 119:209–211, 1970.
30. Pearn, J. H., and J. Wilson. Acute Werdnig-Hoffman disease. Acute infantile spinal muscular atrophy. Arch. Dis. Child. 48:425–430, 1973.
31. Pearn, J. H. Patients' subjective interpretation of risks offered in genetic counselling. J. Med. Genet. 10:129–134, 1973.

VI

PRINCIPLES OF GENETIC SCREENING AND FUTURE RESEARCH NEEDS

The Committee's reviews of current practices in genetic screening revealed a need for easily attainable summaries of legal, ethical, and economic principles as they apply to genetic screening, and for some standardization of procedure in the design and operation of screening programs. In addition, it was evident that there are many unresolved questions that require research. Accordingly, this section of the report consists of four chapters. The first three present appropriate legal, ethical, and economic principles, and the fourth summarizes problems for which answers can be obtained only by research.

10 Legal Principles for Genetic Screening

Genetic screening raises a whole range of legal issues. The commonplace ones, such as physical injuries caused by screening procedures or performance of screening functions by persons not qualified to carry them out, can be judged by standard contract and malpractice doctrines and will not be addressed here.[1] The unresolved questions concern issues in genetic screening where new developments in the law confront new developments in medicine. Attention will be focused here on the following four difficult legal questions:

To what extent must the results of screening be disclosed to the person screened?*

To what extent may the results of screening be disclosed to other persons without the consent of the person screened?

Are there any constitutional barriers to the state's compelling participation in screening programs?

Do any constitutional difficulties arise if screening programs are limited to specific racial or ethnic groups?

THE SCOPE OF REQUIRED DISCLOSURE TO SCREENEES

The aim of genetic screening conducted on a "service" (rather than a "research") basis is to provide information to the person screened.

* For purposes of this legal analysis, references to "the screenee" or "the person screened" should be taken to include the parents or legal guardian of a minor who undergoes genetic screening.

Consequently, in order to fulfill this aim, genetic screening programs should be prepared to report the results of the screening test or tests (i.e., the presumptive genetic diagnosis) to the person screened. Difficulties may arise, however, when screening for one condition turns up information about other, unsuspected traits or disorders about which the screenee had not sought information. For example, as mentioned earlier in this report, Down's syndrome screening may reveal that a child has the XYY chromosome variation, an aneuploidy that some believe may predispose a person toward undesirable intellectual and social attributes. Or screening may suggest the probability that a child's natural father is someone other than his putative parent, a fact that the child's mother may have tried to conceal. Finally, the screener may believe that the screenee is not equipped psychologically to deal with the screening results at the time of the screening. The question thus arises whether the screener has legal authority to withhold the screening results from the screenee under any or all of these circumstances.

The legal principle applicable can be stated succinctly: Information may be withheld if, but only if, the person screened agrees that the information will not be disclosed to him. To be effective, such agreement would probably have to be reached by screener and screenee prior to the test. If the person screened demands otherwise, there is no *legal* justification for withholding information from him.

This emphasis on the screenee's agreement to justify withholding information reflects some developing trends in the law generally governing "informed consent" in physician–patient relations. (Although not all genetic screening will be conducted by physicians, we believe that it is reasonable to compare the screener–screenee relationship with that of physician and patient.) In the past, when disputes have been brought into litigation, the scope of the physician's right to withhold information from his patients has essentially been determined by reference to typical professional practice in the physician's community. Thus, if most physicians would consider particular information about a patient's medical condition or the risks of a contemplated procedure too sensitive to disclose to the patient, such nondisclosure would be considered justified.[2] By this standard, a screener might justifiably withhold results indicating XYY chromosomes, illegitimacy, or other data, on the ground that his fellow doctors would agree that such disclosure would be "antitherapeutic" to the patient.

But this traditional standard has come increasingly under attack both in legal commentary[3] and in court cases.[4-6] The better and more modern rule is that a physician may not withhold any medical information that his patient would need to make an "informed" decision about his medical choices; the adequacy of the disclosure made is to be measured by what lay jurors conclude a reasonable man would have wanted to know, not by what physicians customarily tell. The adoption of this new standard carries the doctrine of informed consent to its logical conclusion. The premise behind that doctrine is that the legal protection given to bodily integrity and self-determination, in medical care as in other social contexts, can be effective only if the consent of the patient is "informed."[2,7] Clearly, then, the requirement of adequate information should relate to what an average person in the patient's position would need to know in order to reach a well-considered decision; to permit the physician to substitute his judgment for the patient's on this point is, in effect, to nullify the patient's right to self-determination.

The application of the modern version of the informed consent rule to genetic screening is both necessary and proper. This does not mean, of course, that all the results of screening must always be disclosed. The primary limitation on full disclosure is that the screener may establish a general rule against it in advance, to which the screenee's assent is required before the screening test is performed. In a research program, for example, screening may be conducted solely for purposes of enumeration, without any obligation to disclose the results to individuals, provided that they are knowing and voluntary subjects of the research. Likewise, if the persons conducting a cytogenetic screening program conclude that disclosure of results of equivocal import (such as the XYY karyotype) is likely to interfere with proper child-rearing practices without bringing any substantial benefits to the child, they should obtain the parents' specific consent at the outset that only certain kinds of information will be disclosed to them and that other information will be deliberately withheld. From an ethical as well as a legal perspective, it is important that this consent be chosen as explicitly as possible, so that the screenee understands not only the specific purpose of the screening and what information will, accordingly, be disclosed, but also what kinds of information (such as equivocal genetic information or prejudicial social information) will not be disclosed.

If these terms are clearly presented to people as they enter a screening program, they will be free to refuse participation or to seek other screening programs where the desired information can be obtained. While some persons may refuse to participate in screening programs on terms of limited disclosure, their refusals should force screeners to reconsider whether the medical benefits to be expected from screening are more important than the possible detriments of disclosing information that is "incidental" or "irrelevant" from the screener's perspective.

If, on the other hand, this issue is not explicitly raised on entering the program, and the screener instead relies on his "medical judgment" alone, or on a fictitiously "implied" agreement to withhold "incidental" information, the screener runs a serious risk of being held liable if the person screened suffers an injury that can be traced to his or her ignorance of the information that was withheld. In most screening programs, where very large numbers of people are tested, a uniform policy on disclosure will therefore be needed. If the issue of disclosure is raised in a face-to-face discussion between screener and screenee before the latter enters the program, it should be possible for them to arrive at an individualized judgment regarding the desirability of disclosing all possible information, based on the data about the specific emotional and social vulnerabilities of the individual for whom disclosure of certain information may or may not be harmful.

THE SCOPE OF PERMITTED DISCLOSURE TO THIRD PARTIES

The consent of the patient is the basic legal requisite necessary for disclosure of medical information to third parties. There are two exceptions to this principle. The first, well-established, exception permits a physician to disclose otherwise confidential information when such disclosure is clearly necessary for the patient's medical care.[8,9] Thus, for example, a psychiatrist is authorized to contact court authorities for civil commitment proceedings when his patient is imminently suicidal. The second exception, which has only scattered approbation in the case law, permits disclosure of information to protect others from risk created by the patient's condition—for example, a highly communicable disease.[9,10]

This second exception would become relevant were genetic screening to reveal a disadvantageous characteristic of such a nature that the screener believes that the screenee's relatives should be warned of the risks they face of developing or passing on a genetic disorder.* Under current law, genetic screeners would be ill advised to contact relatives without the screenee's explicit consent, in view of the sparse case law support for a "public health" exception to the confidentiality rule. Of

* Although reference is made here to the "results of screening" being communicated to third parties by "the screener," a patient–physician relationship would probably have replaced the screenee–program relationship by this point. In many instances, it is to be expected that no diagnosis definite enough to lead to contacting relatives would come from the screening itself. If the presumptive diagnosis of the first test has to be subjected to further study, the screenee will probably come into direct contact with a physician who will confirm or refute the initial diagnosis.

course, in most circumstances, the screenee's cooperation (by way of supplying the names of relatives and so forth) would probably be necessary to permit the screener to act.

There are, however, several possible ways to change this situation. Screening programs might explicitly require screenees to agree before entering the program that any information revealed that in the screener's judgment might be of medical importance to their relatives may be communicated to the relatives or their physicians. Or state legislatures might enact statutes either permitting, or requiring, screeners to disclose the possible existence of harmful genetic characteristics to relatives without the consent of the person screened. An analogy for such a law might be drawn to statutes that now require physicians to report cases of venereal disease (VD) regardless of their patient's consent. The substantial degree of noncompliance with such VD statutes may result largely from the stigma attached to the diseases involved, but it also illustrates the difficulty of enforcing a statute when one must rely on the affected party's voluntarily supplying sensitive information.

As a matter of public policy, however, neither course of action is justified. The policy objections to nonconsented disclosure of genetic information are, at base, similar to the objections to mandatory genetic screening programs. It is true that, in some individual cases, there is likely to be medical benefit from nonconsented disclosure to relatives. But there are broader social reasons that argue against pursuing these individual medical benefits in this way. Genetic screeners who contact possibly affected relatives are, of course, pressing unsolicited information on them. It is likely, in a significant number of cases, that these relatives will not want such information and will not be prepared (for ethical or emotional reasons) to benefit from it. Though relying on the consent of the initial patient screened does not guarantee that any relative contacted will welcome the genetic information, the possibility of benefit is at least increased when someone with personal knowledge of the relative has made the initial judgment that this information will be more useful than harmful.

Further, and even more significantly, a general rule that screenees cannot withhold genetic screening information about themselves from anyone who might possibly be affected implies that the society expects all persons who obtain information either about their own or about their relatives' genotypes to take remedial action in response to that information. This implication would appear to represent a medical–social judgment that genetic "normality" is a prime childbearing goal for the population at large. This is particularly true of screening designed to uncover carriers who themselves are not at risk but who may be at risk for giving birth to children affected by a genetic disorder. It is more important for society to follow a conscious policy of protecting individual autonomy in assessing the social implications of one's individual genotype than to mobilize social resources behind a coercive model of genetic "normality."

At the very least, information relating to the entire range of genetic variability that a human being may manifest is not the proper subject of mandatory disclosure on a "public health" rationale. The analogy to compulsory public health measures fails because there has been no showing that genetic diseases pose a grave and immediate threat to the community in any way comparable to the dangers that have been found to justify other instances of public health intervention.[11]

Thus, it is appropriate at this stage in the development of genetic screening programs and of the public's understanding of genetic variation to preserve the common law protections given to the confidentiality of the results of screening programs. Indeed, should there be any question about the adequacy of such protection at present, since many screening programs will not bring the screenee into a direct physician–patient relationship,[12] a statute giving explicit protection to the confidentiality of screening results may be desirable. Generally, it is proper for the choice of when and how to contact relatives to be left to the person screened, in light of both his concern and knowledge about them and his feelings about sharing personal information with them. Nevertheless, should this policy result in a widespread problem, it would be appropriate for legislatures to consider statutes permitting the conveying of genetic information to persons at risk, without their request and without permission of the person from whom the information is derived. Such statutes ought to be limited to information that would alert a person to a life-threatening or massively disabling condition, however.

CONSTITUTIONAL ISSUES IN MANDATORY SCREENING

Two types of mandatory genetic screening programs have already come into existence. The first, which is best illustrated by PKU screening of neonates, is aimed at the detection of affected individuals who are in need of treatment, particularly where treatment rendered at the asymptomatic stage of the disease is much more helpful than that rendered after the condition has become manifest. The second, such as sickle cell screening, is intended primarily to tell carriers of a recessive deleterious gene that they are at risk for bearing children with a genetic disease if their mate is also a carrier.

A policy analysis of these two sorts of programs clearly leads to differing conclusions; on a number of grounds, the first type of screening appears much more justifiable than the second. If, for example, it is feared that parents and physicians will not make sure that all neonates are tested for PKU, routine screening on a compulsory basis is supportable under the *parens patriae* doctrine that the state acts to protect those who cannot protect themselves. If the detection of affected individuals will lead to their treatment and to the prevention of the burdens of the disease, screening can be justified as a public health measure (akin to preventing the spread of a disease) and as a way of saving public funds (since many, or most, untreated individuals would otherwise require lifelong care at state expense).

These arguments do not, however, support the second type of screening, unless the state's policy is also to intervene in decisions about reproduction so as to prevent certain people from having children. As was suggested in the preceding section, the Committee does not believe that either knowledge about genetics or the threat posed by genetic disease is sufficient at the present time to justify state coercion in reproductive matters. Although statutes permitting the involuntary sterilization of institutionalized mental defectives remain on the books in nearly half the states, the "eugenics" philosophy they embody has been largely abandoned. Thus neither paternalistic nor public health nor public financial grounds seem adequate to support mandatory screening for other than reasons of medical intervention.

But these policy arguments do not readily answer the question of whether mandatory screening of either type violates the Constitution of the United States,* to which we shall now turn. The basic objection to mandated screening is, as noted, founded in respect for individual choice in child-rearing matters. This policy discussion may appear somewhat paradoxical, since screening itself is intended to provide information upon which choices can then be based. But the decision about what information, if any, is to be sought can itself properly be considered a matter of individual choice. Knowing adverse information itself is a powerful impetus toward action, even to the extent of coercing a particular decision. If a woman knows, for example, that she is carrying a Down's syndrome child, that knowledge can press her toward choosing an abortion. If the woman holds ethical precepts against abortion, she might reasonably choose not to have this information so as to defend

* Not treated here are the problems, if any, that genetic screening may raise under state constitutions, since such issues are likely to be very similar to those raised under the federal charter.

her sense of personal morality from the inevitable pressures placed on it by the known temptation to abort a handicapped fetus.

Accordingly, since forced genetic information intrudes on private childbearing choice, an argument can be drawn from recent Supreme Court decisions that this intrusion is impermissible state action.[13,14] Although the Supreme Court in 1927 upheld a state law permitting compulsory sterilization of feeble-minded persons on eugenic grounds,[15] a substantial number of subsequent Supreme Court decisions have undermined that decision, and it seems safe to predict that compulsory sterilization laws (and any extension to compulsory abortion) would withstand current constitutional scrutiny only if the compelled conduct were found to be "necessary" to achieve a "compelling" state objective.[13,16,17]

The question thus becomes one of whether compulsory genetic screening can be equated with compulsory sterilization or abortion. A number of salient differences suggest themselves. First, compulsory sterilization or abortion dictates whether children should be born to particular parents. Compulsory screening of prospective parents before conception or directly of the fetus prenatally forces information on the parents that they may take into account in their childbearing decisions. But, provided that screening is not linked to abortion or sterilization by law, its intrusion into "family privacy" is much less drastic since it does not of its own force forbid anything. Second, its scientific basis is much stronger and it is more precise diagnostically than other techniques that have been used to separate "fit" from "unfit" parents.[18] Further, in the case of screening intended to lead to treatment, the state can plausibly argue that its interest in promoting the well-being of children will be significantly aided by screening programs, and that this overshadows any parental interest in preventing an invasion of their own, or their child's, privacy.

A great deal will thus depend upon the objectives of each particular screening program and the manner in which it is conducted. Programs that involve minimal physical or emotional risk for the screenee, and that offer the prospect of beneficial treatment that the screenee would otherwise not know he needed, are likely to pass constitutional muster. The screening of newborns for inborn errors of metabolism susceptible to medical management would be an example of such a program, since the only physical intrusion on the individual is the taking of a small blood or urine sample, and the likelihood of serious injury is remote. Although mandatory screening for untreatable metabolic errors would also involve little risk, such programs are of more doubtful validity if they offer no benefits to the individual but are conducted only for research or enumeration purposes. Similarly, the interference with personal integrity and autonomy entailed in screening for recessive disease carriers is small and justified by the public benefits accruing from better informed decisions about marriage and reproduction. Mandatory amniocentesis, while probably not subject to the infirmities of a statute compelling abortion, treads very close to, and may even cross, the line beyond which the state may not interfere with family choices without greater justification than the collective judgment that certain children ought not to be born for their own sakes or for the funds it will save the state.[12]

Whether a compulsory screening statute would be constitutional is not, however, the only consideration for a legislature in enacting it. As was previously concluded, it is preferable on policy grounds for screening to be voluntary—except in the case of neonatal screening leading to treatment if it were found that nonmandatory screening leaves many babies unscreened because of parental noncooperation or physicians' ignorance or oversight.

CONSTITUTIONAL ISSUES IN LIMITED-ACCESS SCREENING

Screening programs run by a state agency or supported by public funds would be regarded as "state action" subject to the requirements of the equal protection clause of the fourteenth amendment, even though conducted on a voluntary basis. Would screening services provided, for example, only to Ashkenazi Jews in a Tay-Sachs program or only to blacks in a sickle cell program then be found to be illegal discrimination?

There are two responses to this question, one certainly in the negative and one probably so. First, the mere fact that benefits are not being distributed equally in society is not in itself a ground for invalidating a screening program. The choice of which problems to attack and the manner in which they should be tackled is left to the legislature without court interference, although the distinctions drawn may result in some inequalities.[19,20] A classification will be upheld if it is based on differences that are rationally related to the purposes for which it was made and which are not invidious.[21,22] Since many genetic disorders occur with an overwhelmingly greater frequency in certain ethnic or racial subgroups than others, it would be reasonable to direct screening programs to these populations.

Yet the fact that such groups may be defined on racial lines presents the second aspect of the equal protection question. Classifications based on race are said to be "suspect," and such a finding puts the burden of justification on the government.[23,24] A possible argument in favor of a genetics program for a racial or ethnic group would be that it is intended to benefit the group rather than to expose it to burdens and that the group is in particular need of such legislative benevolence. "Beneficent racial quotas," for example, have been upheld by courts, while "stigmatizing racial exclusions" have been roundly condemned—even though the difference between benign and malignant racial or ethnic discrimination is difficult to assess with confidence. Constitutional scholars have engaged in heated debate, in the decades since *Brown* v. *Board of Education*[25] was decided, about whether the holding of the case (invalidating school racial segregation) necessarily extended to all forms of racial (or ethnic) discriminations.[26,27] That debate has not yet been concluded. But the fact that the question remains unsettled strongly suggests that the courts will not strike down genetic screening laws on these grounds.

The difficulties of the argument can be seen by comparing sickle cell screening programs limited to blacks with special state educational programs limited to blacks (such as lower admission standards for blacks in state colleges, or quotas in public schools to assure "racial balance"). In both cases, the "vulnerable population" in need of special state services is not exclusively black, even though the state for administrative and social reasons chooses to restrict the program to blacks. In both cases, the state program is considered by its proponents and most of its participants as beneficial, notwithstanding that others consider the special programs stigmatizing in many ways. In both cases, the program has stimulated considerable controversy within the society. For special educational programs, the courts have uniformly upheld racial limitations, at least where there is a clear past history of state educational segregation; and even in the absence of such history the trend of the case law favors such programs.[28-30] These courts, in short, have chosen to overlook the possible stigmatization worked by the racial limitations and focused instead on the good intentions of the proponents and the apparent likelihood that more good than harm will come from these programs to the recipient groups. Though the beneficial uses of the racially restrictive sickle cell screening programs may be equally doubtful, their beneficence seems at least as clearly established as minority group special education provisions. Courts eager to preserve the latter programs are unlikely to invalidate the former.

But, as with the discussion of the constitutionality of mandatory screening laws generally, the fact that courts will not invalidate these laws on constitutional grounds does not establish that they are good policy. Constitutional doctrine is not a sufficiently flexible regulatory instrument to achieve the necessary sensitivity for competing social concerns. In this matter, as in many others, legislators and the proponents of state programs must rely more on their own restraint and good judgment than on court superintendence.

REFERENCES

1. Franklin, M. Medical mass screening programs—A legal appraisal. Cornell Law Quart. 47:205–226, 1962.
2. Waltz, J., and T. Scheuneman. Informed consent to therapy. Northwestern Univ. Law Rev. 64:628–660, 1970.
3. Restructuring informed consent—Legal therapy for the doctor–patient relationship. Yale Law J. 79:1533–1576, 1970.
4. Canterbury *v.* Spence, 464 F. 2d 772 (D.C. Cir. 1972).
5. Cobbs *v.* Grant, 104 Cal. Rptr. 505, 502 P.2d 1 (1972).
6. Wilkinson *v.* Vesey, 295 A. 2d 676 (R.I. 1972).
7. Natanson *v.* Kline, 186 Kan. 393, 350 P.2d 1093, *clarified and motion for rehearing denied,* 187 Kan. 186, 354 P.2d 670 (1960).
8. Clark *v.* Geraci, 29 Misc.2d 791, 208 N.Y.S.2d 564 (Sup.Ct. 1960).
9. Barry *v.* Moench, 8 Utah2d 191, 331 P.2d 814 (1958).
10. Simonsen *v.* Swenson, 104 Neb. 224, 177 N.W. 831 (1920).
11. Jacobson *v.* Massachusetts, 197 U.S. 11 (1905).
12. Green, H. P., and A. M. Capron. Issues of law and public policy in genetic screening, pp. 57–84. In D. Bergsma, ed. Ethical, Social and Legal Dimensions of Screening for Human Genetic Disease. New York: National Foundation, 1974.
13. Roe *v.* Wade, 410 U.S. 113 (1973).
14. Griswold *v.* Connecticut, 381 U.S. 479 (1965).
15. Buck *v.* Bell, 274 U.S. 200 (1927).
16. Skinner *v.* Oklahoma, 316 U.S. 535 (1942).
17. Burt, R. A. Legal restrictions on sexual and familial relations of mental retardates—Old laws, new guises, pp. 206–214. In P. F. De La Cruz and G. D. LaVeck. Human Sexuality and the Mentally Retarded. New York: G. D. Brunner/Mazel Publishers, 1973.
18. Ferster, E. Eliminating the unfit—Is sterilization the answer? Ohio St. Law J. 27:591–633, 1966.
19. Richardson *v.* Belcher, 404 U.S. 78 (1971).
20. Semler *v.* Oregon State Board of Dental Examiners, 294 U.S. 608 (1935).
21. Williamson *v.* Lee Optical Co., 348 U.S. 483 (1955).
22. Morey *v.* Doud, 354 U.S. 457 (1957).
23. Loving *v.* Virginia, 388 U.S. 1 (1967).
24. Korematsu *v.* United States, 323 U.S. 214 (1944).
25. Brown *v.* Board of Education, 347 U.S. 483 (1954).
26. Wechsler, H. Toward neutral principles of constitutional law. Harvard Law Rev. 73:1–35, 1959.
27. Bittker, B. The case of the checker-board ordinance—An experiment in race relations. Yale Law J. 71:1387–1423, 1962.
28. Keyes *v.* School District No. 1 Denver, 413 U.S. 189 (1973).
29. Norwalk CORE *v.* Norwalk Board of Education, 298 F.Supp. 213 (D.Conn. 1969), *affirmed,* 423 F.2d 121 (2d Cir. 1970).
30. Fiss, O. The Charlotte-Mecklenburg case—Its significance for northern school desegregation. Univ. Chi. Law Rev. 38:697–709, 1971.

11 Ethical Aspects of Genetic Screening

This chapter is intended to suggest a *modus operandi* for concerned screeners, consumers, and regulators who must answer the difficult ethical questions involved in screening. It should be seen as a means of examining the morally relevant issues that are presented throughout this report and that must be considered by anyone involved in screening.

One view of ethical decision-making, propounded by Firth,[1] is that an action is right if it would be approved of by an "ideal ethical observer" with the following characteristics:

Omniscient, meaning that he has all the relevant facts

Omnipercipient, meaning the ability to vividly imagine the feelings of all parties concerned

Disinterested, meaning impartial or free from self-interest

Dispassionate, meaning free from strong feelings

Consistent, meaning that he uses generalizable principles, applicable to other similar situations

Granting that no mortal possesses all these qualities, the theory proposes that a decision partakes more of rightness the closer the decision-maker comes to emulating the ideal observer. Physicians will see an analogy to the practice of differential diagnosis in clinical problem solving, a technique that does not guarantee the right diagnosis, but that minimizes the possibility that a wrong decision will be due to the failure to consider a relevant factor.

OMNISCIENCE

Getting one's facts straight is the most obvious duty of a decision-maker; yet the failure to achieve this goal may be the most common cause of ethically questionable practices in medicine. Many apparent value conflicts melt away when it is discovered that opponents are in fact in conflict over differing perceptions of the empirical situation.

A recurring presumption in clinical genetics is the belief that useful information is usually transmitted in the course of genetic counseling. While counseling can no doubt be immensely successful in the hands of some experienced people, the few data that exist on the subject cause concern. It is not clear empirically that counseling does "usually" succeed in making the patients better informed and therefore better able to make informed choices.

If the presumed benefit of a screening program depends on genetic counseling, then it is essential to know that counseling is effective; and if such counseling is ineffective in many instances, then each ineffective instance constitutes a situation of risk without benefit. When not merely noncommunication but miscommunication occurs—so that, for example, a person with sickle cell trait either believes he has sickle cell disease or that sickle cell trait is a serious illness and bases major social decisions on this false datum—the makings of tragedy are at hand.

The history of PKU screening and treatment programs discussed in Part III provides another example of decision-making that was ethically questionable because of failure to consider enough facts. The unnecessary and unwise treatment of infants who had a clinically insignificant form of hyperphenylalaninemia, rather than PKU as they were diagnosed, came about because mass screening and treatment were implemented on a broad scale before adequate data were available on the indications and necessity for such treatment.

The Committee has concluded that it would be wrong for a screening program to be predicated on unsupportable assumptions or erroneous data, and that persons initiating screening programs have a duty to minimize the risk of such error. The mechanisms for maximizing the reliability of such information are varied. At the least, a vigorous scientific review by acknowledged experts should be a part of all new programs. This could be accomplished through such existing agencies as institutional review committees for experimentation involving human subjects, state health departments, and federal funding bodies, or through the formation of new bodies such as the Commission on Hereditary Disorders recently established in Maryland.

OMNIPERCIPIENCE

The training of persons in the health care system should make them sensitive to the feelings of others, but other influences and pressures on them may, in fact, interfere with the maximum expression of omnipercipience in their decision-making about genetic screening. For example, the pressures of administering a grant, the earnest desire to help thousands of potential victims, the pressure to publish, and impatience with medicine's limited abilities in discovering and treating much illness—all these may conspire with other forces and incentives to press the decision-maker forward despite potential harm to screenees. The occurrence of psychic and social injuries will seldom be enough to decide against a particular program, but it would be wrong to proceed without ever considering such risks. Unfortunately, it is apparent that well-meaning programs can lead to great unintended harm unless decision-makers carefully attend to their duty of percipience.

Imagine a patient with meningomyelocele, having survived a childhood of suffering and now able to compete in the world, who hears on television a speaker enthusiastically announcing that prenatal diagnosis will soon be available for such a defect. Momentarily unaware of his special listener, he extols the goal of "ridding ourselves forever" of such children, "who are such a burden to their families and society." The language seems especially callous from the perspective of the special listener. Consideration of an affected individual's feelings does not require that prenatal diagnosis be discontinued because of such adverse effects. The requirement is that persons responsible for such programs be as fully sensitive as they can be to the existence of such feelings and regard them as morally relevant data in deciding whether to proceed and how to proceed.

DISINTEREST

No human being is free of self-interest. The potential interests of the would-be screener—advancement of knowledge, advancment of career, a zeal to "stamp out disease"—do not render him incapable of considering the interests of potential screenees. But they may create a conflict of interest placing at risk the screenee, whose protection is dependent on the screener.

An example of the need for greater disinterest is provided by a number of existing screening programs, particularly those with a strong research component. Screeners obtaining samples to be tested for one condition have been known to screen for additional conditions without informing or obtaining consent from the screenee; this procedure also raises problems about the confidentiality of information so obtained. Because the decision to conduct such screening is left to the judgment of the health professionals running the program, who are certainly not disinterested, the interests of the screenee may be consciously or unconsciously ignored or minimized in the decision-making.

The first requirement, then, is for the screener to maximize the opportunity for the interests of the screenee to be expressed. Ideally, as in other hazardous medical interventions, no subject should be exposed to a significant risk without his fully informed consent, freely given and uncoerced.

When the subject matter or type of risk makes it difficult to achieve disinterest through a single decision-maker, better decisions may be reached by involving people whose interests can balance each other. In many genetic screening programs, the risks are not physical but psychological and social. The disinterest of the screener and the informed consent of the screenee may not be adequate in the face of hazards such as loss of self-esteem, loss of insurability or employability, broken courtships and loss of marriageability, or profound and irreversible influences on children's development.[2,3] It may be very difficult to convey information about, or for the screenee to understand, something like a possible loss of self-esteem should he be found to carry a harmful recessive gene. Even with concrete physical risks, the present mode of obtaining consent is seen by many as ineffective in communicating useful information.[4-6] Requirements for speed and efficiency in mass genetic screening programs add another constraint to the ability of the screener to adequately inform subjects of possible risks. Thus, unpredictability of adverse consequences of screening programs argues for consumer participation on a continuing basis in program formulation, administration, and review.

DISPASSION

While the value of dispassion in decision-making cannot be disputed, the failure to cultivate it lies at the root of many ethical objections to past screening programs. For example, the physician who has had to carry family members through the emotional upheaval of caring for a baby with Tay-Sachs disease and watching it die may naturally feel an urgent desire to screen every person of childbearing age, so that another affected infant might never be born. Indeed, such passion is vital for the enormous expenditure of energy required to establish and operate a mass screening program. Yet it is equally likely to inhibit adequate consideration of possible hazards.

Passions may be more difficult to overcome than self-interest, but mechanisms that broaden participation in decisions will also serve here. Such emotions may be managed by exposure to the scrutiny of someone with a competing passion or someone skilled in detecting irrational or emotional reasoning, such as a psychiatrist or ethicist.

CONSISTENCY

The requirement that one search for consistent principles in screening programs will minimize the risk of programs being conducted without sufficient regard for ethical issues. The achievement of a consensus on principles may not be as important as the *process* of trying to find these principles. Such reflection on and formulation of ethical principles is not a skill acquired in the usual medical career. It is an area where the ethicist can be of assistance to physicians and others who are planning genetic screening—not to make decisions for them, or to tell what is right and what is wrong, but to assist in doing the difficult work of arriving at consistent principles and anticipating their application to future genetic, or other health-related, programs.

CONCLUSION

Many of the most troubling problems in genetic screening today are not scientific but ethical. The resolution of such issues, if left to health professionals alone, may be based on a narrow interest and may be in conflict with consumer interest. Consultation with ethicists may not always be practical, but emulation of the ideal ethical observer will maximize the rightness of any decision and minimize the probability that a decision will fail to incorporate ethically relevant data. The essential features of such a process are to pay scrupulous attention to the validity of assumptions and facts on which a screening program is based and to maximize the representation of all possible interests in all significant decisions.

REFERENCES

1. Firth, R. Ethical absolutism and the ideal observer theory. Philos. Phenomenol. 12:317–345, 1952.
2. Stamatoyannopoulos, G. Problems of screening and counseling in the hemoglobinopathies, pp. 14–15. In A. G. Motulsky and F. J. G. Ebling, eds. Fourth International Conference on Birth Defects. Vienna, Austria, Sept. 2–8, 1973. Abstracts of Papers. International Congress Series No. 297. Amsterdam: Excerpta Medica Foundation, 1973.

3. Walzer, S. Personal communication, 1973.
4. Epstein, L. C., and L. Lasagna. Obtaining informed consent: Form or substance. Arch. Intern. Med. 123:682–688, 1969.
5. Ingelfinger, F. J. Informed (but uneducated) consent. N. Engl. J. Med. 287: 465–466, 1972.
6. Fost, N. C. A surrogate system for informed consent. JAMA (In press).

12 An Economic Perspective on Evaluating Screening Programs

Screening programs are typically undertaken for humanitarian, not economic, reasons. The evaluation of such activities, however, involves a consideration of their economic attributes. The economic perspective provides a basis for evaluation that can serve to focus analysis on the means whereby the costs and benefits associated with the program can be evaluated.

The central analytic theme of economics is the basic problem of how to get the most out of the resources available to society, although what "getting the most" really means is subject to considerable discussion. More formally, the object is to optimize the benefits that can be derived from the use of resources, given the fact that such resources are not in infinite supply and that each use of resources implies that other resource-using activities cannot be undertaken. It is this relationship between costs and benefits that the economic perspective is designed to clarify. The purpose of economic analysis is to provide a structure for making specific the dimensions of that general objective.

THE ECONOMIC FRAMEWORK

The market system, particularly the perfectly competitive market structure, is only one device for evaluating the costs and benefits involved in exchange. It yields an optimal result when costs and benefits are considered relevant only when they relate to those individuals directly involved in the transaction. In fact, there are few transactions of this nature. The use of resources for the production and distribution of human services rarely produces benefits solely for the producer and the user. The essential economic and social nature of human services is that they do not fit into a simple market strategy that leaves producers and consumers to their own devices. It becomes all the more essential to be explicit about identifying the expected benefits and the true burden of costs.

Because human services are often public goods, there are additional difficulties associated with the identification of costs and benefits. While private goods as well as public goods may involve cost or benefit to those other than the individuals involved in the transaction (externalities), it is possible in many cases of private goods to ignore the externalities as not being central to the allocative decision; and we are often willing to do so. For public goods, the existence of externalities initiates the public involvement in the first place. Therefore, ignoring them is not feasible.[1-3]

Conceptually, relating costs to benefits as a vehicle for determining the appropriate allocation of resources is not a complicated idea. In actual practice, however, it is difficult. One major difficulty stems from the problem of measuring and valuing the benefits that accrue to different individuals, impact on different sectors of society, or take different forms. Without a convenient measurement device to make possible the quantifying of benefits, it is difficult to make comparisons. For many private goods and services, the market, by establishing a uniform price, provides a yardstick for the measurement of costs and benefits. Because of the externalities noted above, however, prices for public goods in general are less likely to provide an adequate measure of "true" costs and benefits.

Basically, the economic strategies for organizing and structuring the analysis of costs and benefits are of two types: *cost–benefit analysis* and *cost–effectiveness analysis*. Cost–benefit analysis involves establishing a relationship between the value of benefits generated and the costs that must be incurred to obtain these benefits. Cost–effectiveness analysis, on the other hand, evaluates alternative costs associated with the achievement of a given objective. It should be obvious that the latter is less complex since it does not require precise valuation of benefits.[4]

For evaluating screening programs, both these forms of analysis have their place. Often, health screening programs are argued for on the grounds that the benefits generated by these activities are large relative to the costs that need to be incurred. At the least, it is always argued that the benefits are greater than the costs. This is a cost–benefit argument. An example of a cost–effectiveness issue would be an evaluation of how the identified PKU child might most efficiently be served. This type of cost–effectiveness analysis might involve evaluating the use of alternative diets and treatment patterns in order to provide a *given* level of expected IQ score. Such analysis can ignore differences in the relative efficacy of one treatment modality as against another and ask only the general question, "Is there a less costly way to achieve a given result?"

While the distinction between the two types of analyses is clear enough, the difficulty with undertaking such analysis lies in the need to identify and evaluate explicitly the benefits and costs associated with each alternative being considered. Many of these costs and benefits are not immediately evident in the design and conception of the activity. The direct costs and benefits, those that fall upon the actual providers and the users of the service as part of the activity, are usually evident. However, the indirect costs and benefits, though not so visible, might be equally significant in evaluating the program.

For example, screening programs stimulate a certain amount of additional involvement with the medical care system that might produce benefits beyond those directly associated with the disease for which the screening is undertaken. Alternatively, generally widespread fear and uncertainty about relatively rare conditions might generate considerable external costs to some families.

Often it is not easy to determine whether specific indirect impacts are costs or benefits. For example, one of the benefits often attributed to renal dialysis in the home is that it enables the individuals receiving treatment to remain with their families in the home environment. However, there is evidence that sharing a home with the physical equipment required to provide the dialysis to the patient precludes for the family as a whole many dimensions of a normal existence, by providing a constant reminder of the illness around which family life is centered and organized. Experience indicates that, while for some families home dialysis yields benefits, for others the costs imposed will far outweigh those benefits. Many "human services" may generate these kinds of ambiguous costs or benefits, thereby placing an even greater burden on the analyst.

Another significant problem in specifying the costs and benefits associated with a given human service program is identifying the *external impact* of the service. Hinrichs and Taylor[5] have attempted to distinguish between external impacts among production activities when the production of one service imposes additional costs on the production of another and external impacts among consumers of services where a consumption by one individual of a service imposes additional costs on other consumers. An example of this latter would be increases in waiting time for other laboratory services as a result of an extensive screening program. In addition, they note externalities between production and consumption where production activities lead to increased costs to consumers, such as air, water, and noise pollution as a result of the production process.

They also note a fourth direction of external impact where activities by consumers impose additional costs on the production process.

Another major complexity added to the evaluation of costs and benefits is the fact that neither the costs nor the benefits are incurred at a single moment of time. The benefits from many human services programs accrue well after the incurrence of the major costs. The problem of adjusting the evaluation of costs and benefits for their position in time is one that has merited the attention of many economists.[6]

In each case it is essential to determine the present value of a future stream of benefits and often, because human service programs involve a commitment to provide services over time, the incurrence of a future stream of costs. The inherent complexities in a cost–benefit analysis are made more difficult by this time factor.

IDENTIFYING THE BENEFITS FROM SCREENING PROGRAMS

Identifying the benefits from any human service program is a matter of considerable difficulty. The proponents of such programs often start with a presumption that such activities are inherently "good" and therefore ought to be undertaken. Because the economic perspective imposes a consideration of opportunity cost in the decision to undertake a program, however, it is not sufficient that such activities be good; they should be better than alternative uses of the same resources. While such an analysis requires evaluation of costs as well as benefits, examination of aspects of *benefit identification* in the area of screening might be useful.

The identification of benefits is, in the first instance, highly sensitive to the efficacy of the service being provided. A useful analysis would require a certain degree of specificity in the objectives of the service. For programs in screening, it might require a certain reduction in morbidity or mortality from a given disease, or a reduction in the degree of disability associated with various types of illnesses. For other types of human services it might imply a reduction in the level of unemployment or in the incidence of various types of antisocial behavior. In any case, it is essential to identify specifically the anticipated benefits from the program involved.

In specifying the benefits from screening programs, some additional difficulties are encountered. While a considerable amount of effort in some programs (e.g., PKU screening of newborns) is devoted to case identification, the benefits in such programs are generated only by effective treatment. However, changes in benefits from changes in treatment may occur in two ways. On one hand, any general improvement in the effectiveness of treatment in reducing or eliminating the adverse impact of the disease being screened for is likely to increase benefits from the program. Alternatively, however, more effective prevention and improvement in techniques of identifying cases without screening (from symptoms, for instance) may reduce the benefits attributable to the screening program itself.

For programs that only identify potential for obtaining benefits, such as sickle cell testing, estimates of expected benefits are extremely tenuous. Valuing these benefits requires an additional step. Often the benefits from screening programs are valued in terms of the alternative costs foregone as a result of the program. In the case of screening for and treating infants with PKU, benefits in some programs were valued as the average yearly cost of services to the mentally retarded multiplied by the number of expected years of service that would not be needed as a result of the detection program. Such a valuation scheme can be deceptive.

For example, estimates of benefits for California's PKU screening program were based on the following analysis. It cost an average of approximately $5,000 per year to provide residential services for a mentally retarded child or adult. Approximately 1% of the in-patient mentally retarded population in the State of California may be attributed to phenylketonuria. On average, a mentally retarded individual who requires residential care will utilize 25 years of service. This yielded the following estimate of benefits: For each child identified as having PKU and treated in such a way as to eliminate or to preclude the mental retardation, $125,000 ($5,000 times 25 years) is saved. Therefore, the value of the benefit from such a program is put at $125,000 per child identified and treated. Similar estimates have been generated for New York and Mississippi.[7] This tendency to identify benefits as costs foregone or costs that are now being incurred (usually in other programs) that will not need to be incurred if the proposed program is successful in a standard strategy in arguing for the benefits of many service programs.[8]

There are a number of difficulties, however, in this way of viewing the benefits of the program. If only 1% of the in-patient population is the result of PKU, then the elimination of that source of mental retardation would result at best in a 1% drop in the in-patient population of the state institutions for the mentally retarded. Such a relatively small drop in the in-patient population would not necessarily lead to an equivalent drop in the cost of care.

On the one hand, the total cost of service per year in the State of California might be reduced by much less than $5,000 per year per child not admitted since the marginal cost of the foregone service is usually less than the average. On the other hand, PKU-caused mental retardation may generate higher patient needs for care than that from other causes and may, therefore, account for a greater proportion of resources devoted to care of mentally retarded than 1%. However, unless a significant proportion of cases within a single institution were PKU-caused, such effects are not likely to show up. A second difficulty reflects the fact that the incurrence of those benefits takes place over a 25-year time span and that their value at the present time is likely to be considerably less than their total. In any case, such estimates of benefits are likely to be misleading.

IDENTIFYING THE COSTS OF SCREENING PROGRAMS

Identifying the benefits from screening programs is difficult; identifying the costs associated with such programs also requires considerable caution. Typically, screening services occur within the context of other services and depend on the activities of these other services for some of the inputs to their clients. Often only those costs that are imposed directly on the program being evaluated are acknowledged as having relevance. For example, in estimating the cost of screening children for PKU, part of the costs involved represent the actual testing of the newborn infants. In some states the testing is done by state laboratory and the costs of operating that laboratory will be reflected in the state's evaluation of the costs of the service. In other states, the tests are required by law, but the actual laboratory work is done privately by the hospital or outside laboratories. These costs are incorporated into the cost of delivery to the parents. In the latter case, such costs do not show up as part of the state cost of service.

The benefits from PKU screening programs accrue only as a result of finding and treating an infant with PKU. The costs of screening all infants must, therefore, be matched against the benefits to the few, even though for most of those infants screened there will be no direct benefit. The potential cost–benefit relationship of such a program is highly dependent on the incidence of the disease that is being screened for. In the case of PKU, one case is likely to be found for every 15,000 or 16,000 infants screened. In one state that did not provide the laboratory services, the costs of the program were calculated at approximately $5,000 per case identified. Since the average laboratory charge for the screening test in that state was over $2, it is clear that the actual cost had to be closer to $40,000 than to $5,000.

Many of the evaluations of costs and benefits associated with human services programs fail to identify major components of costs, since the source of the evaluation often identifies only those direct costs that would typically show up in the program's budget. In Massachusetts, where the state laboratory does almost all the screening for inborn errors of metabolism, estimates are more readily established. Even in Massachusetts, however, the estimate of $200,000 per year ($2.50 per birth) does not include the costs of the physical facility and the capital equipment needed for testing 80,000 children annually.*

Even beyond the actual costs of the tests, the personnel and other costs associated with drawing blood samples from all newborns are not likely to be insignificant. Typically, such costs are omitted from analysis, but in a study for New York State such costs were estimated to be $1.33 per live birth, over 55.9% of the total costs of the PKU program.[8a]

The same study noted that over 93% of the costs of the program were associated with case finding, with only 6.7% being devoted to treatment. The estimates for treatment and on-going diagnostic evaluations were acknowledged to be low since they omit the cost of any medical, dietary and other social work consultations, the costs of additional hospitalization, or any treatment costs beyond age six. Nevertheless, even with lab costs of 87¢ per test, case finding alone was estimated at $2.40 per live birth, or over $36,000 to identify each PKU infant.

The examination of screening programs provides a useful illustration of some of the complexities of cost–benefit analysis. With the development of the technology of metabolic screening of newborns, it became possible to consider requiring that such screening take place. In the middle and late 1960's, there was a surge of state laws passed that required the screening of newborns for PKU.

In the first rush to pass legislation, little attention was given to any systematic cost–benefit analysis. The development of such screening programs was widely supported by groups interested in the mentally retarded. The major benefit argued in the political arena, as noted above, was avoidance of the burden to society of the costs of caring for the mentally retarded. Another major set of benefits, of course, accrue to the individuals, who, by means of early detection and treatment, avoid becoming mentally retarded.

The benefits to the individual who is *not* mentally retarded but who would have been in the absence of the program accrue continuously over his or her entire lifetime. These benefits are not limited to costs avoided but represent quantitative and qualitative additions to the value of existence. Not identifying the value of such future benefits understates the

* Estimates for Canadian screening programs are directed only at marginal costs (i.e., the additional costs placed on the existing system by the screening activity). It is estimated that in Quebec, costs of the Provincial Health Program are increased by approximately $267,000 ($3 per birth for 89,000 births).

actual benefits that are likely to accrue. There are equally complex problems in identifying the costs. If screening is to be effective, all newborns must be screened. This means that the costs of screening are imposed uniformly, either on society as a whole through a public program or on all parents of newborn infants, by requiring that such tests be performed. Although the costs are borne by all, the benefits are likely to accrue in large measure only to those who are identified as having the disease.

The actual cost of such a program relative to the benefits will depend to a large degree on the incidence. However, the cost is also affected by the sensitivity of the test. How often does the test have to be done? Are there further tests that are required when an infant is found to be positive by the screening test? In the case of PKU, further tests and individual counseling are also required as well as a general physical evaluation of the infant. These represent additional costs that must be calculated as part of the costs of the system.

The costs noted above relate only to the identification of children with PKU. The treatment requires an additional set of costs. Basically, the treatment is dietary. In many computations of the costs of treatment, only the costs of the dietary supplement are identified as being appropriate, the most typical estimate being $2 per day. In actual fact, the maintenance of a child on a strict and rather boring diet requires a significant amount of additional parental and parental substitute time. The additional costs of babysitters and child supervision may be significant, but they are rarely, if ever, considered as part of the costs of such a program. The long period of dietary control imposes certain burdens upon the household, which typically show up in a greater need for counseling services and a higher level of expenditures for physical and medical services for the child. These costs will show up as burdens on other service delivery systems if those services are not found directly within the medical treatment system. (Such costs are equally relevant to the treatment of end-stage kidney failure, where the dialysis regimen also imposes burdens on other service delivery systems if such treatments are not to have significant adverse side effects.)

Some of the difficulties in establishing accurate cost estimates reflect the wide diversity in sources of funds and locus of care in many state programs. It was earlier noted that in California the tests are done in many different labs and paid for by the parents. This makes cost estimates quite speculative. Other costs also often fall outside the formal program. Table 12-1 shows estimates presented to the committee for the State of Oregon screening program. The variety of sources of funds shown here is probably typical of many such programs. (See also Appendix C, Tables C-4 and C-6.)

TABLE 12-1 Cost of Oregon PKU Screening Program[a]

	Known Cost ($)		
	Per Sample	Annual	Approx. Cost ($)
Initial blood sampling in hospital charged to patients	0–2.00		
Follow-up blood sampling in MD's office charged to patients	0–2.00		
State Health Laboratory tests	1.07		
Testing for PKU alone	0.75		
State Health Screening Laboratory (50% from earmarked State Health Division Funds; 50% from special grant)		80,000	
Office of MCH director for provision of special diets		7,000	
Office of MCH director for collection of records, provision of community care by state nutritionist, etc. (100% from general MCH funds)			10,000
Private physicians for patient care			No est.
MD's laboratory for confirmation tests and some clinical follow-up (100% from National Foundation—March of Dimes)			7,500
University of Oregon Medical School for hospitalization (100% from State Hospital budget or insurance)			2,500
Crippled Children's Division for follow-up and developmental assessments, IQ, etc. (100% from general funds)			5,000
Proposed *additional* costs of improved service to provide a medical director, part-time social worker, and geneticist and adequate investigation of currently unfinished business and to provide proper follow-up of abnormal results			30,000

[a] Information provided by Dr. Neil Buist, University of Oregon Medical School.

The above observations can only provide the flavor of the considerations that are relevant to undertaking cost–benefit analysis of a PKU screening program. Nevertheless, they provide an opportunity to point out some additional issues of general consequence. Clearly, changes in the technology of screening can have significant impact on the cost–benefit analysis. If a screening device for PKU were developed that halved the costs of testing—since those costs are spread over 16,000 infants for each identified case—the cost per case might be significantly reduced.

The analysis is also highly sensitive to the efficacy of treatment. Every improvement in the treatment process increases the expected benefits, although such improvements in treatment may also imply the incurrence of additional costs. Each new option requires another round of analysis and evaluation. Often for human services, each technological change that shows any positive benefits at all is regarded as an appropriate addition. Perhaps on closer inspection, the cost of these changes may make them less desirable than they appear at first glance. This points out another item of particular significance in the evaluation of human service delivery programs. While screening is primarily a medical service, it is clear that the costs imposed and the benefits derived are highly dependent on the outputs of other services delivery systems—such as child care, family counseling, and residential services. Each of those service delivery systems is a setting wherein additional costs and benefits of a PKU screening program are found.

PKU SCREENING COMPARED WITH OTHER SCREENING PROGRAMS

It is useful to compare the PKU screening program with two other programs, each of which involves the same technology—that of screening—but yields a very different estimate of both costs and benefits. These programs are those for Tay-Sachs disease and sickle cell disease.

Tay-Sachs disease, as we have seen, is almost entirely restricted to the offspring of Jewish parents of Eastern European extraction. This means that the potential group to be screened is much more readily defined and that many individuals need not be screened at all, thereby reducing the potential cost of such a program. Perhaps more significantly, no treatment exists for Tay-Sachs disease. One child in four of a pair of parents who are carriers is likely to have the disease.

The purpose of screening is primarily to identify such infants before they are born and provide an opportunity for abortion early in the period of the pregnancy if the parents wish it. Here the benefits of the program do not accrue to the child. Rather, the benefits are seen as accruing to the parents and to other family members in the avoidance of the economic, social, and emotional costs associated with the birth, care, and inevitable early death of an affected child.

The purpose of such a screening program is to identify Tay-Sachs carriers, to provide an adequate level of genetic counseling for such families, to provide an opportunity for screening *in utero* and for subsequent abortion if that is what the family desires. Because most of the costs are imposed on the family itself, the decision as to whether or not to have the child is left to the family.

To the extent, however, that the medical, economic, and counseling needs of the family fall upon public programs, some of the costs will be external to the family decision-making unit. In this case, benefits will accrue to the state as a result of a family's decision to abort. The existence of public human service programs will often, as in this case, change the locus of impact and, perhaps, even the valuation of both costs and benefits.

The second program to be compared with the PKU programs is that for sickle cell trait. There has been in recent years a great increase in both mandatory and voluntary programs of screening for sickle cell trait. Who benefits from such programs? Clearly, the individual who has the trait is not necessarily made better off by being aware of it.

The main argument for such programs is that they provide the basis for genetic counseling. Such counseling makes it possible for those who possess the trait either to avoid marrying other carriers, thereby eliminating the likelihood of having children who might develop sickle cell anemia, or to enable those parents who know they both possess the trait either to avoid having children or to watch more closely for signs of the development of the illness. In many ways, this is a rather speculative set of anticipated benefits. Even more significantly, it imposes a tremendous burden upon those who submit to screening, thereby imposing various costs *without necessarily being able to ensure any significant generation of benefits.*

The issues involved in sickle cell screening programs are significantly more complex than those presented here, but this discussion is sufficient to show that such screening clearly involves a different set of impacts from those of the other types of screening programs. In each of the three cases the technology involved is similar, but the costs incurred and the expected benefits to be achieved are considerably different.

A last example from the general area of screening may serve to emphasize the point. Multiphasic health testing is a procedure where individuals are given a battery of medical tests in order to identify potential illness. The first experiments in multiphasic screening were carried out under public auspices through free-standing health testing centers often not in a setting that routinely provided medical services. The early experience with such programs indicated that the identification of illness was often not followed up by proper receipt of service. All the potential benefits from such a screening program depend on the receipt of treatment from other settings in the human service delivery spectrum. Failure to link those services to the screening process or, conversely, to develop screening processes within the service delivery setting, made achievement of the anticipated benefits impossible. More recently, we note a resurgence of interest in multiphasic health testing but, almost invariably, within the context of a setting that provides medical services. We can expect the benefits obtained from such testing services to be significantly greater than those of our earlier experience.

The above examples are all situations that call for the development of cost–benefit analysis. In each case the benefit from screening is dependent on triggering a whole host of responses in other service delivery settings in an effort to utilize and respond effectively to the knowledge generated in the screening process. Without such responses, the quest for benefits may prove futile. Often, however, choices might be most appropriately made by means of cost–*effectiveness* analysis. Very often, cost–effectiveness analysis can be undertaken in such a way as to avoid some of the complexities of evaluation of benefits. For example, a decision about the imposition of new technology will often respond to a cost–effectiveness analysis where specification of an identical set of benefits can be made. The costs of alternative means of achieving those benefits can then be evaluated in order to find the least-cost alternative. One example can be found in the comparison of alternative treatment modalities for end-stage kidney disease.[9]

Two technologies exist, renal dialysis and organ transplantation. In fact, these treatment modalities are not substitutes. A successful kidney transplant is a cure, often enabling a return to normal healthy patterns of behavior. A patient on successful dialysis must maintain a fairly restricted life style, remains ill, and is dependent on frequent medical interventions for continued existence. Qualitatively, a vast difference exists between the benefits to the individual generated by each of these lifesaving treatments for end-stage kidney disease. (Such differences are also significant in evaluating the need for long-term dietary controls for PKU children. The quality of existence for the growing child who avoids mental retardation through dietary control may be quite different from that of the child who obtains the same general benefit through prevention, genetic counseling, or yet-to-be-developed chemotherapy.) Nevertheless, a first approximation to comparing the alternative costs of each technology can be undertaken by estimating the costs for equivalent numbers of years of life saved, while ignoring the differing benefits associated with the quality of existence.

It is important to note one other difficulty in evaluating service programs such as screening. Many service delivery settings incorporate a number of different types of service. The developments of the multi-service center and the neighborhood health center—with medical care, mental health care, counseling, day care, and even job training and consumer services existing side by side—are examples of attempts to incorporate within a single setting a whole host of services each of which may generate its own peculiar set of benefits, which may differ considerably from center to center and from time to time.[10-13] Sorting out the costs and benefits of each individual service may be impossible. The same observation would apply to individual elements of multiple tests within a single screening activity.

CONCLUSION

While the above discussion has been only illustrative, it should demonstrate that, although the concept of relating benefits to costs is simple enough, its actual application involves problems of considerable complexity and difficulty. Nevertheless, the perspective is essential to a systematic evaluation of new opportunities for organizing, structuring, producing, and delivering all human services. The need for such activity reflects the basic economic assumption of scarcity of resources, an assumption well supported by the experience in the area of human services delivery. Given scarcity of resources, it is essential that services be provided in ways that are most likely to generate positive benefits both for the users who avail themselves of those services and for society as a whole.

Many devices for improving the effectiveness of such decision-making have been proposed—formal planning structures, consumer participation, and, often, resort to the marketplace. However, the nature of human services and the large variety of potential benefits and costs involved require a more disciplined awareness of the nature of cost–effectiveness and cost–benefit analysis. The actual analytical mechanics require stepping back from advocacy and mapping out, in a more systematic way, the specific interdependencies among human services in which each new service delivery strategy is dependent.

REFERENCES

1. Steiner, P. O. The public sector and the public interest. In R. H. Haveman and J. Margolis, eds. Public Expenditures and Policy Analysis. Chicago: Markham, 1970.
2. Arrow, K. J. The organization of economic activity: Issues pertinent to the choice of market versus nonmarket allocation, pp. 59–73. In R. H. Haveman,

and J. Margolis, eds. Public Expenditures and Policy Analysis. Chicago: Markham, 1970.

3. Piore, N. Rationalizing the mix of public and private expenditures in health. Milbank Mem. Fund Quart. 46(Suppl.):167–170, 1968.
4. Rothenberg, J. Cost–benefit analysis: A methodological exposition. Prepared for Evaluation of Social Action Programs Conference, American Academy of Arts and Sciences, 1969.
5. Hinrichs, H. H., and G. M. Taylor. Systematic Analysis. Pacific Palisades, Calif.: Goodyear, 1972.
6. Baumol, W. J. On the discount rate for public projects, pp. 273–290. In R. H. Haveman and J. Margolis, eds. Public Expenditures and Policy Analysis. Chicago: Markham, 1970.
7. Steiner, K. C., and H. A. Smith. Application of cost–benefit analysis to a PKU screening program. Inquiry 10(4):34–40, 1973.
8. U.S. Department of Health, Education, and Welfare. Office of the Assistant Secretary for Planning and Evaluation. Delivery of Health Services for the Poor: Program Analysis, Human Investment Programs. Washington, D.C.: U.S. Department of Health, Education, and Welfare, 1967.

8a. Bush, J. W., M. M. Chen, and D. Patrick. Cost effectiveness using a health status index: Analysis of the New York State PKU screening program, pp. 172–208. In R. Berg, ed. Health Status Indexes. Chicago: Hospital Research and Educational Trust, 1973.

9. Klarman, H. E., J. O'S. Francis, and G. D. Rosenthal. Cost effectiveness analysis applied to chronic renal disease. Med. Care 6:48–54, 1968.
10. March, M. The neighborhood center concept. Publ. Welfare 26:97–111, 1968.
11. Foster, J. T. Neighborhood health centers: A new way to extend care. Mod. Hosp. 110:95, 1968.
12. Elinson, J., and C. E. Herr. A sociomedical view of neighborhood health centers. Med. Care 8:97–103, 1970.
13. Feingold, E. A political scientist's view of the neighborhood health center as a new social institution. Med. Care 8:108–115, 1970.

13 Future Research Needs

Earlier sections of the report have recounted the conditions under which genetic screening is now being practiced, pointing out both positive accomplishments and unresolved questions. It remains now to consider what investigations the unresolved questions call for. This unfinished business is grouped into the following areas: the adaptation of genetic screening to modern health care; technology and method; applications to genetic screening of epidemiologic studies and research in population genetics; education, public and professional; and sociologic studies of the impact of screening.

GENETIC SCREENING AND HEALTH CARE

The principal models for genetic screening reviewed by the Committee have been programs for PKU, sickle cell disease, Tay-Sachs disease, and antenatal diagnosis for Down's syndrome. Each of these has been engendered by pressures related strongly to the disorder in question, with only incidental attention paid to its relationship to developments in medical and health care. For the future, however, if prevention of disease and promotion of good health are to assume prominence in the health field, the constrained and narrow base provided by these models must give way to a generalized approach capable of accommodation to qualities and quantities of screening not now envisioned and compatible with the rapid evolution of health care that we are now experiencing. To this end, genetic screening programs should be regarded as experiments testing the hypothesis that they are one among many measures intended to preserve and enhance good health. In this way, the timeliness of screening, its priority, and its benefits and costs, can be assessed in the context of other forms of screening and other preventive measures.

Appropriate Settings

The several models have placed screening in many diverse settings. These settings may have been urged on the various programs by the exigencies of the particular projects together with the necessity to accommodate to popular and professional ignorance, rather than by rational choice. Now, however, the proposition that genetic screening can be done in such conventional health situations as clinics and health maintenance organizations should be tested, and the conditions under which such settings could be made to work best should be examined. If practical, such locations would be economical of space, personnel, and supplies, and would have the advantage of taking genetic screening out of schools and churches and placing it in a more appropriate milieu.

Studies of Operational Details

The Committee's investigations revealed much diversity of detail in the ways in which transactions between screening authorities and screenees were organized—in the prescreening education, the transmission of the results of tests, the delivery of counseling, and the treatment and follow-up. The effectiveness of all of these was dependent upon collaboration between several groups, each of which might itself consist of several persons. The responsibility for specific screenees was therefore, widely dispersed, in antithesis to the personal and individual quality of the conventional doctor–patient relationship; although this dispersed responsibility has not yet been studied in any systematic way, anecdotal evidence suggests that it has many weaknesses.

Studies are needed of the effectiveness of prescreening education, of who submits to the tests and why, and of who rejects them and why; of the efficiency of transmission of information about results; of the quality and context of the counseling and the attributes of the counselors; and of the steps by which a person found to have a positive test result is brought to definitive management. A context and methods for such studies exist in the literature of health behavior and medical sociology—disciplines that have been little employed so far in the elaboration and appraisal of genetic screening processes. In testing the effectiveness of currently employed methods, the investigations must explore the adequacy of medical bureaucracy to fulfill the needs it is being asked to meet and determine whether screening is best done outside or within the conventional channels of patient care.

TECHNOLOGY AND METHOD

Conditions for screening are most favorable when a test is easy to do, reliable, inexpensive, and capable of automation. Progress is being made in the development of new tests and the refinement of old, but in general, such technology has received neither the attention nor the financial support it must have if genetic screening is to thrive. Granting agencies might take note and promote some interest in this field.

Some issues for study are (a) the further extension of the multiplication of tests to be carried out on single specimens; (b) the uses of test materials that can be obtained by noninvasive means, such as saliva, sweat, tears, and other secretions and material from hair and hair follicles, fingernails, and so on; (c) the elaboration of new tests for new inborn errors that employ the techniques of organic chemistry to detect important metabolites that could accumulate as a result of blocks at any one of several enzymatically controlled steps in the metabolic pathway; and (d) the further refinement of miniaturized techniques for assaying metabolic processes in single cells.

There is substantial agreement on the usefulness of regional laboratories, and the reasons for developing such laboratories will become more compelling as the number of tests grows. Experiments in regionalization may be constrained by the awkward necessity of interstate financing, but since in the future such services may be supported by new federal agencies financing, for example, national health insurance, such schemes may flourish.

There is a timeliness about the amplification of screening techniques that is exemplified in Thomas' thoughts about the need for "high-level technology," in which simple, inexpensive, and easily delivered preventive measures eliminate the subsequent need for the costly, complicated, and usually only partially effective measures required to treat overt disease.[1]

APPLICATIONS TO GENETIC SCREENING OF EPIDEMIOLOGIC STUDIES AND RESEARCH IN POPULATION GENETICS

Epidemiologic Studies

The history of screening for PKU reveals that the discovery of cases of hyperphenylalaninemia that were not PKU was unexpected, and that before investigators became aware of this genetic and phenotypic heterogeneity some persons received treatment suitable for PKU but not for them. It is common experience that once an apparently workable treatment for a newly described disease becomes available, it is at first difficult, and later comes to be regarded as unethical, to do a controlled study of its effectiveness. And it is in the nature of medical practice that a treatment may be devised before the natural history of the disorder is well understood. Accordingly, when a disease, even a seriously damaging one, is first described, it is entirely reasonable to screen a population for other cases for purely epidemiologic reasons, even when there is no specific treatment at all. It is only in this way that information can be gathered that can lead to accurate decisions about who will be benefited by a treatment when it is proposed and from whom the treatment should be withheld as inappropriate.

Research in Population Genetics

A good deal of screening is done for nonmedical reasons; data are collected for purposes of studying the genetic composition of human populations and the forces that mold it, as well as to learn the extent and quality of genetic variability. To these ends, samples of cells and blood or other body fluids are collected from hundreds of thousands of people, and genetic variants are characterized and gene frequencies calculated. At a minimum, about 30% of human gene loci have been found to be polymorphic, while the remainder are either invariant or occupied by an occasional allele with a frequency of .001 or less.[2,3] In other studies chromosome variations are the object of search; while most of these are rare, new staining techniques have revealed minor structural variations with frequencies in the polymorphism range, and by combining the techniques for detecting the biochemical polymorphisms with cytologic methods, rapid progress is being made in the geographic location of the gene loci in the chromosomes.[4]

Although all this work may appear to be unrelated, or at best only tangential, to the overtly medical missions of screening, such investigations can provide the markers, or genetic characteristics, for which medically related screening may be carried out. For example, the α_1-antitrypsin *Z* allele was discovered in the course of a population screening and its relationship to obstructive emphysema was only incidentally noted by an alert investigator. There are other genes existing in populations in frequencies of .01 or more that are known to be strongly and directly associated with disease, and there must be many more still undiscovered. If the polymorphic genes represent the major reservoir of human genetic variability, and if disease is represented as homeostatic insufficiency, then the principal genetic contributions to common human diseases must reside among the polymorphic loci.

Thus the extension of the list of these common genes, together with the discovery of their relationships to disease, if any, fulfills at once the research aims of both the geneticist and the clinician. The discovery a few years ago of associations, albeit weak and inconclusive, of ABO blood group types with gastric cancer and duodenal ulcer, and the more recent disclosure of rather stronger but still indirect association of *HL-A* alleles with autoimmune diseases are cases in point.[5] Another more easily interpreted example is the mutant aryl hydrocarbon hydroxylase allele that has been found to occur in a population in the United States with a frequency of .28 and that in homozygotes may be associated with susceptibility to bronchogenic carcinoma.[6] The importance of this kind of research, with its aim of detailing the extent and quality of human hereditary variation and its implications for the elucidation of the causes and variability of common diseases, cannot be overemphasized.

EDUCATION: PUBLIC AND PROFESSIONAL

The success of preventive or other medical programs is measured by the effectiveness of the collaboration between the agency that offers the health care and the people who receive it. Evidence has been presented elsewhere in the report that this collaboration is often impaired by a lack of knowledge of genetics on both sides and by uncertainties with regard to the techniques of persuasion and public education on the part of screening agencies. Some procedural guidance has been offered for the latter (see Part VII, Section 7), but there is need for research in the refinement of the methods and in their evaluation. As for education in genetics, there is a need to enhance public knowledge and to improve the teaching in medical schools of those aspects of genetics most germane to preventive medicine.[7]

Public Education

In Chapter 9 (p. 165) the health belief model was presented to explain current health behavior of the public and to provide the basis for recommending programs designed to increase public participation in screening programs. A logical conclusion to be drawn from that material was that people need to appreciate that their children may be vulnerable to genetic disease or abnormality transmitted by healthy parents. They need to learn that such abnormalities may have serious consequences for the children unless they are properly managed, to believe that the early identification of disease or possible disease often permits effective remedial action to be taken, and to learn that the benefits that accrue from such early detection and intervention outweigh the economic and psychological costs that may be incurred.

In considering the question of how motives and beliefs can be modified, it is useful to distinguish between educational activities directed toward children and those directed toward adults.

Children For the first several years of life, the child has no differentiated cognitive structure concerning the importance of health, his vulnerability to disease, the severity of disease, the benefits of professional intervention, and the costs of such intervention. Since the learning of new beliefs is generally more successful when it does not conflict with already established beliefs, educational activities introduced during this early phase should be more effective than if undertaken later in life. Obviously, by a certain age the child will have acquired relatively enduring opinions on various health matters; Gochman[8] has shown that this may occur by age eight or so. This would mean that primary educational intervention should be initiated sometime before children reach the third year of formal education, and should continue indefinitely. There would seem to be no reason why children could not be introduced very early to basic information about human biology, including genetics and touching on how various diseases are transmitted, how they may be prevented or managed, and the like. The Committee knows of no systematic efforts to design and to study the effectiveness of such educational approaches, but they should be tried.

One argument typically raised against health education in young children is that it naively fails to realize that the child's basic views and orientations toward life are acquired during the socialization process within the family. This, of course, is true, but it is also true that not all the socializing influences in life originate with the family; many come from peer groups, teachers, and the mass media. When these other socializing influences are not consistent with the teachings in the home, they will probably not gain as strong a foothold in the child's cognitive development as when the two sources of influences are mutually reinforcing. Nevertheless, even in such cases of inconsistent education, the child may acquire some beginning knowledge and orientation that will make him more susceptible to subsequent influences later in life, and the subsequent education of his children, in turn, may be rendered that much easier. An effective educational program of the kind described must be regarded as multigenerational; quick solutions are unlikely.

In many cases there will be no deep conflict between such education as is proposed and parental points of view. Many parents will willingly join in a partnership with the educator if they view the outcome as having potential benefits for their children. Even parents whose own dietary practices, exercise patterns, and smoking habits are life-threatening may be eager to join with the educational system in developing different patterns in their children. To be sure, children will always identify with their parents in the course of their development, but there is no reason to believe that they will invariably identify with and adopt the patterns of behavior that constitute threats to health, especially if parent and teacher are joined in an effort to produce different patterns.

Adults An examination of efforts aimed at modifying important motives and beliefs of adults reveals a disappointingly low rate of success. People who are responsible for planning health education programs for adults nevertheless need answers to specific questions: What should we tell people about disease X? Should we frighten them or reassure them, or both? What kind of person will they believe? Where can we reach them?

Decisions about how to answer these questions are usually made on the basis of personal reactions and inferences derived from studies that may bear on the problem at hand. Unfortunately, many of these studies have been done in unrealistic settings (such as classrooms) with atypical groups (such as college students) and using content unrelated to health. Some studies have been done using health content in real-world settings, but scientists are understandably hesitant about extending the findings to topics on audiences other than those actually studied. Thus, the findings so far must be regarded as suggestive rather than definitive; and the questions must now be asked and answered specifically in the context of genetic screening.

Medical Education

The recent attention to genetics in medical teaching is reflected in the survey of doctors' attitudes (see Chapter 9, p. 161); younger physicians are more likely to recognize its pertinence and application than those who graduated more than 10 years ago. But there is evidence that despite this recent emphasis, the congruence of genetics with preventive medicine and primary medical care has not been fully appreciated; the survey of physicians undertaken by the Committee abounds in such evidence. In addition, texts and journals of epidemiology, public health, and preventive medicine give little space to genetic subjects and papers, and those medical schools that emphasize teaching and training in family practice and primary care tend to offer very little genetics in the curriculum.[9]

The genetic knowledge most germane to public health and preventive medicine is population genetics, with its emphasis on the distribution of genes in families and populations and the study of the impact of such factors as mating systems, natural selection, and random drift on the frequencies of genes and chromosomes in ethnic groups and subpopulations. The affinity between population genetics and primary health care has been little stressed, but investigators and workers in both fields should find much of common interest. Perhaps this latent compatibility might be most rapidly and favorably developed in medical school teaching, where representatives of both fields could instruct the students in the application of population genetics theory to medical practice.

THE SOCIAL IMPACT OF SCREENING

Side Effects

The Committee's investigations reveal that screening shares at least one important characteristic with other innovations of modern technology: While conferring undoubted benefits on the many, there are collateral consequences for a few which are at least a nuisance and at worst leave the intended beneficiary worse off than if he had never had the service. These consequences are those transgressions of civil rights and psychological hazards that have been detailed in other parts of the report. They are due to the narrow focus of the screening administrator on the structural and organizational detail of the project and the consequent neglect of the human qualities of the objects of the screening; to delays and imperfections in the fulfillment of the sequential elements of the screening process; and to the ignorance and misunderstanding of the people who offer themselves for testing.

While we know these problems exist, we do not know their extent, nor do we yet have any consensus on how to deal with them. Clearly they should be studied and empirical data should be gathered; and because they are a product of the interaction of the health establishment and the public, of medicine and society, the methods of sociology should be used.[10]

Sociology has so far been insufficiently involved in public health planning and evaluation. The participation of sociology and other social science disciplines in such evaluation is important because their role is to examine the functions of human institutions independently of any value judgments. They can be expected, therefore, to emphasize aspects of those functions that are overlooked by the policymaker—in this instance, the screening agent.[11,12] And in addition to their research tools, social science investigators can bring to screening policy decision-making those attributes of disinterest, uninvolvement, and community representation that, as has been suggested elsewhere in this report, are important requirements for ethical decision-making.

The Social Uses of Genetic Knowledge

The discussion of the social questions raised by genetic screening projects is simply a specific case of a more general debate on the uses of genetic knowledge in the interests of individuals and society. (For an outline of the content of this debate, the reader is referred to the informed and comprehensive review by Motulsky.[13])

The central questions being discussed are, first, the desirability of the innovations suggested and whether medicine and society are ready for them, and, second, whether genetic knowledge should ever be used in ways that subvert the interests of individuals in order to achieve some gain for the whole society; since the answers are many and diverse, it cannot be said that there is yet any consensus (for a representative list of papers and books on the subject, see reference 9).

Perhaps genetic screening is an appropriate context in which to develop that agreement. All of the questions of definition and protection of civil rights, of ethical decisions, and of the balance between the interests of individuals and those of society are exposed by genetic screening, and should it become a widespread and routine practice, it will touch literally everyone. Thus the issues will be forced upon all the interested parties—scientists, physicians, lawyers, ethicists, clergy, politicians, and the public—and assuming that appropriate data are gathered and evaluation is continuous, truly representative decisions should be the result.

REFERENCES

1. Thomas, L. Commentary: The future impact of science and technology on medicine. BioScience 24:99–105, 1974.
2. Harris, H., and D. A. Hopkinson. Average heterozygosity per locus in man: An estimate based on the incidence of enzyme polymorphisms. Ann. Hum. Genet. 36:9–20, 1972.
3. Harris, H., D. A. Hopkinson, and E. B. Robson. The incidence of rare alleles determining electrophoretic variants: Data on 43 enzyme loci in man. Ann. Hum. Genet. 37:237–253, 1974.
4. Ruddle, F. H., and R. S. Kucherlapati. Hybrid cells and human genes. Sci. Amer. 231:36–50, 1974.
5. McDevitt, H. O., and W. F. Bodmer. HL-A, immune-response genes, and disease. Lancet 1:1269–1275, 1974.

6. Kellermann, G., M. Luyten-Kellermann, and C. R. Shaw. Genetic variation of aryl hydrocarbon hydroxylase in human lymphocytes. Amer. J. Hum. Genet. 25:327–331, 1973.
7. Childs, B. A place for genetics in health education, and vice versa. Amer. J. Hum. Genet. 26:120–135, 1974.
8. Gochman, D. S. Children's perceptions of vulnerability to illness and accidents. Publ. Health Rep. 85:69–73, 1970.
9. Childs, B. Garrod, Galton, and clinical medicine. Yale J. Biol. Med. 46: 297–313, 1973.
10. Mechanic, D. Sociology and public health: Perspectives for application. Amer. J. Publ. Health 62:147–151, 1972.
11. Rogers, E. S. Public health asks of sociology. . . . Can the health sciences resolve society's problems in the absence of a science of human values and goals? Science 159:506–508, 1968.
12. Mechanic, D. Politics, social science, and health policy in the United States, pp. 45–57. In Politics, Medicine and Social Science, New York: Wiley, 1974.
13. Motulsky, A. G. Brave new world? Science 185:653–663, 1974.

VII

PROCEDURAL GUIDANCE FOR GENETIC SCREENING PROGRAMS

This section of the report consists of the Committee's suggestions for practical and procedural guidance for those involved in decisions concerning whether and, if so, how to set up screening programs. It is based on lessons learned from the Committee's survey of current practices.

It is self-contained and can be usefully read by itself. It is, therefore, designed to repeat, in concise and summary form, various points made in the earlier parts of the report.

(1) The Aims of Genetic Screening

Genetic screening is carried out to find persons with particular genotypes in order to fulfill such traditional medical objectives as the provision of care for people who are sick and the prevention of disease.

SCREENING FOR MANAGEMENT

A search may be undertaken to find persons (a) with genetic diseases that are potentially fatal or that can cause distortion of development or (b) with genetic predispositions that, under appropriate conditions, may lead to acute illness or, in time, to chronic illness. The disorders screened in fulfillment of this aim should be known to be susceptible to some ameliorative treatment—such as dietary adjustment, the removal of an offensive environmental agent, or avoidance of a certain drug or other provocative substance—or to the provision of supportive care. If supportive management is the best that can be done, then there should be evidence that it is in fact helpful and that it does not engender anxieties or create conditions that themselves hinder development or impair the enjoyment of life.

SCREENING TO PROVIDE REPRODUCTIVE INFORMATION

This kind of screening is designed to discover persons who have a significant probability of producing genetically damaged children. Such persons are most frequently the heterozygous carriers of genes that in homozygotes are associated with serious genetic disease, and they may wish to know their reproductive risks as well as to discuss such alternatives as artificial insemination or adoption. Although the persons counseled in this way are most commonly couples contemplating reproduction, such risks are no less calculable for persons considering marriage or for single persons who are simply seeking information.

Screening is also carried out to find couples who are both carriers of genes associated with diseases susceptible to antenatal diagnosis by amniocentesis. Selected populations may also be screened by amniocentesis for particular abnormalities, for example, older pregnant women, whose risk of carrying a fetus with Down's syndrome is known to be high.

SCREENING FOR ENUMERATION

Screening of this kind is commonly carried out for public health purposes. That is, it may be desirable to know the number of babies born with congenital anomalies in some particular locality over some period of time. This has the virtue of providing incidence and prevalence figures for the community, and in addition, if monitoring is continuous and shows significant changes in incidence in time and place, efforts can be made to discover the causes of such changes. For example, seasonal changes in the incidence of malformations may be associated with infections, while a sudden increase in frequency of a particular anomaly may be the result of the adverse effects of some drug. This kind of screening may also ensure that the identity of affected persons is brought to the attention of health authorities, who may then see that counseling and other services of the appropriate community agencies and programs are made available.

None of these aims of genetic screening are mutually exclusive. For example, it may be of advantage to public health authorities to know the incidence of treatable genetic diseases or of the carrier state for particular disorders that are untreatable and for which screening is carried out to detect carriers for the purpose of offering reproductive information. In addition, conditions will unquestionably move from one category to the other as specific or supportive treatments are elaborated for disorders whose pathogenesis becomes clear as the result of investigations, or as specific treatments are substituted for reproductive information, or reproductive information is substituted for enumeration, and so on.

SCREENING FOR RESEARCH

Screening for research purposes is of two kinds. In one, data are collected to test hypotheses related to human physiology and evolution but not necessarily to health or disease. Such surveys are characteristically done in studies of population genetics in which the investigator wishes to make decisions with regard to selection or drift to account for gene frequencies, or simply to characterize the extent of polymorphism or genetic heterogeneity in man. Such studies may consist of observation and quantitation of physical variations, of biochemical markers, or of chromosomal differences.

The second category of research purposes consists of investigations into feasibility of screening for service. In one kind of research, new methods or new screening procedures may be tried out, or a new genetic marker may be tested in a population to find its frequency and to determine whether it would be useful to consider it as an object for screening.

Another important investigative aim is the description of the natural history of a newly described disorder, for example, an inborn error of metabolism. The elucidation of the pathogenesis of such a disorder often suggests a treatment that makes up for or circumvents the deficiency that is its hallmark; and investigators are often driven by the logic of their reasoning to try such a treatment in a series of cases, neglecting the possibility that the range of variability may embrace both illness and normality. Then, after successes in treating patients who are undeniably sick, others who might never be sick may be brought into treatment after discovery by screening for a biochemical marker unrelated to clinical signs, with the entirely laudable end in mind of treating before irreversible damage can be done.

For such conditions several research aims should be carried out. If no treatment is obvious, data should be collected to discover the full range of abnormality so that by the time a specific treatment becomes available it may be possible to segregate that fraction of patients who will never be harmed by the disease and who should, therefore, be spared a tedious and expensive treatment that may entail some degree of hazard, no matter how slight. If, on the other hand, a sensible treatment is immediately suggested, it should be tried out with appropriate safeguards, and if new cases are discovered by biochemical markers, the strong probability of genetic and clinical heterogeneity should be considered before everyone is subjected to treatments that may be inappropriate for many.

UNACCEPTABLE AIMS FOR SCREENING

Although some of the above objectives might be regarded as unconventional by some physicians, all are clearly related to health or to the study of human differences. That is as it should be, since there are no legitimate nonscientific aims of genetic screening. Screening should be offered to people as a service to them, and no pressures should be applied to persuade them to cooperate out of a sense of public duty. Further, political and eugenic ends must be excluded; and it should be recognized that genetic screening does not aim for the perfectibility of man. It is merely one among many other uses of medical knowledge to improve the adaptive state of genetically threatened persons and to prevent needless suffering and human and economic waste. Rigorous safeguards are required to prevent its perversion to selective discrimination for any other than generally accepted medical or scientific reasons or for such illusory goals as the betterment of mankind.

(2) Genetic Screening in the Context of Existing Screening and Medical Practices

GENETIC AND NONGENETIC SCREENING

Screening for genetic variations is relatively new, and since practices already established for nongenetic screening may not be always appropriate, a comparison of the aims of these two kinds of procedure may help to clarify future plans and thinking.

First, in screening of all kinds, the discovery of one affected person often leads to a search for other affected persons, whether related or in contact by proximity. But for genetic diseases, in contrast to infections, the pattern of dissemination is more precisely definable by kinship, and the population at risk is more readily identified. For example, the discovery of a disease or carrier state in one person may lead to a search for other affected persons among members of a widely dispersed family.

Second, whereas in both genetic and nongenetic screening, a search is made for persons with early disease or showing certain risk factors, the former also seeks persons who will themselves never be threatened but who carry genes that under appropriate conditions may lead to illness in descendants.

Third, screening for nongenetic disorders is usually limited to those that are frequent. Genetic conditions that are the objects of screening are often rare.

Fourth, although new tests are occasionally added to the screening battery for nongenetic conditions, the number of tests capable of detecting genetic conditions is rising exponentially and is ultimately constrained only by the number of mutations whose adverse effects can be detected and whose detection could be of benefit to their possessors.

Fifth, the person to be protected by nongenetic screening is, generally speaking, the person tested. In contrast, a search for the possessors of genetic conditions is often carried out in order to offer information about reproductive options or to provide antenatal diagnosis by amniocentesis so that the birth of a seriously diseased fetus may be prevented. As a result, although it is not a general aim of genetic screening to influence the future incidence of disease, if many persons exercise their option to reject reproduction or to abort affected fetuses, the incidence will be reduced. Nongenetic screening cannot have this effect, since its only object is to find and treat persons with diseases, not to alter the environment in such a way as to change the future incidence.

Finally, nongenetic screening is usually intended to discover people with diseases due to influences outside themselves and for which they may feel no responsibility. But genetic screening discovers something within a person's own makeup that may threaten his self-esteem or cause him to feel guilty of transmitting some "blight" to his children. This raises special social, ethical, and legal questions having to do with consent, privacy, confidentiality, and labeling.

GENETIC SCREENING AND ORDINARY MEDICAL CARE OR OFFICE PRACTICE

While the aims of genetic screening are mainly medical, certain aspects of these objectives are at variance with those of standard medical care and office practice. If genetic screening should become an important aspect of medical care, and especially if it should be carried out mainly under the direction of practicing physicians, standard views and procedures will have to be changed in certain ways. Some examples follow.

The discovery of a person with a genetic disease or carrier state raises the question of whether someone has the responsibility to discover and to inform relatives outside that person's immediate family of their risks. Apart from reporting contagious diseases, physicians are not usually very aggressive in the pursuit of the health care of persons outside their own practices and may find uncongenial the prospect of helping to track down persons unknown to them. In addition, doing so raises legal and ethical problems. The discovery of a genetic variation is information belonging to the possessor of the gene or genes in question, and it cannot legally be transmitted to anyone else without the permission of its owner. Thus a physician can be put in the position of being legally prevented from telling relatives of their risk if the original patient is unwilling to release the information. This may seem unlikely, but it could result in tragic outcomes.

When a patient with a specific complaint consults a physician, the latter is obliged to do what he can to discover the cause of the complaint and to give appropriate advice. If, after doing his best, however, assuming his best is up to a generally accepted standard, he has little of benefit to offer, he cannot be censured for failing to please the patient. On the other hand, the initiator of a screening program does have an obligation to do something beneficial for the screenee, when the latter has submitted to a procedure based on promises of benefit offered by the former. The necessity to observe this ethical requirement is underlined by the public promotion given to screening programs in which potential screenees are often exposed to pressures to be tested. These may take the form of educational programs promoted by nonmedical groups, including churches, and presented in newspapers and by radio and television.

While most people have some comprehension of the need for immunizations, tuberculin tests, Papanicolaou smears, and other prophylactic measures, the object of a genetic screening program usually has no idea of his need for the tests and must be educated. Although physicians should increase their current efforts to educate their patients in matters of human biology, genetics, or even health and disease, new means of changing consumer performance and expectations are badly needed.

Physicians, in daily practice, gain insight into the behavior of persons who are ill and develop skill in interpreting and managing patients, but they have little experience with the psychology of the approach of healthy persons to preventive health measures. This may explain the high degree of noncompliance with preventive (and often also therapeutic) instructions reported in the literature. Physicians should be educated to deal with the vagaries of preventive health behavior.

(3) Screening Methodology

CRITERIA FOR SCREENING TESTS

Criteria for screening tests have been treated at length elsewhere.[1,2] In brief, the test should be reliable, repeatable, and accurate. Its sensitivity and specificity should be defined. It should be capable of automation for purposes of efficiency and economy. The testing procedure should be subject to a minimum of clerical error, and processing and delivery of the sample in the field should not compromise the validity of the test through significant alteration in the biological properties of the sample. It is understood that mass screening is not to be implemented for medical intervention or reproductive counseling (or even for enumeration) in the absence of pilot studies or facilities for follow-up.

ACCURACY AND VALIDITY OF TEST

These characteristics are determined by what the test measures. A specific method that clearly identifies a metabolite, or characterizes a protein, is important as a back-up technique for confirmation of a positive test by a method that may be less definitive but more suitable for large-scale screening methods. It is generally understood that the confirmatory test is applied to a second sample to avoid error from an artifact in the first sample or a clerical error of identification.

PROBABILITY OF CORRECT ASCERTAINMENT

This is an important problem in the use of screening tests for genetic variation. When the test screens for variation in the gene product, it may be possible to recognize the variant state (positive test) with complete confidence. For example, a mutation that produces electrochemical change in protein structure may permit screening for the protein variant by electrophoresis. If the position in the electrical field occupied by the variant molecule is unique, the appearance of material at that position during performance of the screening test is a clear "signal," without "noise" in the system. On the other hand, if the test measures catalytic activity of the mutant gene product, then reception of the signal may be impaired because of normal variation in activity of the species. The latter may further reflect polymorphism at the relevant gene locus (loci) or multifactorial phenomena that escape clear definition and strict control. This normal variation contributes "noise"; the good test simply maintains the highest possible "signal:noise ratio" under the circumstances.

A statistical definition of the signal may be simple but nonetheless unsatisfactory for purposes of efficient screening. For example, a positive test or abnormal value may be defined as one that exceeds two standard deviations from the mean, assuming a Gaussian distribution in the system. If the index trait has a frequency of 10^{-4}, and the population under surveillance is 10^5, the signal:noise ratio is 1:225 at either tail of the distribution curve. When the frequency of the trait is 10^{-5}, the ratio becomes 1:2,250. By raising the cut-off point to three standard deviations, the signal:noise ratios at the two frequencies are reduced to 1:16 and 1:160, respectively.

Noise is contributed by subjects with normal variation but without the index trait who have been detected by the test. Further testing is then required to identify the person with the target mutation(s) among the normal variants.

CHOICE OF TEST

The choice of test is often a compromise between the signal:noise ratio and the cost:efficiency ratio. The terms *specificity* and *sensitivity* define the compromise according to the following matrix:

STATUS	TEST: Negative	TEST: Positive
Healthy	*a*	*b*
Trait or Disease	*c*	*d*

Specificity describes the fraction of healthy subjects with a negative test (a) when the test is applied to the total population of healthy persons ($a + b$). *Sensitivity* is the fraction of at-risk persons recognized by a positive test (d) among those who actually have the trait ($c + d$).

Healthy subjects who yield a false-positive test (b) and subjects with the trait who yield a false-negative test (c) contribute to the "cost" of the screening program; the total cost in testing errors is defined as $(b + c)/(a + b + c + d)$. Power functions can be developed to select the best test and the cutoff point that permit the lowest cost.

The foregoing recognizes that variant genotypes can sometimes be identified only with a probability that should be specified. Simultaneous use of two different tests can enhance discrimination of the mutant trait and reduce the chance of misclassification.[3] The method involves the application of Bayes' theorem to density functions, and it clearly reduces the undesirable consequences of misclassification of subjects. For example, the relative counseling errors have been compared when the density function method and a linear method of discrimination are used to detect heterozygotes for the Tay-Sachs allele; classification errors involving normal subjects and heterozygotes are both reduced with the former method.

CONSISTENCY

Uniformity of standards is a critical factor in the testing system. Two World Health Organization documents[1,2] advocate centralization of laboratory responsibility and regionalization of the testing activity. The Committee concurs with this advice. Efficiency of sample collection and follow-up of positive tests is enhanced by regionalization; reliability and standardization of the test are sustained by centralization. Moreover, flexibility in the testing system is likely to be greatest when only one laboratory is required to respond to new technology that improves performance of the test. Reference samples shared among centers can assure a uniform standard if there is a network of testing centers.

Errors are inevitable in screening. A reasonable goal for a testing program is to eliminate errors of methodology; that is, the reproducibility of the test must be high. However, errors of classification (signal:noise problems) cannot be avoided if the test is truly a *screening* method. Appropriate follow-up and confirmatory testing at a center where expertise in diagnosis is present will reduce classification error due to genetic heterogeneity and quasicontinuous variation. Better statistical methods will also reduce the probability of classification error.

Ethically, the results of the test should be presented to the client in probability form so that his understanding of the problems of screening can be enlisted at a rational level. However, the logistics of explaining probability to large numbers of subjects would appear to be insurmountable, even if deemed desirable. It is generally understood that the logic of probability is used to instruct the counselor in providing the information to the client.

CONTINUOUS EVALUATION

Monitoring the screening methods will uphold the efficiency and accuracy of the testing system. For example, automation of the serum hexosaminidase assay[4,5] has recently increased the efficiency of screening for Tay-Sachs heterozygotes. At the same time, improved statistical analysis of data obtained by accurate hexosaminidase assay can reduce the classification error in Tay-Sachs screening.[3,5]

SUMMARY

It can be said that the quality of screening conforms to the technical accuracy and validity of the test, its specificity and sensitivity, and its consistency when used by different screening laboratories. Constant evaluation is required to upgrade testing methods and to reduce classification errors not only by improved methods but also by the appropriate statistical handling of the test result.

REFERENCES

1. World Health Organization. Screening for Inborn Errors of Metabolism. Report of a WHO Scientific Group. WHO Tech. Rep. Ser. No. 401. Geneva: World Health Organization, 1968.
2. Wilson, J. M. G., and G. Jungner. Principles and Practice of Screening for Disease. Public Health Papers No. 34. Geneva: World Health Organization, 1968.
3. Gold, R. J. M., U. Maag, J. Neal, and C. R. Scriver. The use of biochemical data in screening for mutant alleles and in genetic counselling. Ann. Hum. Genet. 37:315–326, 1974.
4. Lowden, J. A., M. A. Skomorowski, F. Henderson, and M. Kaback. Automated assay of hexosaminidases in serum. Clin. Chem. 19:1345–1349, 1973.
5. Delvin, E., A. Pottier, C. R. Scriver, and R. J. M. Gold. The application of an automated hexosaminidase assay to genetic screening. Clin. Chim. Acta 53: 135–142, 1974.

(4) The Desirability of Regional Facilities

The histories of all the programs reviewed reveal an individual and very different stamp for each. Some states have one screening authority, one laboratory, and one or two follow-up resources. Other states have many. The diversity of approach, efficiency, and costs make recommendations promoting some degree of standardization inescapable. One way of moving toward uniformity, efficiency, and cost reduction might be regionalization, to be discussed in this section.

CURRENT PLANS

A few states have seen the virtue of centralizing laboratory efforts by setting up a single laboratory for several states. This involves pooling of resources to equip one laboratory to do all the necessary tests. Negotiations are under way in the Northwest for half a dozen states to combine in this fashion, and a similar consortium of New England states also has plans.

EFFICIENCY

Any rapid increase in screenable variants may make it difficult for a single laboratory to carry out tests for all. Regional organizations may make it possible for a laboratory in one state, for example, to do one kind of test and another in another state to do others, and for each to have a unique set of expensive equipment, thereby avoiding costly duplication. Precedent for this is given by the experience in Quebec, where one laboratory does tests on all blood samples while another does tests on urine. Such specialization also leads to concentration of experience, which itself promotes efficiency, and cost reductions are likely to follow.

DANGERS

Even while proclaiming the virtues of regional laboratories, the risks of bureaucratic inflexibility must be mentioned. The elaboration of new methods and the improvement of old are perhaps more likely when many laboratories are involved, while the possibility of stifling innovation may be greatest when all procedures are carried out under the direction of a single authority.

AN INTERESTING EXPERIMENT

An interesting and informative experiment is being promoted by the National Genetics Foundation, which has worked out a national network of clinics and laboratories for the disposition of persons with genetic needs. This includes laboratories capable of specialized analyses and genetics centers for counseling. For example, an applicant is referred to a nearby genetics clinic where medical attention and genetic counseling are available. The clinic physicians may send blood, urine, or tissue samples for analysis to a special laboratory, which may be in another part of the country. To send all samples requiring one kind of analysis to one laboratory and all requiring another to another enhances the experience of each laboratory, increases efficiency, and lowers cost. It is a model that should be investigated further.

(5) Auspices and Settings for Genetic Screening Programs

Experience reveals that screening programs are initiated and carried out under the sponsorship of a variety of agencies, each reflecting the special viewpoint of the initiator. Some are designed expressly for service, others mainly or altogether for research. A general description of these agencies follows.

SCREENING FOR PUBLIC SERVICE

Genetic screening for public service has been sponsored by various groups:

- State and city health departments are most frequently involved. Where screening is required by law, the state health department is usually required to implement the regulations. Where not mandated, both city and state departments of health have set up programs according to their own priorities.
- Disease-related foundations have supported screening with money and personnel. They have also pressed for legislation.
- Some genetic screening has been conducted as a matter of policy in certain group practices and health maintenance organizations.
- Interested physicians in university departments and clinics have sponsored screening programs with service to the public as the primary aim, but often including some elements of research.
- Occasional programs have been initiated and conducted by non-medical groups.

Many programs are carried on under combinations of these auspices. For example, state health departments may provide the materials and analysis for screening to physicians who take the test sample in the hospital or office. In others, financial support is provided by the state for the analysis, while a disease-oriented foundation supports the educational effort and supervises mass screening sessions. Each program appears to have taken form without reference to others. This is not surprising, because experience is meager and the literature even more sparse, but the diversity of approach and of organization reflects a need for some coherent scheme for screening that would embrace all the important aspects of planning, organization, achievement of stated goals and evaluation, as well as provide a model for others to copy. It is pointless for each new screening program to evolve spontaneously, repeating past errors.

RESEARCH SPONSORSHIP

The discovery of a new polymorphic protein variant is usually followed by tests in populations to establish gene and phenotype frequencies. If there is evidence that a variant is associated with some disease, the investigation is usually broadened to include physiological and biochemical tests of the effects of the variant on its possessors, sometimes involving hospitalization in clinical research units. The results of these studies may lead to suggestions for changes or regulation of dietary or other personal habits of the persons with the variant phenotypes, and this may or may not be done as a part of the research design. The initiators of this kind of study are usually investigators whose experience and knowledge are closely related to the phenotype in question, and the studies are usually planned to test their circumscribed research hypotheses. Thus the rules under which research in genetic screening is carried out are determined by the questions being investigated, and the lack of experience of the investigator with the sociologic, legal, and ethical aspects of genetic screening may lead to the omission of safeguards more often observed in programs carried out under public sponsorship.

GENETIC SCREENING AS A MATTER OF PUBLIC POLICY

The diversity of the auspices under which genetic screening has been done and the lack of uniformity of approach raise the question of where responsibility for screening programs should lie.

There are many reasons for suggesting that this responsibility should be a matter of public policy. One is that sooner or later genetic screening will affect a large part of the population, perhaps everyone, and the ways in which it differs from ordinary medical practice make it essential that the public be represented in the design and implementation of the programs. If people are to be persuaded to seek genetic preventive measures, they must be involved in the educational measures required, in ensuring that legal and civil rights are not infringed upon, that ethical standards are maintained, and that public resources are appropriately disposed. In addition, because the field is technically complicated and cannot evolve solely in physicians' offices, laboratories and other public facilities are required, both for maintaining existing programs and for devising, testing, and implementing new ones. In fact, genetic screening is already a matter of public policy, since 43 states have laws (mandatory or voluntary) requiring screening for PKU. Testing for sickle cell disease and trait is also being carried out publicly and is in some states legally required.

Proposed Commission to Regulate Screening Practices

The mechanism for executing this public responsibility will no doubt vary from one state, city, or other political division to another, depending upon local wishes and resources, but one instrument for the purpose might be a commission of some kind, including representatives of the medical profession, public health authorities, medical schools, if any, lawyers and legislators, educators, and the general public. The commission might be created by state legislation or might be sponsored by a state health department or by local representatives of some federal agency that may administer some national health scheme or federal insurance program. The commission might function usefully in the following ways:

- The commission might be charged with reviewing and approving all new screening methods and projects receiving public support. This might entail the supervision of pilot studies, making decisions on moving from pilot study to public service, and informing hospitals, physicians, and other agencies in the community of the availability of the service. If all projects in a single state or region were to be subject to such a review, a desirable element of uniformity and economy would be introduced.
- The commission could also set standards of screening practices and quality control for laboratories, treatment procedures, and uses of public agencies and other facilities. Since the commission would be a permanent body even though its membership might change, it would soon become a repository of much experience and expertise, giving its members the knowledge to evaluate new projects in the light of old ones.
- It is probably best to avoid the rigidity inherent in legislation re-

quiring genetic screening, whether for one or for several disorders. There is something repetitious and futile in passing a new law as each new disorder reaches the public consciousness. A public screening commission, on the other hand, may be flexible and may absorb public pressures on legislators, avoiding the passage of coercive laws while serving as a source of information and advice to the lawmakers. If a state is determined to have legislation for genetic screening, such an impulse could be channeled into the creation of the commission, which could then be empowered to promulgate the regulations for new projects.

• As a public agency, the commission could ensure appropriate public participation in decisions about screening. It should have sufficient stature to obtain opinions supporting or opposing the advisability of particular programs on scientific grounds, and should be able to protect the public from those unintended transgressions of the civil rights and sensibilities of the screenees that can occur in projects designed by people who are well-intentioned but whose focus on preventive and medical aspects is so narrow that they neglect these social impacts. Experience of many screening programs suggests that these unexpected side effects are manifold and can seriously dislocate the lives of screenees. Doubtless, new and unforeseen problems will arise as screening expands, and their solution will require the wisdom and knowledge of people of diverse experiences. For this, the weight and visibility of some public and representative agency are needed.

Broad public representation among members of the commission could also protect the community from the pressures of special-interest groups, who, in their preoccupation with their own concerns, may obtain official or even legislative sanction for programs that are not in the general interest.

• A further function of the commission might be to set standards and provide assistance in the design and propagation of educational efforts, directed both at increasing participation in particular screening programs and at educating the general public in preventive medicine and in human biology. There is ample evidence that ignorance blunts the perception of the need for, or the usefulness of accepting, preventive medical measures.

• Genetics has provided so penetrating an understanding of life and development that some scientists have expressed fears that this knowledge might be misused, even by well-meaning persons, to fulfill eugenic aims. They cite the possibilities of genetic engineering or reproductive manipulation that might result in more harm than good. In fact, these possibilities are unlikely to be realized soon, if indeed they ever are; but genetic counseling, screening, and amniocentesis might be perverted to purposes of "improvement of the race" and do, therefore, represent a real threat. A commission with broad professional and public representation would provide the most certain insurance against such misuse.

Questions arise as to the relationship of a public commission to research screening originating, for example, in medical schools and hospitals. It would seem improper for such a commission to exercise control over such investigations, except, of course, if it or the state had funds to grant for support of such research. On the other hand, the commission might exert a strong influence by virtue of its prestige and position in the community, as well as its knowledge and experience in setting standards for screening practices and the availability to it of experts in scientific, social, and legal fields. As an example, the commission might transmit its standards for research to medical school and hospital committees on clinical investigation or to local or national granting agencies, thus exerting substantial moral pressures on the design of research projects. It might be useful also in providing information to investigators on public acceptance of projects, or to judge, if asked to do so, their quality and appropriateness.

The involvement of laymen on the commission could also serve as a link to lay organizations in local communities when mass testing programs are undertaken—for example, screening for Tay-Sachs or sickle cell carriers—in nonmedical settings such as religious, labor, or public facilities. The involvement of lay organizations may help to make the screening program more acceptable to potential screenees, and hence more successful, and to prevent unnecessary harm from being caused by the screeners' ignorance of special customs or other background factors in the community.

Whether a commission should be endowed with coercive powers will, no doubt, be determined by the customs and moods of various states. The history of legislation mandating genetic screening suggests that it is not yet clear that laws requiring screening are helpful, and in some cases they have been shown not to be. One compromise that appears promising is the Commission on Hereditary Disorders created by the legislature of the State of Maryland. This commission is empowered to review new screening techniques and from time to time to issue regulations to the Health Department covering all aspects of new programs.

THE SETTING IN WHICH SCREENING IS DONE

Genetic screening programs are usually carried out in one of two kinds of setting. The first of these is medical and the second includes a variety of nonmedical environments.

Medical Settings

Medical settings include hospital nurseries and outpatient clinics devoted to the care and study of particular diseases. These are satisfactory places that will continue to be employed, especially in conjunction with health department laboratories and other facilities.

Screening for nongenetic conditions is sometimes accomplished in physicians' offices, but there is little genetic screening now going on there. Most doctors are little motivated to do preventive work, and what they do is seldom concerned with genetic traits. The most that can be expected from physicians in private practice today is referral to some center where the tests may be obtained. On the other hand, some screening is already being carried out by large prepaid group clinics, and it is likely that such services will expand. Such institutions may turn out to be the optimal setting for genetic screening.

Nonmedical Settings

Screening tests are sometimes done in church or community buildings or in schools, even in factories or other industrial places. Screening is done under these conditions usually in an attempt to test, in a short time, a large proportion of some group supposed to be at risk, or at least to give the project a massive start, assuming that it will be carried on indefinitely elsewhere, but at a reduced rate.

Conclusions

It is not yet clear which setting, if any single one, is ideal for fulfillment of the aims of genetic screening. The mass technique has not yet been sufficiently studied to know its virtues and defects. It is evident, however, that there are some differences between the people who come forward to be tested and those who do not, despite the aim of such efforts to attract all who are susceptible. In addition, screening in public places may lead to "labeling," with whatever harm that may do. That is, if one is seen being tested in a public place, others in the community may draw incorrect conclusions about one's genotype; but if one is never seen in such a place, no mistakes can be made. If, on the other hand, one is seen in a medical setting, it could be for any one of a variety of ordinary reasons.

Mass screening projects will undoubtedly play an important part in the acceptance of screening, which (together with public education) must precede the inclusion of genetic screening in standard preventive health measures, especially in prepaid group practices.

(6) Populations to Screen

Among the genetic screening programs reviewed, there has been much variation in the choice of populations or groups to test, in the age at which screening is done, and in the size and composition of samples.

GROUPS

It is a fixed purpose of genetic screening that the results of a test should be of benefit to the individual tested, and while this may result in some benefit to society or to some segment thereof, the latter advantage should be incidental. For this reason, any screening test offered for service (as opposed to some research aim) should be offered to everyone; and if it is required, it should be required of everyone.

This has not been a general practice, and the reasons advanced for restricting screening to "high-risk groups" are genetic. It is in the nature of mating systems to cause the concentration of particular alleles in groups of people who share a common history. Some of these genes are mutants, and the examples of diseases associated with them are familiar: Tay-Sachs in Ashkenazi Jews, sickle cell in blacks, and, to some degree, PKU in whites of Western European origin. Logic, then, suggests that screening for these particular genes be limited to the groups in which they abound, omitting those in which they are infrequent. Such a view contributes, no doubt unwittingly, to those discriminating practices that we are at pains to eliminate from our society and that should be permitted to play no part in genetic screening. Such discrimination may operate both ways: that is, by contributing to the sense of inferiority imposed on the members of one minority, or by claiming some superior quality for another. Reasons for limiting screening to one population or another do exist. But wherever such reasons are employed, the initiators of screening programs should be sensitive to the possibilities of discrimination; they should also ensure that the screenees are aware of the arguments favoring focusing on them as opposed to others and that these arguments do not include social discrimination.

The principal constraint favoring selective screening is economic. It is suggested that economy favors limiting the search to "high-risk groups," and this is reasonable, providing risk is related to cost. That is, if a test costs a few pennies, can be automated, and is easy to administer in the mass, then a frequency in a population of 1/25,000 becomes a "high risk." But if each test costs \$10 or more, then "high risk" might be limited to 1/10 or 1/30. So the controlling factor is economic and impersonal and has nothing to do with the selection of race or ethnic minority for eugenic or political reasons. Improvements in technique resulting in reduction in costs may be expected to change the relationship of risk to cost, moving generally toward the ideal of screening all persons for all traits.

AGE

The optimum age for screening depends upon the aim of the test. If the screening is for purposes of treatment, then the best time to screen is sometime before the best time to begin the therapy—that is to say, at a time when the diagnosis is unequivocal but before irreversible damage is done. For inborn errors of metabolism in the newborn infant, the screening becomes a matter of urgency, since permanent damage may be done in a few days, and death may follow in a matter of weeks. For diseases of late onset, however, the choice of time may be more difficult. If treatment is definitive and a potential victim learns of his disease well before its onset, the anxiety induced may be tolerable; but if nothing can be done to avert the onset or to ameliorate the manifestations of a disease, it is better that the future patient remain in ignorance of his fate.

Screening for purposes of counseling is best done at times closely related to marriage and childbearing. The knowledge that one is heterozygous for a gene that is harmful only in homozygotes is useful only in the context of plans for children. Such knowledge will lead to testing of the spouse or intended spouse and (if both are heterozygotes) to discussion about odds and whether to reproduce or to have an amniocentesis, assuming an antenatal diagnosis can be made. But to detect the same gene in a child and to inform him of it is to open up many possibilities for misinformation, misapprehension, anxiety, and fear.

Screening for Down's syndrome by amniocentesis is a special case. Since the risk for the fetus rises with the age of the mother, the general practice is to examine the pregnancies of only older women. The exact age below which an amniocentesis will not be done varies from one center to another but is seldom below 35 and is more usually set at 38–40. This is partly because the risks to the mother, of abortion, or of fetal damage are not yet fully known. Should amniocentesis itself turn out to be a harmless procedure, and should karyotyping become automated and inexpensive, no doubt many more pregnancies will be scrutinized.

If the screening is for enumeration only, then the optimum time is at onset. This ensures the prompt disposition of whatever facilities the community may be able to offer the patient and family at a time when they are most needed.

SIZE

Ideally, the population screened should include everyone who is susceptible or fulfills the aim of the screening. In practice, however, sample size may be determined by a number of factors.

The prescreening educational program may determine how many people are screened. If physicians are not apprised of the availability of the test, or if the efforts to inform the public are minimal or are not easily comprehensible, few screenees may be attracted, and those who are will be only the best educated. Participation will also be influenced strongly by the extent of public determination to have the test and public participation in the planning and execution of the programs. The histories of screening for PKU, sickle cell anemia, and Tay-Sachs disease all indicate this. Economic factors and local priorities may delay or prevent the implementation of new programs, or they may cause the screening to be limited to some "high-risk" group. Finally, the size of a population to be screened may be determined by research aims. For some investigative purposes, relatively small numbers may be appropriate, but research goals do not preclude the collection of very large numbers of observations.

(7) Education of the Public

In the main report the health belief model was presented to explain current health behavior of the public and to provide a basis for recommending the content of educational programs designed to increase public participation in screening programs. A logical conclusion to be drawn from that material was that people need to appreciate that their children may be vulnerable to genetic disease or abnormality transmitted by healthy parents. They need to learn that such abnormalities may have serious consequences for the children unless they are properly managed; they need to believe that the early identification of disease or possible disease often permits effective remedial action to be taken; and they need to learn that the benefits that accrue from such early detection and intervention outweigh the economic and psychological costs that may be incurred.

RESEARCH ON PERSUASION

Some recommendations based on research and experience can be offered to persons planning educational programs. Just as new findings concerning the effects of a drug may require changes or restrictions in the way the drug is used, new evidence about audiences or appeals may alter the conclusions presented here. In line with the traditional question in the field (*Who* says *what* to *whom* through what *medium* with what *effect?*), the recommendations concern the source, message, audience, medium, and effects. The following recommendations will be largely though not exclusively drawn from the summaries of hundreds of research studies reviewed by Karlins and Abelson.[1]

1. A spokesman should be chosen who is likely to be believed by the intended audience. This person should be seen as knowledgeable, unbiased, likable, noncontroversial, similar to the audience in some respects, and having the best interest of the audience at heart. For one group, a black physician might be an ideal spokesman; for another, a schoolteacher; for another, a mother of a child with Down's syndrome; and so on.

In the selection of credible spokesmen, attention should be given to the role of what has been termed the opinion leader. It is useful to recognize that people may be influenced by a communication that never reaches them directly. In a field study, Katz and Lazarsfeld have shown that a person's immediate family is responsible for two thirds of the specific influence attempts on him.[2] A message advocating specific behavior that reaches a person's family may be transmitted to him even though he himself never hears the message.

Starting with this evidence, the investigators have demonstrated that in each community there exist opinion leaders who exert a strong effect upon the opinions and behavior of others. These opinion leaders are the mediators or gatekeepers in any persuasion attempt, standing between the primary source of communications and the eventual target audience. This process is termed the "two-step flow of communication." It asserts that influence attempts are not always or most effectively made as a direct impact of source upon audience; rather the two-step flow shows that a communication source may affect directly only a small number of opinion leaders, who, by virtue of their prestige, influence others to emulate them.

2. The usefulness of the information to the person receiving it should be emphasized. Recommendations should be as specific as possible—e.g., "Get a flu shot on Thursday," rather than "Protect your health"—and should show how a particular action can help.

3. Presenting both sides of an issue rather than one alone will be more effective for people who are initially hostile to one position, or are likely to hear opposing views. Exposing people to "counter-arguments" tends to have two favorable effects: It increases the credibility

of the communicator, and it prepares the audience to resist these arguments when they are encountered at a later time.

4. No general rule can be given concerning the use of appeals to fear. The results depend upon the situation, the audience's initial level of anxiety about the topic, the number of threats posed, the perceived effectiveness of actions that can be taken, and many other factors. It is generally agreed that some amount of fear arousal increases the likelihood that people will act, but specifying (and inducing) the optimum amount is extremely difficult. Strong fear appeals seem to be better when they pose a threat to the audience's loved ones (rather than a direct personal threat), are presented by a highly credible source, deal with topics relatively unfamiliar to the audience, and are directed to people with relatively low income and education, high self-esteem, and low perceived vulnerability to danger. When fear appeals are used, the audience should be placed in a position to take immediate action on the recommendations and should be given explicit instructions to help them do so.

5. Information alone rarely impels people to act. Many people fail to take appropriate health actions despite an awareness of risks, and others, who enjoy taking risks or are immobilized by fear, fail to act *because* of this knowledge. In some cases, there are barriers (psychological, social, and environmental or situational) that keep people from following recommendations that they claim to accept.

Many examples of this belief–behavior discrepancy could be cited, but a few will illustrate the point. In one national survey, 83% of those interviewed mentioned toothbrushing as a way to prevent dental disease, but only 55% said they brushed their teeth after meals. More than 90% of the public believes seat belts are effective, but only one person in four uses them regularly. Most people agree verbally that regular physical and dental examinations are a good thing, but only a small minority actually have such examinations. Of course, many people probably do not obtain preventive medical care because they believe the probability of detecting serious disease is small, or that most detectable conditions are self-limiting and therefore not serious, or that early detection of disease confers no special benefits. This behavior may be reinforced by physicians who publicly express doubts about the utility of checkups.

Even in an unusually well-informed group there will be some people who (despite awareness of the risks) are overweight, some who smoke, some who have not had tests for TB or diabetes or glaucoma, some who avoid periodic physical or dental checkups, and so on. This fact reinforces the belief that educational programs that succeed in increasing people's knowledge about health may still achieve only limited success in affecting health behavior. This is not to question the value of providing information about health hazards and adaptive behavior, but rather to suggest that programs should devote greater effort to emphasizing the payoff of preventive behavior and to undermining the barriers that keep people from following recommendations.

There are important uses for information programs. Undoubtedly, they strengthen the views of those already committed to the desired position and provide them with a means of verbalizing their views. In addition, for those desiring to take particular action, information can tell them how and where to take the action.

6. The active participation of the audience should be elicited. Active participation facilitates both learning and recall of message content.

7. The group influence can reinforce messages. Existing group norms relevant to the proposed behavior should be ascertained. Since perceived norms can either reinforce or undermine a set of recommendations, it is crucial to identify them early and plan accordingly.

8. Repetition of messages is desirable. Communications are always competing with many others for attention. While it is theoretically possible to repeat a message too often, of course, there is very little danger of excessive exposure with public service messages. The problem is how to get enough time or space to be noticed at all.

9. Using multiple channels of communication is advisable whenever possible, since no single medium will reach everyone. To convey complex material, print media should be included so readers can control their own rate of exposure. However, many people of below-average education make little use of printed materials; consequently, they need to be reached through personal contact or through broadcast media with simplified content. The mass media reach far more people than personal contact, but the latter is more effective—and the use of both is better than either alone.

10. It is always desirable to assess the characteristics of the audience before making critical choices regarding media and content. Examples of failure to do this are easy to find: Almost 2,500,000 Americans, most of them nonwhites over 45 years of age, are illiterate, yet much health information is still directed to this relatively high-risk group in printed form.

The point has been made repeatedly that the public is not a homogeneous mass. There are many ways of dividing it into smaller segments—for example, by level of education, family income, age, and health status. Some of these ways of dividing the public into various categories are of greater use than others to the health professional; some provide data that can be used in designing information programs for specific groups.

Persuasion is most likely to succeed when the underlying reasons for the attitude or behavior one is trying to change are taken into account—for example, the health motives of the audience, their perceived vulnerability to problems deemed serious, and their perception of the benefits and costs of following recommendations.

Everyone's motives and beliefs are resistant to change by external pressure. A common defense against persuasion is avoidance, which may take the form of selective exposure to information and forgetting or distortion of material one is exposed to. Messages in the mass media are easy to avoid or forget, but they may be quite effective in triggering a response in persons who are initially receptive to the content. Knowing in advance the beliefs and attitudes of the potential audience can give the communicator a crucial advantage in designing messages to reach those who normally avoid health information.

11. Media and formats should not be limited to the traditional ones. Children are now reached through games, coloring books, and comic books on such topics as drugs, smoking, and safety. Clients of a planned parenthood clinic paid little attention to the usual pamphlets but read birth control information when it was presented in a confession-magazine format.

12. Assessments of program impact should include measurements taken at several points in time because the effects (both intended and unintended) can be very complex and can change over a period of weeks or months. Some effects of communications occur immediately after exposure. Some may not appear until after several weeks have passed. Most wear off very rapidly. Some having only a slight connection with the message may turn up. In any case, the practitioner should be aware that the effects of a persuasive message, if any, may not be fully revealed until some time after the communication.

13. Whenever possible, the intended outcomes of an educational effort should be stated explicitly and in behavioral terms. Unless this is done, the effects of the program are not likely to be assessed properly and thus any claims of success will be questionable. Are people being asked to take a specific action? If so, is it to be taken once, or repeated at intervals, or engaged in continuously? Does the action involve *doing* something or *not doing* something? Merely stating that an attempt will be made "to inform mothers of grade schoolchildren about a vision screening program," or "to inform voters of the benefits of fluoridation," is not of much value in planning a program or in arranging to evaluate its effectiveness.

14. No single message or campaign is likely to produce major changes. Mass communications tend to reinforce existing views and rarely change deep-seated attitudes or opinions. Many people who are

targets of communications will not be in the audience, and some of those who are will distort or forget the message. These factors will limit the success of the program no matter how well it has been planned.

A number of conditions must be met in order for any message disseminated through the mass media to have the desired effect: opportunity for exposure, actual exposure, attention, learning, acceptance, perceived self-relevance, engaging motivations to act, recall, and opportunity for action. For example, a health message presented on television will not directly reach those who are not watching TV (or are watching other stations) when it is shown; some of those who have the opportunity to see it will not be paying attention; some who pay attention will not learn to accept the content of the message; some who learn and accept it will not believe it applies to them; some who think it does will not be motivated to take the action recommended; some who intend to act will forget the message before they have the chance to act; and some who remember it may be in a situation which precludes their following the recommendation. The same series of conditions applies in the case of pamphlets, posters, lectures, and other channels of communication commonly used to convey health information.

It would not be fair to conclude from this discussion that the mass media serve little useful purpose. With respect to any health proposal, there are likely to be a great many people prepared to take action by virtue of their attitudes and beliefs about the efficacy of the action. For them a message transmitted by the mass media may serve as the necessary trigger or cue for behavior. Others may lack only specific information about an action, such as the location of a service or the hours during which it is to be available; for them the mass media are likely to be an efficient means for communication of information. But, as regards long-lasting attitudinal and behavioral change, it seems fair to conclude that the mass media are far more effective in informing than in inducing change.

SURREPTITIOUS FORMS OF PERSUASION

Occasionally, "new" forms of persuasion appear and temporarily attract considerable public attention. If these methods are effective in producing political defections or selling products, it is asked, why can't they be used in persuading people to practice good health habits? Apart from the ethical questions involved the available evidence does not support the conclusion that people can be made to act against their will.

During the Korean War, *"brainwashing"* (based on interrogation, isolation, information control, and use of various rewards and punishments) received a lot of publicity but in fact had little impact—even though its users had almost complete control over their prisoners. In the 1950's, *subliminal advertising* was developed on the theory that messages presented below the threshold of awareness (such as on a movie or TV screen for only 1/30 of a second) would influence people without arousing their defenses against persuasion. Controlled experiments showed this technique to be ineffective, and it is no longer being used. (At least we think so. . . .) Many people believe that *hypnosis* can be used, even on a mass basis, to control behavior—but again, the facts do not justify this belief. The same is true of other methods that have been tried experimentally, such as controlled administration of *drugs, sound, light patterns,* and *electrical stimulation* of the brain.

Research is continuing in all these areas, and new evidence may alter at any time the negative conclusion stated here. For the moment, however, the methods described briefly above are not used in the health field for three reasons: They don't seem to work, we can't exercise the degree of control that might make them work, and ethical considerations preclude our attempting to circumvent free and informed choice on the part of our clients.

CONCLUSIONS

Favorable attitudes toward and participation in screening programs depend in part on a combination of motives and beliefs:

- A *health motive* that makes health, including genetic risks and disease, a salient matter to the individual
- A perception of *vulnerability* to a disease, condition, or trait, believed to have actual or potential *serious* consequences for oneself or one's offspring
- The belief that intervention is *beneficial* in reducing vulnerability to or seriousness of the condition
- The belief that the economic and psychological *costs* of screening are small relative to the perceived benefits of screening

While there is some evidence that behavior can be modified without prior modification of underlying motives and beliefs, for example, through the modification of the social and physical environment and the use of group dynamics, there are good grounds for continuing efforts to teach the desirable health motives and beliefs. In this effort attention should be devoted to the unmatched opportunity for original education in young children who have not yet developed ingrained fallacious views of biological processes; but attention must also be given to continuing efforts to persuade adults to adopt informed views and to act on them. Despite the dearth of firmly established principles concerning persuasion, a number of rules of thumb based on prior research have been reported in this section relating to each component of the traditional mass communication problem. These include guidelines concerning the selection of the *source* of a message, characteristics of various segments of the *target population,* the strengths and weaknesses of various *media,* the *content* of a communication, and the duration of communication *effects.*

REFERENCES

1. Karlins, M., and H. I. Abelson. Persuasion: How Opinions and Attitudes Are Changed. 2nd ed. New York: Springer, 1970.
2. Katz, E., and P. F. Lazarsfeld. Personal Influence: The Part Played by People in the Flow of Mass Communications. Glencoe, Ill.: The Free Press, 1955.

(8) Informed Consent

The doctrine of informed consent governs both therapeutic–diagnostic and experimental procedures, as was demonstrated in the legal and ethical discussions in Chapters 10 and 11. The obtaining of the screenee's free and understanding consent is thus required in genetic screening programs, whether conducted for the screenee's benefit or for other purposes.

The person's agreement to the intervention is necessary to preserve his freedom and autonomy in either instance, but there are a number of additional reasons for requiring it in the case of experimental procedures. First, the person's implied consent to anything done by the physician cannot be assumed on the basis that the physician would conduct only beneficial procedures, because an experimental procedure is by definition one in which the physician's objective is to use the subject to gain knowledge and only in some instances to be of possible benefit to the subject as well. Second, experimental procedures as a rule entail greater risks than established procedures; at the least, the risks are less well known. And finally, the physician's interest in the outcome of the experiment cannot help but interfere with a disinterested and dispassionate appraisal of whether these uncertain risks are outweighed by the uncertain benefits that the subject may wish to bestow upon himself or others through his participation.

Since new genetic screening programs are experimental, both in technique and medical and social outcome, these additional reasons argue strongly in favor of taking care to obtain informed consent from all screenees.[1]

PROCEDURES FOR OVERCOMING DIFFICULTIES OF CONSENT

It is widely acknowledged[2,3] that informing a patient fully is an ideal often unattainable in the real clinical setting. The best mechanism for improving on the present system is not obvious, but the difficulty of communicating information to the average subject suggests that any procedure should err on the side of extra care and effort. The proper attitude for the consent-seeker, as articulated by Beecher,[2] should be to

> . . . seek increased respect for the individual by providing him with opportunities for self-determination . . . (and seek) to reduce assaults on the integrity of man through hidden interventions by others, however benevolent they may be. The final decision as to the degree of acceptable risk belongs to the subject.

A number of procedures have been developed to help assure informed consent, particularly for research programs. In addition to review of both the protocol and the procedures to be used in obtaining consent by a committee of professionals and laymen (including, if possible, some drawn from the pool of potential screenees), the Department of Health, Education and Welfare[4] has specified the requirements of the consent procedures, all of which seem appropriate to genetic screening. These include:

1. fair explanation of the procedures to be followed and their purposes, including identification of any which are experimental;
2. description of risks and benefits to be reasonably expected;
3. disclosure of appropriate alternative procedures that might be advantageous to the participant;
4. offer to answer inquiries;
5. instruction that the participant is free to withdraw at any time without prejudice; and
6. documentation of the consent.

The need for care in obtaining consent is emphasized by the nature of the hazards that have been experienced in screening programs; these include stigmatization, loss of employment or insurance, and family discord, as was discussed in Chapter 5. In addition, the persons being screened should be made fully aware of the limitations of the particular screening program, such as the risk of false-positive or false-negative findings and what can be done to minimize this risk. To avoid having people become "informed" about such hazards only after they have gone through screening, particularly when the program is conducted as a "community campaign" (e.g., many Tay-Sachs and sickle cell screening programs to date) outside usual medical channels, it is important that the hazards and benefits be adequately and realistically conveyed in the educational and promotional literature. Since certain hazards, as well as the possible irrelevance of some profferred benefits for some persons, might lead these individuals to avoid being screened, each possible participant must be made aware of these factors, orally or preferably in writing, before he becomes so enmeshed in the screening process that it is difficult to get out.

ADVENTITIOUS FINDINGS

In most large-scale screening programs, a uniform policy on the disclosure of findings, including those considered "adventitious" to the program's primary mission, will be needed. In other settings, where the person in charge has an opportunity to discuss the program personally with each screenee and evaluate his or her emotional and social vulnerabilities, an individualized judgment on the scope of disclosure may be possible. In either case, it is necessary that the agreement of the person screened be explicit about what information the screener is obliged to reveal to the screenee as well as about what will *not* be revealed. A clear presentation on this point will enable people to refuse participation or seek other screening programs if the policy on disclosure is not to their liking. For example, if the persons in charge of amniocentesis at a particular hospital conclude that in pregnancies screened for Down's syndrome the parents will not be told about results of equivocal import (such as the XYY karyotype) because of the possible adverse social effects of such disclosure, they should so inform the parents *before* conducting the procedure.

CONSENT FOR FUTURE USE OF SAMPLES

Genetic screening programs often involve large groups of people, and the availability of the samples obtained from them presents opportunities for research in areas perhaps unrelated to the purpose for which the sample was obtained. Such research is important if knowledge about genetic disease is to increase. Indeed, it may be essential to conduct such research before treatment programs are instituted; otherwise, reliable base-line data on the natural incidence and variation of the condition will be lacking. But such use of samples should not proceed without the consent of the persons involved. There is no question that an individual may permit a sample taken for one purpose to be used for additional specific purposes by the usual consent procedures. Yet, since it would be nearly impossible to contact all the people who were screened and obtain their permission for a new use of the specimens, consent will have to be obtained at the time the specimen is taken.

If a future use other than the primary diagnostic one is contemplated, the persons from whom samples are taken must at the minimum be informed of such additional uses (e.g., diagnostic tests that are still at the research stage) and given an opportunity to permit or refuse such use of samples taken from them. If the future tests involve conditions that are very different from those presently being screened for or if they may reveal information of a very troubling nature, the person consenting should be informed *specifically* of the disorders for which the screeners will be looking and of the medical significance of a positive finding in his or her case. Thus, for example, if a heelstick blood sample is obtained for PKU screening, it would be sufficient for the person giving consent to agree that the sample may also be examined on an experimental basis for "additional metabolic defects as tests for them are developed and tried out"; but if the blood sample were to be used for chromosome testing (which might reveal sex chromosome aneuploidy of potentially great medical and social impact) or for a Huntington's chorea screen (which might reveal a devastating degenerative disease of late onset), specific consent for these procedures would be needed.

Consent must be sought not only for the research use of a sample drawn for another purpose but also for the use of the information obtained through such procedures; the same principles apply here as in the disclosure of adventitious findings. Having been informed about the kind of information that could be turned up, the person giving consent can then decide whether he or she wishes to be informed of the results or whether the data produced should be used solely by the investigator for his scientific purposes (e.g., statistical reports on the incidence of condition X in a given population). It is clear that much of the hazard inherent in the use of such samples would disappear if there were no way to identify the donor. While any possible benefit to a particular donor would also disappear under this proscription, much meaningful research could be carried out on samples not easily obtainable otherwise. Destruction of identifying marks on such samples, therefore, might make more acceptable a practice of procuring general consent in advance for such investigations.

Clearly, the consent given in these circumstances is not as fully "informed" as the ideal standard would have it—either as to the research use of the sample or the disposition of the information revealed—because the exact conditions being looked for will in some cases be unknown at the time consent is given. But if the risks involved in the screen are comparable to those of the primary condition for which the test is being conducted, or if all greater risks are spelled out, the person giving consent will be in a position to accept or reject the uncertain risks that are involved in any experiment.

WHEN INFORMED CONSENT IS NOT ENOUGH

The premise of the foregoing discussion is that in most circumstances genetic screening will be conducted on a voluntary basis. In such a setting the basic requisites for a program to go forward are the professional judgment of the screeners and the informed consent of the screenees. As mentioned at the outset of this section and in greater detail in the section on auspices and setting (p. 236), however, there are additional limitations on a program besides the mutual agreement of screener and screenee. Since screening may impose costs on society, or may harm individuals in ways that society believes they are unable to anticipate or evaluate adequately, mechanisms of prior review by multidisciplinary committees are required.

Another situation in which consent may not be sufficient to permit an intervention to go forward is when children are to be tested and consent is sought from their parents. If the diagnostic procedure is intended to yield results of potential benefit to the child, the consent of the parent (or other guardian) is sufficient. But where the intervention will not benefit the child, as for example an experimental procedure conducted solely for scientific benefit, the legal authority of the parent is not well established, and if substantial hazards are involved, there are strong arguments against the parents' being allowed to consent. The National Institutes of Health are presently formulating policy guidelines[5] on this difficult and much debated topic.[6,7]

REFERENCES

1. Lappé, M., J. M. Gustafson, and R. Roblin. A report from the Research Group on Ethical, Social and Legal Issues in Genetic Counseling and Genetic Engineering of the Institute of Society, Ethics and the Life Sciences. Ethical and social issues in screening for genetic disease. N. Engl. J. Med. 286:1129–1132, 1972.
2. Beecher, H. K. Research and the Individual: Human Studies. Boston: Little, Brown, 1970.
3. Ingelfinger, F. Informed (but uneducated) consent. N. Engl. J. Med. 287: 465–466, 1972.

4. Protection of human subjects. Fed. Reg. 39:18914–18920, 1974.
5. Protection of human subjects—Policies and procedures. Fed. Reg. 38:31738–31749, 1973.
6. Curran, W. J., and H. K. Beecher. Experimentation in children. A reexamination of legal ethical principles. JAMA 210:77–83, 1969.
7. Capron, A. M. Legal considerations affecting clinical pharmacological studies in children. Clin. Res. 21:141–150, 1973.

(9) Confidentiality

Release of data to third parties (that is, to persons other than the screenee) is justified only when the screenee has specifically given consent to such release. This principle should apply whether the third party actively seeks screening information or the screener wishes to contact third parties and provide this information; it should also apply whether or not the screening information identifies the person screened.

In general, the practices for obtaining consent for release should be governed by the principles regarding informed consent discussed in the preceding section. In particular, because consent for release of information must be adequately informed, blanket consents should not be used (e.g., consents that screening information may be released to "any insurance company at any time"). Rather, the third party to whom release is authorized must be sufficiently identified for the screenee to intelligently weigh the specific risks and advantages of disclosure to that third party. There may be occasions when third parties will obtain court orders requiring divulgence of screening information. Before the screener discloses such information, however, he should contact the screenee to inform him of the court order and give him an opportunity to obtain legal counsel and to contest the propriety of the court order if he chooses.

In some circumstances, the effect of this rule against unconsented disclosures might appear unduly harsh. Some screeners, for example, might strongly believe that information produced by screening should be disclosed to blood relatives who might be affected by a serious, treatable genetic disorder. For the reasons discussed in Chapter 10, the impulse for disclosure in this circumstance is outweighed by considerations of principle dictating that individuals should have power to control the intensely intimate information concerning their individual genotypes. Adherence to this principle does not bar screeners from counseling screenees in favor of disclosure, and from offering supportive services to assist them in reaching this result. Such counseling and support must, of course, rest on the premise that the individual screenee's ultimate power to choose will be scrupulously respected.

RELEASE OF INFORMATION REGARDING CHILDREN

Where children are screenees, the rule governing disclosure becomes more complex. In most states, both parents (while married) are presumed by law to share custody of their children. This presumption would appear to imply, first, that screening information about children belongs equally to both parents and, second, that both parents must agree before any release of screening information to a third party. Genetic screening programs can, however, put particular stress on this principle when, for example, screening information casts unexpected doubt on the child's true paternity. Disclosure of this information can be forestalled if, as discussed in section 8, above, the screener has obtained advance consent from the parents that they will not obtain certain kinds of information which may be developed about the child (such as information bearing on paternity or XYY karyotype). But if such advance consent has not been obtained, screeners would appear legally obligated to share information with both parents.

Where screening information likely to be revealed may harmfully disrupt family life, it is accordingly essential that screeners anticipate these problems in designing the initial screening protocol. If a screener has not anticipated this problem and is legally bound to disclose disruptive information to both parents, it is nonetheless legally permissible to communicate this information in a manner best designed to minimize disruption—for example, by extensive initial counseling with the mother before revealing the information casting doubts about paternity to the father.

RELEASE OF INFORMATION REGARDING RESULTS OF AMNIOCENTESIS

The question of whether the father is legally entitled to share information provided the mother following amniocentesis appears unsettled. On one side, the general legal rule that parents share equally in the custody of their children and have joint authority in medical decisions about their children points toward shared information. On the other side, recent Supreme Court decisions establishing the mother's constitutional right, in consultation with her physician, to decide on abortion point toward a legal rule excluding the father from any necessary role in prenatal decisions likely to be affected by the results of amniocentesis.

Because of this uncertainty about the applicable legal rule, screeners would appear best advised to obtain the mother's consent, before amniocentesis, to sharing the resulting information with the father. This practice would not necessarily settle the issue, since a father might argue that the mother had no authority to deprive him of his right to information about the fetus. Ultimately, however, this question can be conclusively resolved only by litigation or by legislation. The prospects for sensible ultimate resolution would be enhanced if screeners established a practice of obtaining the mother's consent on this question in order to present clearly the issues at stake for litigation or legislation.

RELEASE OF INFORMATION BY LAY SCREENING GROUPS

Where screening programs are carried out under medical auspices, the rules governing confidentiality of information will be derived from general professional norms codified in statutes or court decisions in each jurisdiction. Those norms, as discussed, militate against unconsented release of information. But where such programs are conducted solely under lay auspices, no such traditional sources of authority will clearly apply. Accordingly, it is particularly important that the protocols establishing lay programs clearly specify that the rules against unconsented release of information will be respected.

(10) Transmission of Results, Counseling, and Follow-up

The act of taking a sample of blood or urine for a test is only the first of a series of steps that constitute the screening process. Some result or other, whether positive or negative, must emerge; the result then must be transmitted to the subject, who must be instructed as to its meaning and given direction in regard to further steps to be taken, if any. In addition, there must be some continuity in the care of patients, some assurance that the information transmitted has been received and retained in the form in which it was given, and some assessment of the usefulness of the counseling in the life of the screenee. Consideration should also be given to the inclusion of a caveat concerning the limits of the reliability of the particular test.

TRANSMISSION OF RESULTS

Information should be transmitted promptly, in understandable language, and under conditions that maintain confidentiality, allow opportunity for counseling, and ensure follow-up. A caveat concerning the limits of reliability of the test results should also be included in the information provided.

Time of Communication

The results of the test should be communicated to the screenee or his family as soon as possible so as to minimize the duration of anxiety which may have been engendered by the test. This means that analytical and clinical procedures should be streamlined for rapid completion of the job. Speed is even more essential when the screening is intended to detect newborn babies with diseases of early onset which threaten life or development. If the analysis or transmission of the results takes many days or weeks, babies with galactosemia or maple syrup urine disease, for example, may be dead or irreversibly damaged before anything can be done. This precludes saving up samples for analysis every so often and is an argument favoring automated procedures in continuous use.

Content of Communication

A positive test result usually leads to confirmation of the diagnosis by more definitive tests, and to counseling and treatment. The information to be transmitted, therefore, should be appropriate for the next step in the procedure, whichever that may be. If the next step is to perform a more definitive diagnostic test, the screenee may be told simply that the first test was unsatisfactory and that it has been found necessary to repeat it; if counseling or treatment is the next step, then more complete information will be appropriate.

When the screening test result is negative, the obligation to transmit that information is neither so clearly defined nor so often observed. Yet there are some people who, aware that they have been tested but without any very profound understanding of the nature of the test or of how often the result is positive, have unpleasant fantasies about it. There is surely an obligation to avoid that; but when, for example, hundreds or even thousands of tests are done before a positive result is met, the trouble and expense of notifying all persons with negative results may preclude its being done. Perhaps the decision whether to notify should depend upon the incidence of positive test results, the resources available to the screening agency, and the cost. When the frequency of positives is high, resources are ample, and it is economically feasible, all participants should be notified of the result of their tests. But when there are few positive results, resources are slim, and the cost is prohibitive, the obligation to persons with negative results may be fulfilled if all screenees are told that no news is good news, that if after a specified time they have heard nothing, they will know the result was negative. At the same time, it should be made clear that those in charge of the program stand prepared at any time to answer questions and to clarify doubts or uncertainty, and appropriate facilities should be provided to make this promise a reality.

Occasionally in the course of a screening program, unexpected characteristics are discovered, and the proper disposition of such adventitious information is not always clear. This issue is dealt with in an earlier section (p. 253).

Means of Transmission

The conditions under which the information is given should facilitate the next step. That is, if a sample for a more definitive test is needed, then the screenee should be apprised of that need when he is told the result of his first test, and the setting for this transaction should maximize the probability that the second sample will be obtained. For this, a physician's office is suitable, or a public health nurse may visit the screenee at home. Possibly the telephone might do, although if the news is frightening to its recipient, a telephone message may be too abrupt. A letter may be adequate for some situations, but for others it may not carry a sufficient sense of urgency. Perhaps each characteristic screened for requires a different means of contact; but whichever is chosen, it should be linked to whatever subsequent steps are appropriate, whether it be a second sample, counseling, or follow-up and treatment.

Experience suggests that information should be given out as uniformly as possible, since when special attention is given only to some persons, for example, those with positive results, it may be noticed and a confidence is inadvertently breached. A visit by a public health nurse, for example, may be identified with a positive test for sickle cell trait. On the other hand, a visit by such a messenger to tell a family of a positive test for PKU or galactosemia would be so infrequent in any neighborhood that it would not be associated with any particular disease or genotype.

As in other aspects of screening, all this suggests that methods for information transfer cannot yet be standardized, if indeed they can ever be. Since different methods are likely to be used in the fulfillment of different screening aims, it is essential, here as elsewhere, to evaluate the success of the measures used. The knowledge and satisfactions of the screenees should be tested with the intention of obtaining information leading to the improvement of technique and the maintenance of high standards.

COUNSELING

While it is permissible to carry out screening for research aims that have no medical connotation without providing facilities for counseling, no program (whether for service or research) that is in any way related to health should fail to offer such support.

Definition of Counseling

Counseling involves information about the disorder or characteristic in question, its frequency, and its manifestations, if any, and about the probabilities for transmission to the next generation. It also includes answers to all questions and assurance that the screenee understands fully the meaning of the information given as well as any actions that would be in his interest—for example, reproductive options, the uses of community agencies, or information to transmit to other members of his family. Counselors must also be alert to the emotional impact of the discovery that one has a particular genotype and must be able to provide some positive support to those affected.

Counseling thus defined is to be distinguished from prescreening education or discussions preliminary to informed consent; it deals with all the consequences of the discovery of the genotype. When the result of the screening test is positive, the counseling will necessarily be more extensive and will require more elaborate facilities than when the result is negative; but even the latter event may require explanation, and programs should not neglect their obligation to ensure that all participants know how and where to obtain the service.

The Counselors

Counseling should be given by suitably qualified and trained persons. For many purposes these need not be physicians; indeed, many physicians are not qualified by training or inclination. But neither should the counselors be enthusiastic lay people, veterans of 1-week crash courses in counseling and with little knowledge of genetics. Although nonmedical counselors may handle most questions, however, there remain some complicated conditions that are best handled by an experienced medical geneticist in the setting of a genetics clinic. Such clinics do not abound, but they are to be found in most university medical centers, and screening authorities should be in close touch with them.

In addition to the medical and genetic aspects of characteristics for which screening is being done, nonmedical counselors should be taught to detect signs of overemotional or irrational responses in the screenees, and some medical facility should be available for referral of persons showing these manifestations.

There is a serious lack of trained counselors, and this deficiency may act as a brake on the development of new screening programs. How to increase their number, what the qualifications should be, the content of the training program, who should be responsible for it, and where it should be given, are all questions for which answers are wanting. Certainly, qualifications and training standards should be set, and perhaps the new schools of allied health sciences may see this need as a responsibility they should assume.

The Time and Setting for Counseling

It has been shown repeatedly that counseling is most likely to be understood and retained when the recipient is relaxed and motivated to listen. This means that when the news of the result of the screening test is disturbing, the counselor should attend to those elements of most immediate concern for the screenee, leaving definitive counseling to some more opportune time. It is also clear that retention of the counseling message is, for most people, directly related to the extent of reinforcement. Thus, to be successful, the counseling sessions must take place when the screenee is in a receptive frame of mind and they must be repeated.

The ideal setting for counseling is a physician's office. Confidentiality is easily maintained, since one goes to the physician for a variety of purposes, none of which is easily identified. Such public places as schools and churches, on the other hand, expose the counselee to the risk of identification. For example, a person seen entering a room known to have been set aside for counseling persons with a genetic trait discovered in some screening program is soon "labeled," no matter why he entered the room.

Evaluation

Since human beings vary so widely in intelligence, educational attainment, experience, and personality, it is no surprise that uniform counseling procedures are not uniformly successful. Yet the success of screening programs is strongly dependent upon the use the participants make of the information gained by submitting to the test. If these uses are to be sensible and in the interest of the participant, evaluation of counseling must be a part of standard procedure. Although such evaluation may seem only to complicate the screening process, adding to the work of counselors and clerical staff, it is a critical step in the chain of events that constitute the screening process.

The extent and kind of such evaluation will depend upon the aims of the particular screening program and will differ according to whether a test result is positive or negative. It may take the form of studies to determine who comes for screening and who does not; of testing how much a screenee has learned from a counseling session, and of its meaning in the context of his own life; of efforts to determine the outcomes of actions the participants may have taken as a result of the counseling. Failure to include such evaluation in the structure of a screening program risks the investment of sizable public resources in inefficiency and failure.

FOLLOW-UP

A positive result of a screening test should be the signal for follow-up with a definitive test. If the result of the latter is positive, then some arrangements for management are in order. If the positive result is the detection of a harmless heterozygous state, the management is counseling; but if it is a disease, appropriate medical care should be made available. It is vital that a close relationship exist between the screening authority and the follow-up facility, especially for disorders in which it is essential that treatment follow discovery as rapidly as possible. This has proved to be a complex logistic problem in PKU screening in some states, and unfortunate experiences have been the result of disassociation of the screening and treatment organizations.

Local details vary from one state to another, but the simplest and most successful mechanisms for PKU have involved the assumption by the state of the responsibility to communicate the discovery of a new case to a limited number of PKU clinics located in teaching hospitals and run by physicians with experience in the disease. Many of the states also assume the cost of the special diet on the dual assumption that if treatment is not supplied without regard to ability to pay, the screening itself is better left undone, and that it is to the state's financial advantage to prevent mental retardation.

This model of an intimate association between the screening authority and the organizations capable of giving appropriate treatment is a good one to follow. Details will differ, depending upon the disorder or characteristic under consideration; but the success and usefulness of any screening program to the people to whom it is offered will hinge upon the efficiency of the measures taken to follow through to some definitive disposition of the information gained in the screening.

(11) Costs of Screening Programs

In earlier sections of this report, a number of common difficulties associated with identifying the costs of screening programs were discussed. This section presents a brief synthesis of such issues as a guide for undertaking such activities.

At the most general level, there are really only two activities to be costed: *identifying* at-risk individuals and *serving* individuals so identified.

The first category includes the cost of acquisition of samples as well as the cost of the tests conducted. In addition, the cost of follow-up testing must be included, since few if any screening procedures operate with sufficient precision to effectively eliminate all false positives and false negatives.

COLLECTION

Costs of collection vary considerably among different types of screening programs. For newborn screening programs, such as PKU, the population to be screened is well identified. However, a large number of samples must be obtained to identify a single case. This means that even if the collection cost per sample is small, the cost per case is high. In some studies, the actual cost associated with obtaining blood samples and getting them to the lab represented over 50% of the cost of the entire screening program. For programs of targeted screening, such as sickle cell anemia and (perhaps even more appropriately) Tay-Sachs disease, the sample cost per identified case is smaller. However, in those settings, the populations being screened are not immediately at hand, e.g., in the hospitals. Such programs require incurring costs for outreach, public information, and solicitation of participation. For most such programs, these costs are not trivial. Typically, however, they tend to be omitted in estimates of program costs.

TESTING

In many cases, tests are paid for by the individuals. Actual expenditures may vary considerably within a given program. More important, when such costs are not borne directly by the program, it is often tempting to act as if they did not occur. It is essential to realize that the cost of such a program includes more than the costs that fall directly on the particular screening organization. For tests that require the presence of the individual, such as amniocentesis as a test for Tay-Sachs, the test procedure itself may involve significant cost.

FOLLOW-UP TESTS

Follow-up testing also imposes costs on the program. In particular, follow-up testing for newborns requires special access to physician services, since the child is no longer within an institutional setting. For some programs, the cost of follow-up testing may be quite sensitive to the type of test, and the cost of testing may offset or influence in other ways the cost of follow-up activities.

TREATMENT

Most attempts to estimate the cost of treatment, particularly with regard to PKU programs, have limited themselves to the direct therapy. In the PKU case, this means that the cost of treatment is estimated as being equal to the cost of the dietary supplement. Such an estimate omits many significant costs that prove to be far greater than those associated with diet alone. For example, children under such a treatment regimen require significantly greater access to medical services, partly because of reduced resistance to general illness and partly because of a need for greater monitoring than is necessary for other children.

In addition to direct treatment costs, children in such a program require greater supervision, both parental and otherwise, need more child care services, and probably have higher hospital rates than do similar children without such illness.

For other programs, treatment costs may be influenced by other considerations. As a general rule, it is essential to include the costs of increased utilization of health and counseling services. Since those costs must be incurred, they should be included in the estimates of the costs of treatment.

For certain programs, other costs are important, although significantly more difficult to measure. For example, those forms of genetic screening that serve to identify risk but not illness, such as sickle cell trait screening, may impose personal costs of greater significance, although such costs tend to fall on the individuals involved in nonmonetary ways.

As a last caveat, it seems important to note that screening and treatment programs typically involve a degree of ongoing interaction on the part of such individuals with the health care system. This relationship may generate significantly different patterns of health service utilization and expenditures quite separate from those related to the disease itself. It is also essential to note that for some types of programs, the treatment itself will have varying degrees of success, and the cost of such a program must include the cost of dealing with some of its failures as well as the cost of dealing with its successes.

(12) Conditions for New Genetic Screening Programs

As new screening tests are devised, they should be carefully reviewed. If the exponential rate of discovery of new genetic characteristics means an accelerating rate of appearance of new screening tests, now is the time to develop the medical and social apparatus to accommodate what later on may otherwise turn out to be unmanageable growth.

When responsibility for genetic screening is vested in a commission or other screening authority, it should be the recipient of suggestions for the use of a new test and should carry out the review prior to employment of the test for service in the community. This review should go step by step, beginning with an assessment of need and of public interest and acceptance, followed then by a study of feasibility and after that by a pretest or field trial to determine whether the new test can be fitted into already existing molds or whether something new is needed. The pretest would also evaluate how useful the new test is and how well it is being accepted. The final step is to make the test available as a public service. Figure 12-1 outlines the procedure.

Suggestions for new tests may come from investigators in nearby medical schools or hospitals, or they may be generated within the authority itself. For some disorders the preliminary studies may be already well advanced, so that the commission's review might consist mainly of adapting the text to local conditions. Thus, new tests, already evaluated and in use elsewhere, could be brought into the review process at any level consistent with the rules set by the screening authority.

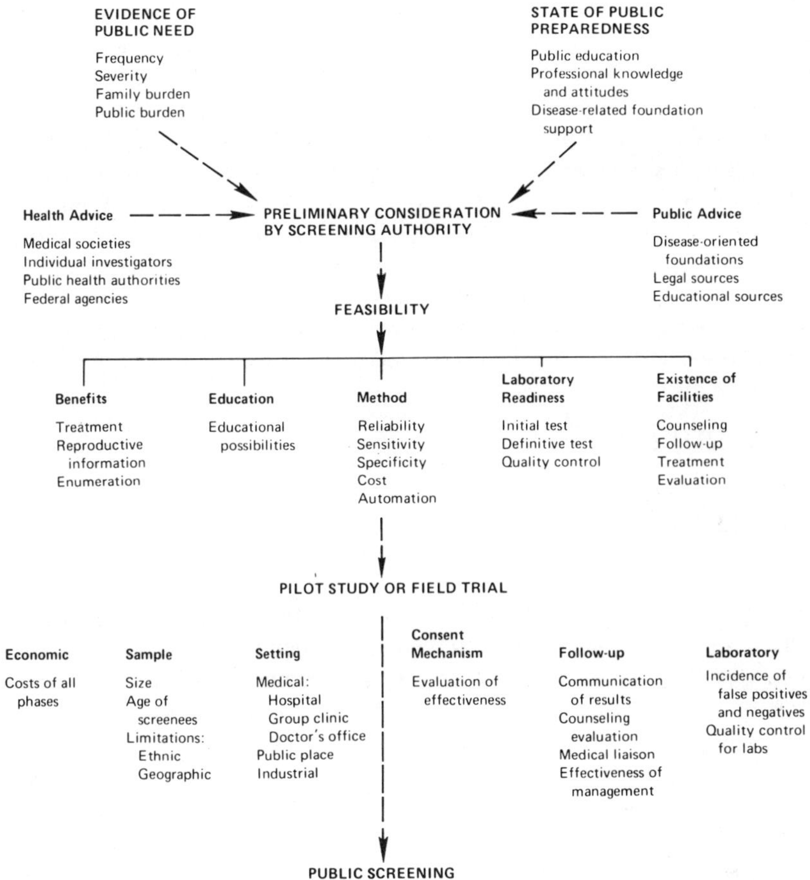

FIGURE 12-1 Procedure for evaluating proposed genetic screening program.

PRELIMINARY CONSIDERATION BY SCREENING AUTHORITY

A request to consider screening for a new disease or characteristic should initiate a review of the condition to establish the degree of public interest and acceptance and the need to invest public resources. The review should include evidence of the frequency and severity of the disorder, of its burden on patients and members of the family, including parents and sibs, and of the implications of the carrier state. It should also involve an assessment of the burden on the public in the form of costs of long-term care and of the maintenance and use of public facilities.

The screening authority will also wish to know the state of public preparedness to support the new screening program and should investigate whether, or how much, public education is needed, whether legal or ethical questions will be raised, and whether there are public or private interests that would be likely to support or oppose it.

Finally, it will be important to discover the extent of interest or concern of the medical profession, including the local medical societies, medical schools, public health authorities, and appropriate local and federal agencies. Advice on all these points should be obtained from appropriate sources. Such consultation with both the medical community and the lay public cannot fail to promote the effectiveness of any new screening program and to enhance the quality of old ones.

FEASIBILITY

Assuming a decision is made to consider a new genetic screening program, its feasibility must be investigated.

Benefits

These may be in the form of treatment or supportive management and reproductive information, or it may be decided that there is some public benefit to be had in simply enumerating the incidence or prevalence of the condition.

Education

The details of the prescreening education may depend upon the population to be screened, the age of the screenees, and whether the test is to be given in a physician's office, in a hospital, or during a mass screening in a school, church, or industrial setting. The possibility and effectiveness of exposure through newspapers or television or other public agencies should be considered, as should appropriate uses of school health education.

The Method

Alternative methods, if any, should be reviewed and one should be chosen for its reliability, sensitivity, specificity, and cost; the possibility of automation should be considered. A definitive follow-up test is also required when the screening test allows for false positives.

Laboratory Readiness

The readiness of the laboratory facilities to do both initial and definitive tests must be established. This may be no problem if a single state laboratory is responsible for all analyses, but if many laboratories are to be employed, the question of feasibility is complicated. Possibly, a single reference laboratory might be required; in any case, some form of quality control is necessary.

Facilities

No new screening program can be set up without provision for counseling, follow-up, treatment, and evaluation. Some assessment should be made of the numbers and qualifications of counselors needed and, for example, it should be determined whether some new training is required for counselors already dealing with screening for other characteristics.

If it is intended to screen a population for a disease, the issue of whether there is some form of treatment and, if so, how effective it is should come under review. If, for example, treatment appears to be successful but has been so little tried as still to be experimental, further investigation is required before screening for that disease should be instituted as a service. In addition, it will have to be determined whether the necessary means and manpower exist and can be disposed for reinforcement and evaluation of the counseling and for continuous supervision and evaluation of the treatment.

PRETEST OR FIELD TRIAL

Assuming the conditions are judged to be favorable for the institution of a new screening service, the whole system should be tried out in a pretest, which should be seen as experimental and which should be entered into with the express intention of determining whether the condition should be added to the list of those for which screening is done in the community. Such a pretest should, insofar as possible, meet all the requirements of a carefully controlled clinical trial.

Sample

For the pretest, some decision will have to be made as to the size and composition of the sample—e.g., the age, ethnicity, race, and sex of the screenees. A possible outcome of the pretest might be a decision not to limit the screening to any one group.

Setting

It will have to be decided whether the screening is to be carried out in physicians' offices, or periodically at schools or other convenient public centers, or on appointed days in mass screenings held in such public places as churches or schools. The pretest may reveal that one is better than another, thus determining which setting will be permanently employed.

Education

It is essential that whatever educational efforts are made be evaluated and amended from time to time. The pretest will offer opportunities to try various educational techniques in order to settle on those that are seen to be most effective in alerting the public and in increasing their knowledge and that can be shown to be associated with maximum public participation.

Consent

It will be important to test the workability of the proposed method for obtaining informed consent. This might best be developed in conjunction with the educational program so that the screenee will perceive that what he is consenting to do is closely related to what he has learned in the educational offering.

Follow-up

Facilities for communication of results, institution of treatment, and counseling must be arranged and their effectiveness evaluated. This is perhaps the most fallible part of the whole procedure, involving as it does many people who must work in concert. On the other hand, it is essential that no part of it fail, since weakness in any of the links may lessen the impact of the whole program.

Laboratory

If the test is a new one, time will be required to establish the reliability of the method. If many laboratories are to be used, the job of quality control is magnified. Careful review will have to be given to the incidence of false positives and especially of false negatives before the test can be finally approved.

Costs

The cost of implementation of a new test should be carefully calculated, including not only marginal costs but actual new expenditures required.

PUBLIC SCREENING

The final step in the process involves a decision by the screening authority to offer, or not to offer, the test as a service to the public. This decision will be determined in part by the successes or failures observed in the pretest, but also in part by those evidences of public and medical acceptance and sense of need that were considered in the beginning.

APPENDIXES

APPENDIX

A Work of the Committee

The National Research Council Committee for the Study of Inborn Errors of Metabolism held its first meeting in August 1972. During that meeting the Committee discussed its charge in detail and heard papers by Dr. Arno G. Motulsky, Committee member, who reviewed various categories of screening and discussed the interplay of genes, environment, and drugs, and by Dr. Charles R. Scriver, Committee member, who traced the development of screening for single-gene defects, for chromosomal anomalies, and for multifactorial malformations that produce morphologic or visible defects.

During the Committee's second meeting in October 1972, Dr. Neil A. Holtzman, Committee member, reviewed the history of the phenylketonuria screening program in the United States. At that same meeting, Dr. Robert F. Murray, Jr., Committee member, described the current screening programs for sickle cell anemia, and a third paper was given by Dr. Orlando J. Miller, Committee member, who discussed prenatal and neonatal screening methods and programs for the purpose of detecting chromosomal abnormalities.

The Committee had examined existing screening programs broadly at its first two meetings. At the third meeting, in December 1972, PKU was covered in detail. Speakers from five states were present: Dr. George C. Cunningham, Bureau of Maternal & Child Health, California State Department of Public Health; Dr. Robert A. MacCready, Massachusetts Department of Public Health; Dr. Lynn Maddry, Director, Laboratory Division, State Board of Health, North Carolina; Dr. Ronald Scott,

Professor of Pediatrics, University of Washington; and Dr. Benjamin D. White, State Health Department, Maryland. In addition, the Committee heard Dr. Harvey L. Levy of the Massachusetts Metabolic Disorders Screening Program, Massachusetts Department of Public Health, speak on the feasibility and costs of testing for a number of other metabolic disorders, using the same blood specimen as that for PKU.

In February 1973 the Committee met for the fourth time. At this meeting the Committee reviewed the data collected by the staff on PKU laws and state regulations. Dr. Judith P. Swazey, Consultant for the Brain Sciences Committee, NAS–NRC, Winchester, Massachusetts, discussed the historical development of PKU laws; Mr. Gary Clarke, Member, Eagleton Institute of Politics, Rutgers University, discussed the development of legislation; Mr. Alexander M. Capron, Committee member, discussed the PKU laws and the state regulations; Dr. Neil A. Holtzman, Committee member, discussed the proposed change in the Maryland bill and the establishment of a commission on hereditary disorders.

The fifth meeting of the Committee, in March 1973, dealt with the economic aspects of the PKU programs and the state of the art of registries in the United States. Dr. Gerald Rosenthal, Committee member, spoke on costs of screening in general and of PKU screening in particular. Registries, as they exist in the United States, were discussed by Dr. William J. Schull, Committee member.

During its sixth meeting, in May 1973, the Committee was addressed by Dr. Robert Guthrie, Research Professor of Pediatrics in Microbiology, Childrens Hospital, Buffalo, New York, who spoke in depth on PKU screening both in the United States and abroad and on the development of the tests for PKU and other disorders. Dr. Richard Koch, Principal Investigator, PKU Collaborative Study, Division of Child Development, Childrens Hospital of Los Angeles, explained how the program in California operates and gave the background of the development of the PKU Collaborative Study. Drs. Malcolm Williamson, Co-director, and James Dobson, Director, PKU Collaborative Study, Division of Child Development, Childrens Hospital of Los Angeles, spoke further on the Collaborative Study: its principal function, criteria for diagnosis and management, and success with data collection.

During the Committee's deliberation, it was decided to examine the management of PKU in the United Kingdom. Dr. Neil A. Holtzman, Committee member, carried out a study on PKU in the United Kingdom, personally visiting the various centers involved in the study.

During the first year of the Committee's work, it became apparent that there was a need for a field study and personal interviews in order to collect first-hand information and data on the evolution of the PKU laws and the role that was played by the medical societies, state health departments, state legislators, the NARC, and the local and state ARC's. The Committee employed Ms. Marilyn Jahn, a doctoral student in Sociology of Science and Medicine at the University of Pennsylvania, to carry out such a study. She collected data from Alabama, Arizona, Delaware, Florida, Illinois, Maryland, Massachusetts, Nebraska, New York, North Carolina, Texas, and Washington. Ms. Jahn was guided by the Chairman and staff during the study.

The Committee also developed a questionnaire to study and evaluate attitudes of physicians toward screening. This study was directed by Dr. Irwin M. Rosenstock, Committee member, with support from the Chairman and staff, and was conducted by the Commission on Human Resources of the NAS–NRC. (The questionnaire appears in Appendix G.)

During the first 6 months of the second year the Committee operated as three subcommittees and held five meetings.

The Subcommittee on Screening for the Purpose of Reproductive Advice held a 2-day meeting during July 1973. Chaired by Dr. Arno G. Motulsky, Committee member, the Subcommittee was addressed by directors of several of the sickle cell screening programs in the United States. Speakers and their topics were Dr. Robert B. Scott, Associate Professor of Medicine, Medical College of Virginia—"Sickle Cell Trait Screening and Counseling in Virginia"; Dr. Doris L. Wethers, Acting Director of Pediatrics, St. Luke's Hospital Center, New York—"Current Sickle Cell Screening Programs in New York City"; Dr. Donald L. Rucknagel, Professor of Human Genetics, University of Michigan Medical School—"Techniques in Sickle Cell Screening and Retention of Counseling by the Screenees"; Dr. George Stamatoyannopoulos, Research Professor of Medicine, Division of Medical Genetics, University of Washington School of Medicine—"Evaluation of a Sickle Cell Screening Program"; Dr. Robert F. Murray, Jr., Committee member—"Preliminary Data on Information Transfer in Genetic Counseling for Hemoglobinopathies"; and Dr. James E. Bowman, Professor of Pathology and Medicine, University of Chicago—"Sickle Hemoglobin Programs, Legal, Ethical and Economical Issues." The Subcommittee was briefed by the following people on the following topics: Dr. Richard T. O'Brien, Assistant Professor, Department of Pediatrics, Yale University School of Medicine—"Screening for Thalassemia Minor"; Dr. George Stamatoyannopoulos—"Screening in the Thalassemias"; Dr. Haig H. Kazazian, Jr., Assistant Professor of Pediatrics, Johns Hopkins University School of Medicine—"Hemoglobin Synthesis in the Developing Fetus"; Dr. Michael M. Kaback, Associate Professor of Pediatrics and Medicine and Associate Chief, Division of Medical Genetics, University of California, Los Angeles—"Experiences with Fetoscopy and Fetal Blood Sampling *in utero*"; Dr. Carlo Valenti, Full Professor of Obstetrics and Gynecology, Downstate Medical

Center, State University of New York—"Seven Years of Prenatal Genetic Diagnosis"; Dr. John S. O'Brien, Professor and Chairman, Department of Neurosciences, University of California School of Medicine, San Diego—"Pitfalls in the Prenatal Diagnosis of Tay-Sachs Disease"; Dr. Michael M. Kaback—"Psychosocial Studies in a Tay-Sachs Screening Program"; Dr. Harold M. Nitowsky, Professor of Pediatrics and Genetics and Director, Genetic Counseling Program, Albert Einstein College of Medicine—"Experiences with a Community Genetic Screening Program (Tay-Sachs)"; Dr. Charles J. Epstein, Committee member—"Prenatal Counseling and Diagnosis of Chromosomal Disorders"; Dr. Aubrey Milunsky, Director, Genetics Laboratory, Eunice Kennedy Shriver Center for Mental Retardation, Waltham, Massachusetts—"Prenatal Diagnosis—Current Experience and Future Practice"; Dr. Carlo Valenti—"Endo-amnioscopy and Fetal Blood Sampling"; Dr. Arno G. Motulsky—"Problems of Secondary Case Detection in Hereditary Disease—Family-Oriented Screening"; Mr. Robert A. Burt, Committee member—"Legal Comments." The Subcommittee met again in October 1973 to discuss its report to the parent committee.

The Subcommittee on Screening for the Purpose of Enumeration met in August 1973. At this meeting, speakers were Dr. Stanley Walzer, Assistant Professor of Psychiatry, Harvard Medical School, and Senior Associate in Clinical Genetics, Childrens Hospital Medical Center, Boston—"A Chromosomal Survey and the Related Behavioral Studies—Decisions, Details, and Dilemmas"; Dr. Arthur Robinson, Professor and Chairman, Department of Biophysics and Genetics and Professor of Pediatrics, University of Colorado Medical Center—"The Epidemiology of Chromosomal Abnormalities and the Prognosis of Newborns with Abnormalities of the Sex Chromosomes"; Dr. Herbert Lubs, Associate Professor of Pediatrics, University of Colorado Medical Center—"Surveys of New Haven, Connecticut, and Grand Junction, Colorado, Newborns"; Dr. Herbert Lubs—"Chromosome Studies in Seven-Year-Olds in the Collaborative Study of Cerebral Palsy and Mental Retardation: Abnormalities and Variance"; Dr. Digamber S. Borgaonkar, Associate Professor and Head of the Chromosome Laboratory, Johns Hopkins University School of Medicine—"Chromosome Study of Maryland Boys"; Dr. John L. Hamerton, Professor of Pediatrics (Human Genetics) and Director, Department of Genetics, Health Sciences Centre, Winnipeg, Manitoba—"Chromosome Abnormalities in a Canadian Neonatal Population—Three Years' Experience"; Dr. Herbert Lubs—"Present Status of Automated Chromosome Analysis at the National Biomedical Research Foundation."

The Subcommittee met once more in October 1973. At this meeting, it examined the studies that have been and are being carried out in the

United States merely for the purpose of collecting information. Dr. J. William Flynt, Jr., Chief, Birth Defects Section, Bureau of Epidemiology, Center for Disease Control, described the Center for Disease Control Study carried out in Atlanta and the combined study by CDC, The Commission on Professional and Hospital Activities, the National Institute of Child Health and Human Development, and the National Foundation. Dr. Gilbert W. Mellin, Associate Professor of Pediatrics, Columbia University, described the Fetal Life Study of the Columbia–Presbyterian Medical Center. Dr. James Miller, Professor and Head of the Department of Medical Genetics, University of British Columbia, described the British Columbia Registry for the delineation of birth defects, and Dr. Ronald Bachman, Chief, Division of Genetics, Department of Pediatrics, The Permanente Medical Group, Oakland, California, described the registry for the delineation of birth defects that he developed for the use of the Kaiser-Permanente Group.

The Subcommittee on Screening for the Purpose of Medical Intervention held a 2-day meeting in September 1973. The members discussed extensively the screening for α_1-antitrypsin deficiency, its historical development, and its methodology. Speakers for the first session were Dr. Richard C. Talamo, Associate Professor of Pediatrics, Harvard Medical School—"Alpha-1-antitrypsin Deficiency—Background Information"; Dr. Chester A. Alper, Scientific Director, Center for Blood Research and Associate Professor of Pediatrics, Harvard University—"Methods of Screening for "Alpha-1-antitrypsin Deficiency and Other Protein Deficiencies"; Dr. Robert H. Schwartz, Associate Professor of Pediatrics, University of Rochester School of Medicine and Dentistry—"Alpha-1-antitrypsin Screening in a Large Population"; Dr. Charles Mittman, Director, Department of Respiratory Diseases, City of Hope National Medical Center, Duarte, California—"Alpha-1-antitrypsin Screening in an Industrial Population"; Dr. Donald S. Fredrickson, Committee member—"Introduction to the Problem of Familial Hyperlipidemia/Hyperlipoproteinemia in Relation to Premature Atherosclerosis"; Dr. Joseph Goldstein, Chief, Division of Genetics, Department of Internal Medicine, University of Texas Southwestern Medical School—"Detection and Segregation of Familial Hyperlipidemia (with Emphasis on Familial Hypercholesterolemia)"; Dr. Peter O. Kwiterovich, Director, Lipid Research Clinic, The Johns Hopkins Hospital—"Neonatal Detection of Familial Hyperlipidemia"; and Dr. E. H. Kass, Professor of Medicine, Harvard Medical School and Director, Channing Laboratory, Boston City Hospital—"Familial Hypertension."

On the second day of the meeting, the Subcommittee considered the background and present status of screening in Canada, as well as specific programs supported by health departments in the province of Quebec and the states of Massachusetts and Oregon. On the second day the speakers and their topics were Dr. Charles R. Scriver, Committee member—"Genetic Services for Diagnosis, Counseling and Treatment in Canada"; Dr. Claude Laberge, Associate Professor of Genetics and Medicine and Director, Human Genetics Unit, Université Laval—"Integrated Multiphasic Screening and New Methodology"; Dr. Neil Buist, Associate Professor of Pediatrics and Medical Genetics, University of Oregon Medical School—"The Oregon Screening Program for Inborn Errors of Metabolism"; and Dr. Harvey L. Levy—"Newborn Screening in Massachusetts for the Inborn Errors of Metabolism."

The full Committee met again in December 1973. The speakers and topics for that session were Dr. Marshall H. Becker, Assistant Professor, Departments of Pediatrics and Psychiatry (School of Medicine), Behavioral Sciences (School of Hygiene and Public Health), and Social Relations (Arts and Sciences), Johns Hopkins University—"Factors Associated with Participation in a Tay-Sachs Screening Program"; Dr. Don P. Haefner, Professor of Health Behavior, School of Public Health, University of Michigan, and Dr. John P. Kirscht, Professor of Health Behavior, School of Public Health, University of Michigan—"Communication and Persuasion—Possible Applications of Research to Genetic Screening"; and Mr. O. Lynn Deniston, Lecturer, School of Public Health, University of Michigan—"Issues in the Evaluation of Screening Programs."

During subsequent meetings in February, May, and September of 1974, the Committee discussed the arrangement and contents of its final report. Committee members and staff prepared papers on the various subjects to be incorporated into the final report. These papers served as the foundation for the report, and a Writing Subcommittee was established to develop and edit the report. This Subcommittee met on June 26 and August 12, 1974. Members of the Writing Subcommittee were Dr. Barton Childs, Dr. Charles R. Scriver, Dr. Irwin M. Rosenstock, and Mr. Alexander M. Capron. The full Committee met September 9, 1974, to discuss the final draft of the report.

CONSULTANTS (PERSONS WHO ATTENDED THE COMMITTEE'S MEETINGS AND WORKSHOPS)

Dr. Chester A. Alper, Scientific Director, Center for Blood Research, and Associate Professor of Pediatrics, Harvard University

Dr. Jonathan Amsel, Post-doctoral Research Fellow in Pediatrics, The Johns Hopkins University

Dr. Ronald Bachman, Chief, Division of Genetics, Department of Pediatrics, The Permanente Medical Group, Oakland, California

Dr. Marshall H. Becker, Associate Professor, Departments of Pediatrics and Psychiatry (School of Medicine), Behavioral Sciences (School of Hygiene and Public Health), and Social Relations (Arts and Sciences), The Johns Hopkins University

Dr. Digamber S. Borgaonkar, Associate Professor and Head of the Chromosome Laboratory, The Johns Hopkins University School of Medicine

Dr. Joseph H. Boutwell, Chief, Clinical Chemistry, Hematology & Pathology Branch, Center for Disease Control

Dr. James E. Bowman, Professor of Pathology and Medicine, University of Chicago

Dr. George E. Brosseau, Jr., Project Officer, Program Manager, Exploratory Research and Problem Assessment, National Science Foundation

Dr. Neil Buist, Associate Professor of Pediatrics and Medical Genetics, University of Oregon Medical School

Mr. Gary Clarke, Member, Eagleton Institute of Politics, Rutgers University

Dr. Bernice Cohen, Professor of Genetics and Epidemiology, The Johns Hopkins University

Dr. George C. Cunningham, Bureau of Maternal and Child Health, California State Department of Public Health

Mr. O. Lynn Deniston, Lecturer, School of Public Health, University of Michigan

Dr. James Dobson, Director, PKU Collaborative Study, Division of Child Development, Childrens Hospital of Los Angeles

Dr. J. William Flynt, Jr., Chief, Birth Defects Section, Bureau of Epidemiology, Center for Disease Control

Dr. Joseph Goldstein, Chief, Division of Genetics, Department of Internal Medicine, University of Texas Southwestern Medical School

Dr. Robert Guthrie, Research Professor of Pediatrics in Microbiology, Children Hospital, Buffalo, New York

Dr. Don P. Haefner, Professor of Health Behavior, School of Public Health, University of Michigan

Dr. John L. Hamerton, Professor of Pediatrics (Human Genetics) and Director, Department of Genetics, Health Sciences Centre, Winnipeg, Manitoba

Dr. Frank Hoppensteadt, Associate Professor, Courant Institute of Mathematical Sciences, New York University

Mr. Rudolf P. Hormuth, Specialist in Services for Mentally Retarded Children, Maternal and Child Health Service, Health Services and Mental Health Administration

Ms. Marilyn Jahn, Doctoral Student in Sociology of Science and Medicine, University of Pennsylvania

Dr. Michael M. Kaback, Associate Professor of Pediatrics and Medicine, and Associate Chief, Division of Medical Genetics, University of California, Los Angeles

Dr. Yuet Wai Kan, Associate Professor of Medicine and Clinical Pathology and Laboratory Medicine, Chief, Hematology Division, San Francisco General Hospital

Dr. E. H. Kass, Professor of Medicine, Harvard Medical School, and Director, Channing Laboratory, Boston City Hospital

Dr. Haig H. Kazazian, Jr., Assistant Professor of Pediatrics, The Johns Hopkins University School of Medicine

Dr. John P. Kirscht, Professor of Health Behavior, School of Public Health, University of Michigan

Dr. Richard Koch, Principal Investigator, PKU Collaborative Study, Division of Child Development, Childrens Hospital of Los Angeles

Dr. Peter O. Kwiterovich, Jr., Director, Lipid Research Clinic, The Johns Hopkins Hospital

Dr. Claude Laberge, Associate Professor of Genetics and Medicine, and Director, Human Genetics Unit, Université Laval

Dr. David Levy, Professor of Biochemical and Biophysical Sciences, The Johns Hopkins University

Dr. Harvey L. Levy, Massachusetts Metabolic Disorders Screening Program, Massachusetts Department of Public Health

Dr. Herbert Lubs, Associate Professor of Pediatrics, University of Colorado Medical Center

Dr. Robert A. MacCready, Former Director of Diagnostic Laboratories, Massachusetts Department of Public Health

Dr. Lynn Maddry, Director, Laboratory Division, State Board of Health, North Carolina

Dr. Gilbert W. Mellin, Associate Professor of Pediatrics, Columbia University

Dr. James Miller, Professor and Head of the Department of Medical Genetics, University of British Columbia

Dr. Aubrey Milunsky, Director, Genetics Laboratory, Eunice Kennedy Shriver Center for Mental Retardation, Waltham, Massachusetts

Dr. Charles Mittmann, Director, Department of Respiratory Diseases, City of Hope National Medical Center, Duarte, California

Dr. Harold M. Nitowsky, Professor of Pediatrics and Genetics and Director, Genetic Counseling Program, Albert Einstein College of Medicine

Dr. John S. O'Brien, Professor and Chairman, Department of Neurosciences, University of California School of Medicine, San Diego

Dr. Richard T. O'Brien, Assistant Professor, Department of Pediatrics, Yale University School of Medicine

Dr. Gilbert S. Omenn, White House Fellow and Staff Assistant, U.S. Atomic Energy Commission

Dr. Arthur Robinson, Professor and Chairman, Department of Biophysics and Genetics, and Professor of Pediatrics, University of Colorado Medical Center

Dr. Donald L. Rucknagel, Professor of Human Genetics, University of Michigan Medical School

Dr. Robert H. Schwartz, Associate Professor of Pediatrics, University of Rochester School of Medicine and Dentistry

Dr. Robert B. Scott, Associate Professor of Medicine, Medical College of Virginia

Dr. Ronald Scott, Professor of Pediatrics, University of Washington

Mr. Arnold H. Spellman, Manager, Information Services Department, Commission on Professional and Hospital Activities

Dr. George Stamatoyannopoulos, Research Professor of Medicine, Division of Medical Genetics, University of Washington School of Medicine

Dr. Charles Stark, Chief, Epidemiology Branch, National Institute of Child Health and Human Development, National Institutes of Health

Dr. Judith P. Swazey, Consultant for the Brain Sciences Committee, NAS–NRC, Winchester, Massachusetts

Dr. Richard C. Talamo, Associate Professor of Pediatrics, Harvard Medical School

Dr. Carlo Valenti, Full Professor of Obstetrics and Gynecology, Downstate Medical Center, State University of New York

Dr. Stanley Walzer, Assistant Professor of Psychiatry, Harvard Medical School, and Senior Associate in Clinical Genetics, Children's Hospital Medical Center, Boston

Dr. Doris L. Wethers, Acting Director of Pediatrics, St. Luke's Hospital Center, New York

Dr. Benjamin D. White, Assistant Secretary for Programs, Department of Health and Mental Hygiene, State Health Department, Maryland

Dr. Malcolm Williamson, Co-director, PKU Collaborative Study, Division of Child Development, Childrens Hospital of Los Angeles

APPENDIX

B Glossary

Allele One of two or more alternative forms of the same gene.

Autosome Any chromosome other than the sex chromosomes (there are 22 pairs of autosomes in man).

Carrier Often used as synonymous with heterozygote; commonly, a nonmanifesting heterozygote.

Chromosome A darkly staining, rod-shaped body consisting of nucleic acids and protein and containing the genes.

Diploid An organism (like man) in which each type of chromosome except the sex chromosome is represented twice.

Dominant A gene is dominant if its phenotypic effect is fully expressed in the heterozygous state (in single dose).

Eugenics The study of methods to improve the hereditary constitution of a species.

Gene The unit of heredity. It is composed of deoxyribonucleate, is self-reproducing, is located in a definite position on a particular chromosome, specifies a particular biological function, and can mutate to various allelic forms.

Genetics The scientific study of heredity; the study of how particular qualities or traits are transmitted from parent to offspring.

Genetic drift Changes in gene frequency that are the result of random events; such changes are much more evident in small populations.

Gene frequency The frequency with which a particular allele occurs in a defined population.

Genotype The specific genes at a particular locus and/or the total genetic constitution of an individual, in both instances as distinct from the physical appearance (phenotype).

Heterozygote A diploid individual with dissimilar alleles at the same locus. A heterozygote will not breed true (See homozygote).

Heterogeneity Composed of dissimilar elements. May be applied both to genetic or phenotypic heterogeneity.

Homozygote Possessing an identical pair of alleles at a particular locus. A homozygote will breed true.

Homeostasis State of physiological and biochemical equilibrium.

Linkage The association of two or more genes (which are not alleles) during transmission to the next generation more often than expected by independent assortment. Linked genes are located on the same chromosome; the closer they are to each other on the chromosome, the more often they are transmitted together.

Locus The position a gene occupies on a chromosome.

Mutant A gene or chromosome that has undergone a transmissible structural change. By extension, an individual showing the effects of such a change may also be referred to as a mutant.

Mutation A transmissible change in the structure of a gene or chromosome.

Natural selection Discriminatory forces in the environment that determine the differential survival and, more important, the differential reproduction of individuals with certain genes in that population. This differential is caused by the different degrees of adaptation of various genotypes to their environments and accounts for the frequency of genes in populations.

Nondisjunction The failure of segregation of paired chromosomes.

Phenotype The appearance resulting from the interaction of the genotype with the environment.

Polymorphism The occurrence in a population of two or more different alleles each with a frequency above .01.

Recessive A characteristic requiring the simultaneous action of both alleles (homozygosity) for manifestion (see *Dominant*).

Sex chromosome The X and Y chromosomes, as distinguished from the autosomes.

Trait A characteristic or phenotype. The word is sometimes used to designate a heterozygous phenotype.

Translocation Transfer of a fragment of one chromosome into another, whether homologous or nonhomologous.

Variant A variation of the usual phenotype.

NOTE: For terms not included above, see King, Robert C. *A Dictionary of Genetics,* 2d rev. ed. Oxford University Press, New York, London, and Toronto, 1974.

APPENDIX

C Historical Aspects (Socioeconomic and Legislative) of the PKU Screening Program in the United States

TABLE C-1 History of PKU Laws [a]

State	Events in Development	Events in Passage	Writer	Introducer
Alabama	1964 screening begun by state laboratory because of publicity of Guthrie trials	AARC and Univ. of Alabama Med. Center recommended a law	Dr. J. McKee, Rehabilitation Research Foundation	Sen. C. Carter in Sena 65 cosponsors in th House
Arizona	No organized PKU program for screening or treatment; no Guthrie trial participation; 1967 state analysis offered for 1 year when federal funds stopped	Not passed	Sen. Sam Lena and NARC	1965 State Senators Ji Young and Sam Le (latter with retarded child) introduced mandatory law; Le conducts survey ea year and if screeni is down, he reintroduces bill
Delaware	No law; full cooperation of 10 hospitals in screening since 1962	None	—	—
Florida	1965 FARC pressed for mandatory law and continued after passage of voluntary law; 1967 Administrator of PKU program pushed for it; 1970 Fla. State White House Conference on Children and Youth recommended mandatory screening	Child with PKU had been missed by screening; mother pushed for bill	Mrs. Maxine Baker	Introduced by Mrs. Maxine Baker Rep. from Miami; both 1965 and 1971 bills
Illinois	1961 letter from parent of PKU child to Governor asking for assistance in supplying Lofenalac [b]; educational programs by state	1963 proposed law; 1965 IARC and Governor's Commission endorsed law	Governor's Commission on PKU	Rep. E. Chapman, Sen. Sapterstein

Lobbiers and Discussion	How?	Debate?	Outcome?	Action to Amend or Repeal?
Health Dept. identifies with Medical Assoc.; both apathetic	—	Not much; Health Dept. didn't oppose, but not supportive	1965 law passed; mandatory	State considering dropping program because of doubts on cost–benefit ratio
—	—	State Health Dept. and MD groups opposed; AARC supported; pediatricians' group opposed specifying a test	No PKU law; passed House, stopped in Senate	—
—	—	—	No PKU law	—
Opposed by State Medical Assoc. by direct contact behind-the-scenes; supported by FARC and some physicians dealing with retarded children; opposition only behind-the-scenes	—	Little debate	1965 passed as voluntary law but didn't work well enough; 1971 mandatory law, includes mandatory reporting of results (see Table C-4)	None now
1963–1965 IARC and Governor's committee for compulsory law passage; Medical Assoc. against requiring physician to screen	Letters, media	Opposed by Illinois State Medical Assoc.; much debate on mental retardation in media; support of IARC	First withdrawn, but 1963 voluntary bill passed; passed 1965 as compulsory	None known

TABLE C-1 (*Continued*)

State	Events in Development	Events in Passage	Writer	Introducer
Maryland	Limited screening begun 1960 by Dr. Benjamin White; MARC went to legislators to sponsor bill	State Health Dept. asked Medical Society to support screening in order to avoid law; they refused, laws were passed	Sen. Gore with State Health Dept.	Sen. Gore
Massachusetts	Dr. Guthrie introduced Dr. MacCready to test in 1962 and screening was begun; the finding of 3 positives in the first 8,000 tests stimulated interest	Supported by Dr. MacCready; sponsored by MARC officer; supported by State Medical Assoc.	Don't know	Mr. D. Pasciucco; Sen. G. Kenneally; 2 legislative members
Nebraska	Guthrie field trials 1963; 1966 educational effort to screen; NARC sought out legislators	1965 NARC initiated efforts. Academic Medicine, American Legion, AFL-CIO, Omaha Health Dept., all supported it; as did respected MD now dean of medical school	—	Sen. Fern Orme and others 1965 and 196[illegible]
New York	Impetus from bio-medical scientists: (1) Guthrie test development; (2) improved diet for treatment	NYARC promoted it; Dr. Guthrie was advocate	Sen. Wm. Conklin	Sen. Wm. Conklin, 1964

Lobbiers and Discussion	How?	Debate?	Outcome?	Action to Amend or Repeal?
Mrs. E. Shriver was refused official Health Dept. support; parents' groups lobbied by meeting with legislators	—	Some prominent pediatricians spoke in favor; medical society against	Passed 1965	Amended 1967: Medical Chirurgical Society Committee had strong negative feelings but could not foresee repeal of law; screening was just good medical practice; 1973 law was replaced with intent to future repeal; Commission on Hereditary Disorders formed by legislative mandate to (1) protect public from misplaced screening efforts; (2) avoid separate law for each genetic disorder. New laws to include: voluntary participation; nondirective genetic counseling; informed consent; confidentiality protection; decisions by committee of legislators, physicians and lay people
Department of Health representative supported bill	—	Very little	1963 mandatory	None
ARC, AFL-CIO, American Legion supported; pediatric chief from U. Nebraska Medical school supported	Meetings, media	MD's (including pathologists) and medical society objected; Christian Scientists wanted to be excluded; 2 legislators opposed	1965 bill withdrawn; mandatory law passed 1967; no provision for quality control but test result must be on birth certificate	None known
ressure by parents' groups; medical society against it	Testimony and publicity	No	Passed 1964, mandatory	Amended 1973 by Sen. Conklin to include 6 more inborn errors

TABLE C-1 (*Continued*)

State	Events in Development	Events in Passage	Writer	Introducer
North Carolina	No participation in 1962–1963 Guthrie trials; waiting for automated blood analysis procedure; main impetus from NCARC	Resolution and funding bill in 1966 by Dr. T. Scurletis of State Board of Health	None	None
Texas	1961 legislator with funds looking for suggestions on legislation	1963 State took part in Guthrie trials; 1963–1965 voluntary program; 1965 TARC shepherded bill	Rep. Steve Burgess: modified by TARC	Galveston legislator Maco Steward, 1961; later, Rep. Burgess
Washington	Participated in Guthrie trials; Children's Bureau encouraged legislation	1965 Joint PKU Committee (MD's and special interest groups) to advise legislature	Executive request bill	Sen. Frank Atwood and others

[a] ARC = Association for Retarded Children; State association is designated by first letters of state name
[b] Artificial diet low in phenylalanine.

Lobbiers and Discussion	How?	Debate?	Outcome?	Action to Amend or Repeal?
—	—	NCARC pressured for law in early 60's; State Board of Health member who was advisor to NCARC said compulsory screening not best approach; objections of private MD's	No PKU law (one of 7 states), but since 1965 has had State Board of Health screening program (voluntary). State Board of Health is controlled by Medical Society which publicized liability of MD for not screening, following up, and treating PKU	—
1964 Texas Plan to Combat Mental Retardation recommended screening; TARC lobbied for it	—	State Medical Society said urine test no good; Medical Society opposed law as precedent for other diseases	1961 bill withdrawn; 1965 bill passed (mandatory); compromise between TARC and Medica Society; follow-up of positive tests by county (not state) to maintain physician control on treatment; burden for screening on MD's; decentralized; therefore, counties without health officers or physicians not covered; no quality control on labs	—
WARC pressured; also some MD's, especially at University Medical School	—	Opposition from Medical Society because rigid law considered unresponsive to changes in clinical knowledge; no debate; resembles Texas and Alabama	1967 voluntary compromise law; decentralized labs; no quality control	—

TABLE C-2 Evaluative Questions

State	Respondent	Has the Law Helped?	Problems Left?	Who Follows up on Screening Issues?	Who Follows up on Diagnosis and Treatment?
Alabama	Physician, Univ. Alabama Medical Center	Yes, to screen, treat, counsel	Should have urine screen at 6 weeks	Health agency	Health agency
Arizona	Chief, Maternal and Child Health	No law	Some hospitals do not screen	No one	Health agencies
Delaware	Director of Maternal and Child Health	No law	State does not supervise screening at 4–6 weeks	State Board of Health	A. I. duPont Institute
Florida	Bureau of Maternal and Child Health	Yes, in administration and screening	Yes, compliance by outlying hospitals	Health Dept.	Health Dept.
Illinois	Pediatrician, Consultant to Association for the Mentally Retarded	Yes, in all ways	—	PKU Advisory Com., State Dept. Health	Same
Maryland	State Health Department	Yes, in all ways	—	State Dept. Health and State laboratories	2 medical centers

Massachusetts	Dr. R. MacCready	Made no difference	Maternal PKU genetic counseling	Peer review through Center for Disease Control in Atlanta	Children's Hospital
Nebraska	Director of State Laboratories	Somewhat, especially in screening	Quality control of labs poor, administration lax	Health agency	Health agency and medical centers
New York	Professor, State University Medical School	Yes, in all aspects	Fund raising	State health agencies	Health agencies and the medical profession
North Carolina	Director, Crippled Children's Branch, State Board of Health	Resolution—not law—did help	Lack of follow-up at level of county health dept., also maternal PKU	State laboratory	Health agencies and 2 treatment centers
Texas	Administrators, State Health Department	Yes, in all areas	No quality control on labs; need stronger regulations	PKU screening division of health agency	No one
Washington	Former Director of Maternal and Child Health	Yes, all aspects, but moderately	No quality control on labs; only 70–80% screening	Health dept. and medical society committee	Health dept. and PKU clinics

TABLE C-3 Attitudes [a]

State	Should There Be a Law Mandating Screening?	Should Treatment Be Required by Law?	Who Should Decide on Passage of Such Laws?
Alabama	Physicians at the Univ. of Alabama Med. Center: Yes, but only for PKU; other disorders too rare	Yes, for PKU	Only MD's and experts; not legislators or pressure groups
Arizona	AARC says yes	AARC says yes	AARC says medical professio and pressure groups
	Chief of MCH says no, it is unnecessary	MCH says no	MCH says medical community should have strongest say
Delaware	Child Diagnostic Center—duPont says no; so does MCH	No	Medical profession, public and pressure groups—not lawyers
Florida	FARC: Yes, voluntary didn't work	Not sure	Lawmakers with input from other groups
	PKU law sponsor: Yes, for PKU	No opinion	No opinion
	MCH: Yes, for PKU, since treatment available	No, but give free treatment	Medical profession, experts, pressure groups
Illinois	MD consultant to IAMR: Yes	No, not necessary	Medical, public, pressure groups
	MD Director PKU Clinic, Children's Memorial Hosp: Yes, if treatment available, as in PKU	No, not necessary, refer to treatment center	Specialists, experts, lawmakers, pressure groups
Maryland	Physician at Health Dept.: No	No, malpractice threat is enough	Experts and pressure groups
Massachusetts	State Health Dept. Lab: Yes, for PKU, but better for health departments to make regulations	No, threat of malpractice is enough	Medical profession and experts
	Ex-senator and sponsor of PKU law: Yes	If necessary	All groups
Nebraska	Dean, School Med., Univ. Nebraska: Yes, for PKU	No information	No information
New York	Dr. Guthrie: Yes, for PKU and other genetic problems	No	All groups: medical, legal and public
	Another pediatrician: No, regulations better than laws	No	Leaders should advise
North Carolina	Physician at the State Board of Health: No	Yes, parent should not decide	Medical profession, experts
	Professor of Pediatrics, Univ. N.C.: No	No answer	Not a proper area for laws
Texas	Health Dept.: Yes, for PKU and genetic diseases which can be treated	No opinion for PKU	All groups, especially medic and public health
	Legal counsel for Medical Assoc.: No	No	Medical profession
Washington	Practicing pediatrician: No	No	All—medical, expert and public groups
	Physician, Director PKU Clinic, Univ. Wash.: Only if there is no other way to get job done	Yes, if there are laws for screening	Medical and specialist group primarily, also others

[a] ARC = Association for Retarded Children; state association is designated by first letters of state name MCH = Office of Maternal and Child Health.

Should Government Be Involved?	Responsibility for Monitoring Screening	Was PKU Screening Premature?
Yes, but so far only for PKU	Experts and related professionals, not the public	No
Don't know	AARC says all professionals and the public	No
MCH says no	MCH says all professionals but not the public	No
Yes, for information and research only	All groups with vested interests (duPont); experts in field (MCH)	No
Yes, in all aspects except state gov't	Professional, public and pressure groups	Don't know
Yes, for PKU	No information	No information
Yes, for PKU	Experts in the field	Yes
Yes, for screening laws, information, research	Experts, government representatives	Perhaps
Yes, to assume cost	PKU committee and government representatives	No
Yes, for education	A special commission	Yes
Yes, especially for information and research	Prefer informal advisory group, primarily experts and professional medical groups with lay people represented	No
Yes, in all areas	A commission involving all groups	No
Yes, but not for treatment	No information	No
Yes, in laws, education, and research	There should be a special commission; citizens, professionals and experts should participate	No
Yes, for information and research	"High power" commission of experts and lay representatives	No
No answer	Should have advisory group for genetic disorders with input from all groups	No
Yes—only information and research	Experts—professional, medical	No
State yes for screening, education, research	Government and informal commission	Yes, needed more education first
Medical community should take lead	State Health Dept.	Don't know
Only on information through Medical Society	Not the government	No
Yes, for screening, treatment, information and research	Technical experts, plus the public	Probably in some places

TABLE C-4 Statistics and Economics

State	% of Newborns Screened before and after Law(s)	Source of Funds	Charge per Test ($)
Alabama[a]	No figures	Federal and state	0.49
Arizona[c]	75–80% in 1967; 66% in 1970	No information	3.00
Delaware[c]	97%	Maternal and Child Health services	1.12
Florida	75% vs. 85% in 1965[b]; 95+% in 1971[a]	Federal	0.75
Illinois[a]	60% vs. 97+% in 1973	Parents and third-party coverage	3.97
Maryland[a]	85% vs. 100% after 1966	State Health Dept.	0.26
Massachusetts[a]	100% before and after	State Health Dept.	0.50
Nebraska[a]	1966—majority of newborns; law stimulated screening but no figures; 99% is estimate	State Health Dept.	No information
New York[a]	85% vs. 100%	No information	0.66
North Carolina[c]	75% in 1966; 80% in 1967; 96% in 1968	Insurers	3.00
Texas[a]	No figures vs. 75% in 1971	No information	0.40
Washington[b]	50% vs. 78%	Federal grant and state funds	3.00

[a] Mandatory law.
[b] Voluntary law.
[c] No state PKU statute.

TABLE C-5 Preliminary Results of Screening for PKU

State	Births per Year[a] (1966)	White Births (% of Total)	No. of Neonates with Confirmed Positive PKU Test/ No. Tested	Incidence of PKU in White Neonates
Alabama	65,808	45	0/85,589 tested by 1972	—
Arizona	32,176	78	3 cases in 5 yr	—
Delaware	10,203	75	7/102,767 in 10 yr	1/10,000
Florida	101,643	63	19 in 5 yr (1966–1970)	1/16,000
Illinois	200,290	76	55/967,950 in 5 yr (1966–1970)	1/14,000
Maryland	63,756	70	26/360,000 in 6 yr (1965–1971)	1/10,000
Massachusetts	101,827	94	66/1,000,000 (1962–1972)	1/15,000
Nebraska	25,450	96	3 since 1966	—
New York	322,765	79	116 in 5 yr	1/11,000
North Carolina	92,863	56	3/68,993 in 1966	1/17,000
Texas	212,271	87	73 found in 9 yr; 9 found in 1st yr (1965)	1/17,000
Washington	50,116	92	15 in 7 yr (1965–1971)	1/19,000

[a] Data from *Statistical Abstract of the United States, National Data Book and Guide to Sources, 1967–1970*; 1966 was chosen because the laws for PKU screening were evolving in most states at that time.

TABLE C-6 Screening for PKU Compared with Nonfederal Maternal and Child Health Financial Effort

State	Estimate of % of Neonates Screened Currently	Type of Law	Date of Passage	Births[a] (1966)	Nonfederal MCH[b] Funds[c] ($) per Live Birth (1966)	Births[d] (1972)	Nonfederal MCH[b] Funds[e] ($) per Live Birth (1973)
Maryland	100	Mandatory	1965, 1967	63,756	35.53	51,059	154.8
Massachusetts	100	Mandatory	1963	101,827	7.84	79,522	12.22
New York	100	Mandatory	1964	322,765	28.52	254,431	11.15
Illinois	97+	Mandatory	1965	200,290	14.43	175,604	7.88
Delaware	97	None	—	10,203	17.82	8,867	24.81
North Carolina	96	None	—	92,863	18.72	89,491	19.13
Florida	95+	Mandatory	1965, 1971	101,643	35.43	108,985	75.00
Washington	78	Voluntary	1967	50,116	18.84	47,148	13.80
Texas	75	Mandatory	1965	212,271	9.17	219,822	9.90
Arizona	66	None	—	32,176	20.68	37,258	23.62
Nebraska	No information	Mandatory	1967	25,450	7.6	23,500	10.85
Alabama	No information	Mandatory	1965	65,808	11.24	61,869	18.46

[a] Statistical Abstracts, 1968.
[b] MCH = Maternal and child health.
[c] Unpublished state record books.
[d] *World Almanac*, 1974.
[e] Bureau of Community Health Services, Public Health Service State Health Dept. Budget or Expenditures Report for Formula Grant Programs, HSM 561-2, Fiscal Year 1973.

APPENDIX

D Statements by the American Academy of Pediatrics on Screening

Screening of Newborn Infants for Metabolic Disease*

COMMITTEE ON FETUS AND NEWBORN

An opportunity to establish screening procedures for case-finding in a number of metabolic diseases now exists in the United States, because most infants are born in hospitals where appropriate screening can easily be carried out. Case-finding in the neonatal period facilitates early inauguration of therapy, genetic counseling, and improved understanding of the natural history and incidence of metabolic diseases.

The Committee on Fetus and Newborn considered four types of screening programs: (1) screening of all newborn infants, (2) screening of specific groups of neonates with increased risk of certain disorders, (3) large-scale, pilot-screening programs, designed primarily for research and acquisition of knowledge about the natural history of disease, (4) screening of expectant mothers, particularly using tests of amniotic fluid.

The Committee did not consider screening of older children. However, it is emphasized that a number of important diseases, e.g., Wilson's disease, cannot be detected by screening in the first few days of life.

In evaluating screening tests for specific diseases, the Committee based its recommendations on the following criteria:

1. Does the seriousness of the disorder justify screening?
2. Is therapy for the disease in question available?

* Reprinted with permission from *Pediatrics* 35:499–501, 1965.

3. Is there a clearly identifiable segment of the population with an increased incidence of this disease?
4. Is it possible to perform reliable screening during the first few days of life?
5. Can the screening test be performed in a routine service laboratory?
6. Is the test acceptable to the physician and to a majority of parents?
7. Is the cost of the test acceptable?
8. Are there acceptable medical facilities prepared to confirm diagnosis and consult about the institution of therapy?

RECOMMENDATIONS

At the present time the Committee believes the following recommendations on screening programs are justified:

Phenylketonuria

A blood test for elevated concentration of phenylalanine performed no sooner than 24 hours after onset of milk feeding and prior to discharge is recommended for all newborn infants.*

A second blood test at 4 or 6 weeks of age is recommended for all infants. This will detect infants who had borderline or low plasma concentrations of phenylalanine in the first few days of life. It will also confirm a positive initial test.

Particular attention should be given to newborn infants in families in which another member is already known to have phenylketonuria, with these infants tested daily during the hospital stay. If results are negative at discharge, the infant should be tested at 1, 2, and 6 weeks of age.

Because of the difficulty of interpreting blood tests and the hazard of unwarranted dietary restrictions, it is recommended that the screening tests be performed in a large central facility, such as a state health department, or at least regional, laboratory. Only a very large facility will experience a sufficiently large number of tests positive for this rare disorder to acquire skill in diagnosis.

It is also most important that the laboratory have a close working relationship with a medical center where the diagnosis can be confirmed, the treatment diet chemically monitored, and the therapy supervised.

* Particular care must be exercised in interpreting results of tests in low birthweight infants for the accumulation of phenylalanine and the urinary excretion of reducing substances because positive findings may not indicate an inherited metabolic disorder in this group of neonates.

Mellituria

Every neonate* should have a test for reducing substances (i.e., not utilizing glucose oxidase) in the urine on the day of discharge from the hospital.

The test should be carried out by the individual hospital laboratory.

It should be noted that metabolic disorders involving galactose and fructose (e.g., hereditary fructose intolerance) will not be detected in infants who have not been exposed to the substance in their diet, e.g., fructose excretion will appear only if sucrose or fructose were present in feeding of an infant with fructose intolerance.

For newborn siblings in families of known galactosemics the following test is recommended: heparinized cord blood should be obtained for measurement of galactose-1-phosphate uridyl transferase activity.† The infant should be placed on a lactose-free milk substitute until galactosemia can be ruled out. If cord blood cannot be examined, a heparinized specimen of blood should be obtained as soon after birth as possible.

Other Metabolic Diseases

After considering a number of other possible screening programs for diseases including maple syrup urine disease, fibrocystic disease, succinylcholinesterase deficiency, glucose 6-phosphatase dehydrogenase deficiency, cretinism, and gargoylism, the Committee believes that at the present time screening tests for these disorders are not ready for application to *all* newborns. All infants born into a family in which an inherited metabolic disorder has been recognized previously should be carefully evaluated in the neonatal period and appropriate screening tests should be performed wherever possible.

The Committee urges that large-scale, research-oriented screening programs be undertaken at several centers; that several methods, including multiple inhibition assay, the newer chromatographic techniques developed for screening purposes, etc., be used in parallel, on blood samples; that all infants studied in the immediate neonatal period be studied again at 4–6 weeks. In this way, incidence and natural history of a large number of inheritable metabolic diseases may be investigated. In

* See footnote on page 302.

† If local facilities are not available, information concerning this determination may be obtained by phoning one of the following institutions: Children's Hospital of Los Angeles, Los Angeles, California (Dr. George N. Donnell); The Children's Hospital Research Foundation, Cincinnati, Ohio (Mrs. Helen K. Berry); Babies Hospital, New York, N.Y. (Dr. Ruth C. Harris).

addition, the most appropriate and efficient screening techniques can be determined. As knowledge accumulates such tests might become applicable to *all* newborns or older infants on a routine basis.

There is insufficient evidence at the present time to warrant screening of all expectant mothers.

COMMITTEE ON FETUS AND NEWBORN

William A. Silverman, M.D., *Chairman*
Alice Beard, M.D.
J. Edmund Bradley, M.D.
Moses Grossman, M.D.
Peter Gruenwald, M.D.
David Y. Hsia, M.D.
Joseph A. Little, M.D.
Jerold F. Lucey, M.D.
Jack Metcoff, M.D.
Henry K. Silver, M.D.
Samuel Spector, M.D.
Aldo Muggia, M.D. (*Corresponding Member*)

CONSULTANTS

William R. Bergren, Ph.D.
Helen K. Berry, M.A.
Robert W. Deisher, M.D.
Robert A. MacCready, M.D.
Fred Rosen, M.D.
Charles Scriver, M.D.
Irmin Sternlieb, M.D.

Statement on Treatment of Phenylketonuria*

COMMITTEE ON THE HANDICAPPED CHILD

In response to many requests from individuals and agencies, the following statement on the present status of treatment of phenylketonuria (PKU) has been prepared. The Committee on Fetus and Newborn has reviewed

* Reprinted with permission from *Pediatrics* 35:501–503, 1965.

the present status of neonatal screening for inborn errors of metabolism (e.g., PKU and related problems) and is reporting separately.

There is considerable discrepancy of opinion regarding the treatment of phenylketonuria. The enthusiasts say that with adequate mass screening, diagnosis, and early treatment, phenylketonuria can be eliminated as a cause of mental retardation; the doubters believe that there is need to improve screening procedures and that the efficacy of treatment leaves much to be desired.

AREAS OF AGREEMENT ON TREATMENT

In spite of discrepancies in the available data, certain facts appear to warrant acceptance, namely:

1. If PKU is detected early, and the infant is started on the proper diet *before 6 months of age,* and then is "adequately" maintained, the child usually will demonstrate borderline to average intelligence at 5 years of age. The earlier treatment is begun, in general, the better the result.
2. For the infant being treated with a diet low in phenylalanine, the acceptable concentration of phenylalanine in the serum probably lies above 3 mg/100 ml and below 8 mg/100 ml. Some insist that it be kept below 4–6 mg/100 ml. Concentrations over 12 mg/100 ml are almost certainly too high to achieve best results.
3. For optimum results the diet must be maintained rigidly and constantly, and at the same time the parents must also offer the child the usual affection, stimulation, discipline, and security necessary for normal behavioral development.
4. Wide individual variations exist in the dietary intake of phenylalanine (20–40 mg/lb in the newborn, and 8–20 mg/lb in the older child) which will result in acceptable levels of phenylalanine in the serum.
5. Frequent accurate determinations of the concentration of phenylalanine in the serum appears to be an integral part of management in order to maintain phenylalanine at a level which will permit normal physical growth without interfering with the development and function of the brain. Such determinations may be needed daily at the onset, then weekly or monthly, depending on the parents' ability to carry out prescribed dietary therapy.

Because of these and other problems of diagnosis and management, most clinics attempting optimal service to children with PKU utilize a multidisciplinary team. The co-ordination of pediatric, social work, psychological, nutritional, and nursing skills in such a team, together with the assistance of a qualified biochemical laboratory, facilitates good care of these children as well as studies of possible improvements in diagnosis and treatment. Since many pediatricians complete their training without ever seeing a case, and/or without the opportunity to supervise the care of children with the disorder over a period of time, it is recommended where possible that physicians take advantage of centers combining these multidisciplinary skills for assistance in diagnosis, treatment, follow-up care, and study of patients with phenylketonuria.

REASONS FOR CONFUSION ABOUT TREATMENT

Because an adequate and reliable diet first became available in this country only in late 1958 and because early screening tests have only recently come into general use, only a few patients have been discovered within the first month of life. Even they have been treated for less than 6 years, and this period of time is inadequate for assessing child development and projecting eventual intellectual ability on optimum treatment. The picture is further confused by the fact that there are rare individuals who biochemically have PKU (i.e., have an elevated concentration of phenylalanine in the blood, or fail adequately to convert a load of phenylalanine to tyrosine as compared to both normals and carriers) and yet are of normal intelligence. Intelligence quotients in twelve such patients so far reported ranged between 96 and 120. At least one infant, identified at birth and placed on the diet for only one year, probably falls into this category. Possibly he would have been entirely normal without any therapy. Although serum levels of phenylalanine in early life are undoubtedly critical, information about them is not available in most reports of such cases. Lack of recognition of the infrequency of such cases may lead to false conclusions that the diet may never be necessary or helpful.

Another difficulty in attempting to interpret results lies in the complete lack of uniformity of opinion as to what constitutes adequate control of dietary intake and what blood levels of phenylalanine should be maintained. Resolution of this difficulty is not aided by inclusion in reports of results of dietary treatment, of patients discovered late, i.e., after approximately 9 months of age, and of those discovered earlier and treated with a "low phenylalanine diet" as prescribed by books and tables, but without benefit of frequent determinations of the concentration of phenylalanine in the blood. Even if one pooled all existing data, it is doubtful that there would be sufficient evidence to judge what level of phenylalanine in the serum constitutes satisfactory control. The available evidence strongly suggests that the correlation of amounts of dietary phenylalanine per pound of body weight with serum levels of amino acid varies not only from age to age in the same child, but from child to child within the same family, and even more so from case to case in unrelated children. It is not yet established whether the serum level of phenylalanine in a patient with PKU needs to be as low as that found in the average unaffected child or adult (i.e., below 4 mg/100 ml) or only in the range of the normal-appearing parent and sibling carriers which may vary between 8 and 12 mg/100 ml after a meal of high protein content.

Lastly, because of the difficulties of maintaining the diet, it is impossible to be sure in any particular patient that the diet was consistently maintained on a day-to-day basis or was merely resumed before known testing periods, so that the child regained the desired serum concentration for the test only.

PROBLEMS IN DIETARY TREATMENT

It is the experience of those working closely with this disease that maintenance of the diet is easy during the bottle-feeding period. Difficulties arise when the child, who should be eating all foods, begins to forage himself. Here is where parental guidance, discipline of the child, and knowledge of the nutritional content of foods and food substitutes become of crucial importance. Utilization of accurate data on the phenylalanine content of all foods is a necessity for easier and better management.[1,2] A particular problem is that, as yet, there are no truly palatable bread substitutes with consistencies similar to actual bread or toast. Availability of satisfactory bread substitutes would make maintenance of the diet a much simpler task for mothers. Other good food substitutes low in phenylalanine are also urgently needed.

It is also generally agreed that severely retarded children first discovered to have PKU after the age of 2 years cannot be brought up to normal intelligence levels, but they usually can be helped. The changes wrought by the diet in these patients include amelioration of objectionable symptoms and behavior patterns, e.g., convulsions, irritability, destructiveness, short attention span, rocking, peculiar hand patterns, and eczema. It has been noted that some of the older children in the initial stages of treatment are temporarily made more hyperactive and difficult to manage, but this subsides and they ultimately become more tractable. The difficulty encountered in changing a child accustomed to eating what he wants, to a very restricted diet, as he simultaneously becomes more active and irritable, has led, in many cases, to the abandonment of the diet before beneficial effects have had a chance to manifest themselves. In older children, more than a year of therapy may be necessary before improvement is evident.

CONCLUDING COMMENT

Any objective evaluation of the results of dietary treatment of children with PKU must take into consideration a multiplicity of uncontrolled variables affecting the outcome. Included are the differing initial levels of intelligence and phenylalanine tolerance in each child, the differing heredities of each child (even in the same family), and the differing abilities and motivations of parents in maintaining the diet. However, it is clear, as stated earlier, that children with PKU can be helped if the problem is detected early enough and adequate treatment is begun promptly and maintained adequately.

This conclusion must not lead to unrealistic expectations or to overenthusiastic application of treatment programs. Some parents are either unwilling or unable to maintain dietary treatment. Over-rigidity of dietary management has led to early death, presumably from insufficient protein intake or hypoglycemia. Over-hospitalization for rigid control has deprived children of the normal stimulation and affection of home and family, thus preventing normal psychological maturation. Exaggerated predictions for normal development regardless of the age of discovery and irrespective of the strictness of the diet or of the hereditary endowment have led to frustration and discouragement on the part of both pediatricians and parents.

Much more data, taking into account all the known variables, must be accumulated and carefully analyzed before definitive statements can be advanced regarding the precise value of diet in preventing or ameliorating phenylketonuria. This will require considerable time. A collaborative study to evaluate management of this disease would be valuable.

COMMITTEE ON THE HANDICAPPED CHILD

Edward Davens, M.D., *Chairman*
C. M. Bielstein, M.D.
Robert W. Collett, M.D.
Sterling D. Garrard, M.D.
Robert Jaslow, M.D.
Robert G. Jordan, M.D.
Richard Koch, M.D.
Robert B. Kugel, M.D.
Thomas L. Nelson, M.D.
J. William Oberman, M.D.
Austin R. Sharp, M.D.
Richard L. Sleeter, M.D.
Melvin Sterling, M.D.

William T. Green, M.D., Consultant
Robert Warner, M.D., Consultant
John Bartram, M.D., Consultant

REFERENCES

1. Black, R. J., and Weiss, K. W.: Amino Acid Handbook, Methods and Results of Protein Analysis. Springfield, Illinois: Charles C Thomas, 1956.
2. Church, C. F., and Church, H. N.: Food Values of Portions Commonly Used (Bowes & Church), 9th Ed. Philadelphia and Montreal: J. B. Lippincott Co., 1963.

Phenylketonuria and the Phenylalaninemias of Infancy*†

COMMITTEE ON CHILDREN WITH HANDICAPS

In 1965 this Committee issued a statement outlining the responsibilities of the physician to the child with phenylketonuria, an inherited abnormality of amino acid metabolism.

A lack of knowledge about the disorder and about the results of treatment placed constraints on the 1965 statement. The Committee therefore feels that, with recent advances in knowledge about the disorder, a new statement is needed.

An increased level of phenylalanine in the blood can occur under sporadic and transient conditions in the absence of disease, with or without a concomitant elevation of serum tyrosine; it is always present in the disorder now called phenylketonuria. Because of incomplete information, simple classification of a specific case of phenylalaninemia is often not possible.

Screening programs allow for the detection of infants with elevated blood levels of phenylalanine. Screening programs should be encouraged and supported because they are the best available means for identifying all infants with abnormalities of protein metabolism resulting in serum phenylalanine elevations.

Two important, unresolved issues need clarification: (1) the effect of a persistently elevated blood level of phenylalanine on the intellectual

* Reprinted with permission from *Pediatrics* 49:628–629, 1972.

† This statement has been reviewed and approved by the Academy's Council on Child Health.

growth of the child when there are no other indications of disease, and (2) the possibility of harmful effects of a diet low in phenylalanine.

The basic treatment of phenylketonuria is to reduce circulating phenylalanine by dietary restriction; and, because a spectrum of disorders causes an elevation of that amino acid, differing approaches in management seem indicated.

The relative rarity of phenylketonuria precludes the opportunity for individual physicians to gain widespread experience and expertise in management outside of a hospital specialty clinic setting. Furthermore, it is desirable to group children with phenylketonuria and related disorders in a clinical setting because these children need the skillful management possible in a therapeutic environment with supportive laboratory and dietary care.

There is a definite need for continuing research and for clustering cases of the disease so investigators in the field will have access to adequate clinical material.

The management of a youngster with an elevated blood level of phenylalanine is complex, and controversy often arises about the appropriate course of action to be taken by a physician attempting treatment. There is no simple solution to the problem. Therefore, after careful consideration of available information, this Committee recommends that, wherever feasible, a child with phenylketonuria should be followed regularly in a clinic or university setting by physicians with expertise in the field, as well as by the child's primary physician, who should be encouraged to participate fully in the treatment program. The needs of the child and the physician, as well as the research needs of the discipline, will best be served by this approach.

COMMITTEE ON CHILDREN WITH HANDICAPS

Robert B. Kugel, M.D., *Chairman*
John Bowman Bartran, M.D.
Roger B. Bost, M.D.
James J. A. Cavanaugh, M.D.
Virgil Hanson, M.D.
John H. Kennell, M.D.
Jean McMahon, M.D.
Paul H. Pearson, M.D.
Roland B. Scott, M.D.
Theodore D. Scurletis, M.D.

Liaison:

J. Albert Browder, M.D.,
National Association for Retarded Children

Daniel Halpern, M.D.,
American Academy of Physical Medicine and Rehabilitation

Edwin W. Martin, Ph.D.,
Bureau of Education for the Handicapped, DHEW

APPENDIX

E American Academy of Pediatrics Statement on Compulsory Testing of Newborn Infants for Hereditary Metabolic Disorders, 1967

Statement on Compulsory Testing of Newborn Infants for Hereditary Metabolic Disorders*†

AMERICAN ACADEMY OF PEDIATRICS

The American Academy of Pediatrics recognizes the continuing impact of medical research on the care of infants and children and assumes responsibility for conveying newly acquired scientific knowledge to pediatricians to improve child care. The Academy encourages the passage of wise legislation, advises government and industry of health needs, and develops programs for improving the health care of infants and children. Out of these concerns for dissemination of information and advice on programs, the Academy believes a further statement on the compulsory testing of newborn infants for hereditary metabolic disorders is appropriate.

The rapid progress of scientific research makes available an ever increasing number of potentially useful diagnostic and therapeutic techniques. New and complex information is often disseminated to the general public in an over-simplified manner by the mass media. As a result, there

* Reprinted with permission from *Pediatrics* 39:623–624, 1967.

† Prepared with the assistance of an ad hoc committee of scientists and representatives of the Committee on Nutrition, the Committee on Fetus and Newborn, and the Committee on the Handicapped Child of the American Academy of Pediatrics, meeting on September 5, 1966, in Evanston, Illinois.

is often pressure to move with a sense of urgency when a new laboratory observation may have therapeutic benefits. Recognition of the reality of such pressure relieves neither the scientist nor the physician from responsibility to guide the translation of scientific observations into public policy.

New awareness of the molecular nature of hereditary metabolic disease, and the realization that medicine can use this knowledge to benefit the patient, may change the prognosis for these diseases. This spirit of optimism has prompted several legislative actions designed to benefit those affected. Statutes have been formulated in either permissive or compulsory terms to promote widespread screening programs for the early detection of certain heritable metabolic diseases. Legislative activity in this area is now almost nationwide.

On the one hand, some authorities are impressed with scientific and public health benefits that have accrued from these programs. On the other hand, some physicians believe that such legislation may not always operate in the best interest of affected children and could even work harm to the normal population. Failure to achieve expected health benefits as a result of premature and injudicious legislation may do irreparable harm to the orderly development of mass screening techniques for the early identification of disease and undermine public support of further research. In consideration of the current state of scientific knowledge and opinion, the principles enumerated here have been prepared to identify the present position of the American Academy of Pediatrics on this issue. These principles are, in part, a reiteration of those advocated previously by the Committee on Fetus and Newborn of the Academy. They are based on medical and scientific principles and on experience gained from the current programs for detection of phenylketonuria in newborn infants.

1. A clear and precise distinction must be made between interpretation of scientific research and evaluation and formulation of public policy. Science, by its nature, demands precise measurement for evaluation and must be judged by those with skill, knowledge, and judgment derived from scientific training. The mechanism of evaluating public policy is less precise since it is derived from political, social, and humanistic criteria.

2. The results of research may eventually lead to enactment of legislation to the end that a significant segment of the public will live in better health or greater comfort. However, such legislation will be inappropriate unless it is already supported by a sizeable body of scientific fact obtained through well designed experiment, suitable numbers of observations, critical scientific evaluation, and general acceptance of the results by the scientific community. Legislation must not be a mechanism for obtaining a large-scale test of any program.

3. In the public interest, legislation for compulsory screening programs must consider the availability of adequate techniques and facilities for the confirmation of the diagnosis and for therapy.

4. It is appropriate to consider the effect of such laws upon the utilization of available scientific and community resources. While lay groups with particular interests may appropriately inform government of unmet human needs, government must evaluate such needs in relation to the commitment of available scientific resources.

5. The Academy recognizes and encourages the efforts of governmental agencies and private groups to foster research into the nature of metabolic disease. However, it wishes to emphasize that such research must be allowed to proceed in whatever direction seems most fruitful to the individual investigator within broad guidelines and should not be hampered by legislation. Certainly, legislation should not hamper the continuation of further scientific research into the nature of metabolic disease.

At this time, the American Academy of Pediatrics favors neither the extension of current compulsory legislation nor passage of new legislation for the compulsory testing of newborn infants for the presence of congenital metabolic disease. The phenylketonuria program is already launched, and evaluation and the results may justify what has been done and offer guidelines for the future. No other diseases currently under study warrant similar legislation. The Academy believes that new scientific information can be applied most rapidly and most effectively by means of professional and public education operating in conjunction with adequate financial support for research.

APPENDIX

F American College of Obstetricians and Gynecologists: Maternal Phenylketonuria*

BACKGROUND

Phenylketonuria (PKU) is an inborn error of metabolism due to an autosomal recessive trait causing a deficiency in the enzyme phenylalanine hydroxylase with resultant inability to metabolize phenylalanine to tyrosine. In classic or infantile PKU, the affected infant is apparently normal at birth since its mother, although a heterozygous carrier of the trait, has normal phenylalanine metabolism and therefore, maintains normal phenylalanine levels in both herself and her fetus during pregnancy. Following birth, the metabolic defect in the infant results in hyperphenylalaninemia with its attendant neurotoxic sequelae, the severity of which depend on the blood phenylalanine level as well as other unknown factors. Recognition of this sequence, along with the demonstration that its deleterious effects may be prevented by a diet low in phenylalanine during infancy, has led to widespread use of screening procedures to detect PKU during the first few days of life. In many states, laws have been adopted requiring mandatory testing of newborn infants prior to discharge from the hospital.

Maternal PKU (i.e., PKU in the pregnant woman) has recently been recognized to have deleterious effects on fetal development. In this condition, the situation is in many ways the exact opposite of that with infantile PKU. The pregnant woman is homozygous for PKU while her fetus

* Reprinted with permission from ACOG Technical Bulletin No. 25, December 1973.

is heterozygous. Her elevated maternal blood phenylalanine levels during pregnancy are reflected in fetal hyperphenylalaninemia, further enhanced by the normal tendency of amino acids to be in greater concentration on the fetal than on the maternal side of the placenta. Thus, in contrast to the infantile form which causes neurologic damage *after* birth, maternal PKU exerts a deleterious effect *before* birth. The first report of the effects of maternal PKU appeared in 1963 (1) and numerous subsequent studies (2, 3, 4) have confirmed the dismal outcome in children born to women with the condition. All exhibit intrauterine and postnatal growth retardation, and mental retardation is virtually universal. At least 25 percent have major congenital malformations, involving a variety of organ systems.

The incidence of PKU is estimated to be approximately 1:20,000. Its importance lies, not in its frequency, but in its preventability as a cause of reproductive casualties (5).

RECOMMENDATIONS

Detection

A screening test should be considered in any woman of the childbearing age who (a) is mentally retarded, (b) has a family history of PKU, mental retardation, or microcephaly, or (c) has a child with intrauterine or postnatal growth retardation, mental retardation, or congenital anomalies. The appropriate screening test for PKU is determination of the blood phenylalanine level, a determination available in many laboratories. Normal values in the fasting state are less than 5 mg percent. Levels of 15 mg percent or greater are distinctly abnormal. Intermediate values (i.e., 5 to 15 mg percent) are of uncertain significance at the present time.

Management

A woman with documented PKU (or, in the case of minors or incompetents, her parents or guardian) should be apprised of the deleterious effects of the condition in pregnancy. Contraception, including permanent sterilization in particular, should be strongly advised. In patients already pregnant when first seen, abortion should be considered. For those in whom contraception or abortion is inapplicable, or unacceptable, a low phenylalanine diet should be maintained throughout pregnancy. It must be noted, however, that the value of dietary management of maternal PKU, while theoretically sound, is unproved. Moreover, for any beneficial effect, it should be initiated prior to pregnancy.

REFERENCES

1. Mabry, C. C., Denniston, J. C., Nelson, T. L., and Son, C.D.: Maternal phenylketonuria: Cause of mental retardation in children without the metabolic defect. N. Eng. J. Med. 269:1404–1408, 1963.
2. Frankenburg, W. K., Duncan, B. R., Coffelt, R. W., Koch, R., Coldwell, J. G., and Son, C. D.: Maternal phenylketonuria: Implications for growth and development. J. Pediatrics 73:560–570, 1968.
3. Fisch, R. O., Doeden, D., Lansky, L. L., and Anderson, J. A.: Maternal phenylketonuria: Detrimental effects on embryogenesis and fetal development. Amer. J. Dis. Child. 118:847–858, 1969.
4. Hsia, D. Y-Y.: Phenylketonuria: Clinical, genetic, biochemical aspects. Proceedings of the Second Congress of the International Association for Scientific Study of Mental Deficiency, pp. 105–113, 1970.
5. Johnson, C. F.: Phenylketonuria and the obstetrician. Obstet. Gynec. 39:942–947, 1972.

The Committee on Technical Bulletins wishes to thank the Committee on Nutrition, Dr. Roy M. Pitkin, FACOG, Chairman, for preparing this Technical Bulletin.

This Technical Bulletin is prepared (with consultation from appropriate experts) by the Committee on Technical Bulletins of The American College of Obstetricians and Gynecologists. It describes methods and techniques of clinical practice that are currently acceptable and used by recognized authorities. However, it does not represent official policy or recommendations of The American College of Obstetricians and Gynecologists. Its publication should not be construed as excluding other acceptable methods of handling similar problems.

G Data on Physicians' Knowledge and Attitudes

A mail questionnaire was developed (see p. 000, below) and sent to a probability sample of board-certified pediatricians, obstetricians/gynecologists, and family physicians. These three categories were selected because it was believed that physicians in these specialties would encounter patients with genetic disease or those at risk of transmitting genetic disease more frequently than physicians in other specialties.

The list and sampling fractions were

Every 15th name listed in the American College of Obstetricians and Gynecologists (1972)
Every 12th name listed in the American Academy of Pediatrics (1973)
Every 33rd name listed in the American Academy of Family Physicians (1973)

In each case, where the directory showed membership distinctions, physicians were eliminated who were unlikely to be board-certified or currently in practice—such as "emeritus," "correspondent," "honorary member," "candidate." The first eight questions on the survey instrument were included as a further screen to eliminate nonpracticing physicians.

The sampling fractions were planned to yield samples of approximately 800 in each of the three major specialties. Provision was made for two follow-up letters for nonrespondents. A final nonresponse rate was predicted to be about 35%, which would have yielded at least 500 specialists in each category. The response rate turned out to be 57.0% for pediatricians, 41.5% for obstetricians, and 34.8% for family practitioners—constituting an overall rate of 44.6% representing 1,092 respondents. Except for the differential response rates by specialty, only minor differences were found between respondents and nonrespondents on demographic characteristics such as geographic location and sex.

Detailed tables follow, to substantiate the general description of the survey results reported in Chapter 9. A full presentation of the study findings will be published independently, because the full scope of the study will go beyond the requirements of the present report.

TABLE G-1 Physicians' Reported Experience with Potential Genetic Disorders

Frequency of Contact with High-Risk Patients	Pediatricians		Obstetricians		Family Practitioners		Total	
	N	%	*N*	%	*N*	%	*N*	%
I have never had such patients	18	10.8	11	3.3	31	11.1	60	7.7
I have rarely had such patients	32	19.2	89	26.4	106	38.1	227	29.0
I have occasionally had such patients	65	38.9	179	53.1	115	41.4	359	45.9
I have had quite a few such patients	29	17.4	48	14.2	21	7.6	98	12.5
I have had a great many such patients	23	13.7	10	3.0	5	1.8	38	4.9
Total	167	100.0	337	100.0	278	100.0	782	100.0
Not applicable, no response	301	—	3	—	6	—	310	—

TABLE G-2 Physicians' Reported Experience with Actual Gentic Disorders in Children

Frequency of Contact	Pediatricians		Obstetricians		Family Practitioners		Total	
	N	%	*N*	%	*N*	%	*N*	%
Never	2	0.4	71	46.7	27	11.8	100	11.8
Extremely infrequently	77	16.6	40	26.3	100	43.7	217	25.7
Infrequently	203	43.8	40	26.3	94	41.0	337	39.9
Significantly frequently	181	39.1	1	0.7	8	3.5	190	22.5
Total	463	100.0	152	100.0	229	100.0	844	100.0
No response	5	—	188	—	55	—	248	—

TABLE G-3 Perceived Frequency of Genetic Defects in Live Births, by Specialty

Perceived Frequency of Defects	Pediatricians		Obstetricians		Family Practitioners		Total	
	N	%	*N*	%	*N*	%	*N*	%
Less than 1%	150	34.9	122	40.1	128	51.6	400	40.7
1–5%	240	55.8	163	53.6	108	43.5	511	52.0
6–10%	30	7.0	15	4.9	9	3.6	54	5.5
More than 10%	10	2.3	4	1.3	3	1.2	17	1.7
Total	430	100.0	304	100.0	248	100.0	982	100.0
No response	38	—	36	—	36	—	110	—

TABLE G-4 Proportion of Physicians Believing Each of Four Special Actions Is Warranted by Inborn Errors of Metabolism

Special Actions	Pediatricians		Obstetricians		Family Practitioners		Total	
	N	%	*N*	%	*N*	%	*N*	%
More emphasis on metabolic errors in medical education	313	76.0	222	78.4	193	81.4	728	78.1
Continuing medical education	408	95.8	286	96.0	232	93.5	926	95.3
Community-wide screening programs for selected genetic conditions	247	61.6	161	58.3	137	60.1	545	60.2
Prenatal screening programs for inborn errors having no postnatal therapies	214	54.9	148	54.6	124	55.4	486	54.9

TABLE G-5 Physicians' Subjective Opinion of Risk of Hemophilia, Given a Stated Objective Probability of Occurrence of 1/4 for Child of Unknown Sex or 1/2 for Male Child

	Pediatricians		Obstetricians		Family Practitioners		Total	
Subjective Risk Is Believed to Be	*N*	%	*N*	%	*N*	%	*N*	%
High	415	90.8	280	85.6	201	78.2	896	86.1
Medium	34	7.4	38	11.6	37	14.4	109	10.5
Low	8	1.8	9	2.8	19	7.4	36	3.5
Total	457	100.0	327	100.0	257	100.0	1041	100.0
No response	11	—	13	—	27	—	51	—

TABLE G-6 Physicians' Subjective Opinion of Risk of Tay-Sachs Disease, Given a Stated Probability of Occurrence of 1/4

	Pediatricians		Obstetricians		Family Practitioners		Total	
Subjective Risk Is Believed to Be	*N*	%	*N*	%	*N*	%	*N*	%
High	392	86.0	255	78.2	176	70.7	823	79.8
Medium	57	12.5	64	19.6	62	24.9	183	17.7
Low	7	1.5	7	2.1	11	4.4	25	2.4
Total	456	100.0	326	100.0	249	100.0	1031	100.0
No response	12	—	14	—	35	—	61	—

TABLE G-7 Physicians' Subjective Opinion of Risk of Down's Syndrome, Given a Stated Probability of Occurrence of 1/100

Subjective Risk Is Believed to Be	Pediatricians		Obstetricians		Family Practitioners		Total	
	N	%	*N*	%	*N*	%	*N*	%
High	67	14.7	74	22.8	46	18.5	187	18.2
Medium	206	45.2	126	38.9	80	32.3	412	40.1
Low	183	40.1	124	38.3	122	49.2	429	41.7
Total	456	100.0	324	100.0	248	100.0	1028	100.0
No response	12	—	16	—	36	—	64	—

TABLE G-8 Physicians' Subjective Opinion of Risk of Cleft Lip/Palate, Given a Stated Probability of Occurrence of 1/25

Subjective Risk Is Believed to Be	Pediatricians		Obstetricians		Family Practitioners		Total	
	N	%	*N*	%	*N*	%	*N*	%
High	96	21.1	74	22.7	39	15.2	209	20.2
Medium	239	52.6	165	50.6	122	47.7	526	50.8
Low	119	26.2	87	26.7	95	37.1	301	29.1
Total	454	100.0	326	100.0	256	100.0	1036	100.0
No response	14	—	14	—	28	—	56	—

TABLE G-9 Reported Genetic Disorders Encountered in Practice[a]

	Pediatricians		Obstetricians		Family Practitioners		Total	
Condition	*N*	%	*N*	%	*N*	%	*N*	%
Single-gene defects	724	39.2	42	22.0	105	24.9	871	35.5
Chromosomal defects	541	29.3	54	29.5	131	31.0	726	29.6
Malformations	242	13.1	60	32.8	102	24.2	404	16.5
Multifactorial conditions	158	8.5	7	3.8	40	9.5	205	8.4
Subtotal	1665	90.1	163	89.1	378	89.6	2206	90.0
Conditions of unknown origin	73	4.0	3	1.6	12	2.8	88	3.6
Nongenetic conditions	5	0.2	2	1.1	3	0.7	10	0.4
Response too vague to be coded	105	5.7	15	8.2	29	6.9	149	6.0
Subtotal	183	9.9	20	10.9	44	10.4	247	10.0
Total responses	1848	100.0	183	100.0	422	100.0	2453	100.0

[a] The denominator for this table is number of responses rather than physicians; multiple responses were often given.

TABLE G-10 Beliefs about Assertion That Many Metabolic Disorders Are Genetically Determined

	Pediatricians		Obstetricians		Family Practitioners		Total	
Agreement with Assertion	*N*	%	*N*	%	*N*	%	*N*	%
Clear agreement	358	77.0	210	62.5	144	52.4	712	66.2
Partial agreement	84	18.1	81	24.1	87	31.6	252	23.4
Uncertain	18	3.9	41	12.2	37	13.5	96	8.9
Partial disagreement	4	0.9	4	1.2	6	2.2	14	1.3
Clear disagreement	1	0.2	0	—	1	0.4	2	0.2
Total	465	100.0	336	100.0	275	100.0	1076	100.0
No response	3	—	4	—	9	—	16	—

TABLE G-11 Perceived Impact on Affected Children and Families If All Treatment for Genetic Disorders Were Discontinued

	Pediatricians		Obstetricians		Family Practitioners		Total	
Perceived Impact	*N*	%	*N*	%	*N*	%	*N*	%
Extremely serious	255	56.0	150	45.2	82	29.3	487	45.6
Moderately serious	137	30.1	106	31.9	111	39.6	354	33.2
Not serious	22	4.8	16	4.8	20	7.1	58	5.4
Of unknown severity	35	7.7	44	13.3	49	17.5	128	12.0
No opinion	6	1.3	16	4.8	18	6.4	40	3.7
Total	455	100.0	332	100.0	280	100.0	1067	100.0
No response	13	—	8	—	4	—	25	—

TABLE G-12 Referrals of Patients for Determination of Genetic Disorders within Past 5 Years, by Specialty

	Pediatricians		Obstetricians		Family Practitioners		Total	
Referrals	*N*	%	*N*	%	*N*	%	*N*	%
Single-gene defects	334	67.2	128	25.8	35	7.0	497	100.0
Chromosomal defects	409	50.3	212	31.3	57	8.4	678	100.0
Malformations	44	41.5	51	48.1	11	10.4	106	100.0
Multifactorial conditions	20	44.4	16	35.6	9	20.0	45	100.0
Conditions of unknown origin	41	67.2	15	24.6	5	8.2	61	100.0
Nongenetic conditions	3	75.0	1	25.0	0	—	4	100.0
Response too vague to be coded	87	50.6	62	36.0	23	13.4	172	100.0

TABLE G-13 Preferred Modes of Management for Each Class of Genetic Condition—All Medical Specialties Combined

	Genetic Condition													
	Single-Gene		Chromosomal Defects		Malformations		Multifactorial		Cause Unknown		Non-genetic		Too Vague To Be Coded	
Preferred Management Mode	*N*	%	*N*	%	*N*	%	*N*	%	*N*	%	*N*	%	*N*	%
Counseling	252	28.8	74	20.8	19	48.7	23	45.1	12	35.3	2	20.0	17	31.5
Abortion	157	17.9	129	36.2	8	20.5	1	2.0	4	11.8	2	20.0	8	14.8
Therapy	176	20.1	23	6.5	3	7.7	13	25.5	10	29.4	3	30.0	6	11.1
All of the above	31	3.5	17	4.8	—	—	—	—	2	5.9	—	—	5	9.3
Counseling and abortion	103	11.8	61	17.1	2	5.1	4	7.8	2	5.9	3	30.0	6	11.1
Therapy and abortion	42	4.8	27	7.6	1	2.6	1	2.0	1	2.9	—	—	6	11.1
Counseling and therapy	115	13.1	23	6.5	4	10.3	9	17.6	3	8.8	—	—	6	11.1
Referral	—	—	2	.6	2	5.1	—	—	—	—	—	—	—	—
Total	876	100.0	356	100.0	39	100.0	51	100.0	34	100.0	10	100.0	54	100.0

TABLE G-14 Perceived Probability of Effective Management of Genetic Conditions—Management Modes and Specialties Combined

	Genetic Condition													
	Single-Gene		Chromosomal Defects		Malformations		Multifactorial		Cause Unknown		Nongenetic		Too Vague To Be Coded	
Probability of Success	*N*	%	*N*	%	*N*	%	*N*	%	*N*	%	*N*	%	*N*	%
High	510	58.2	236	66.2	18	46.2	23	45.1	16	47.1	7	70.0	26	48.1
Medium	242	27.6	88	24.7	12	30.8	13	25.5	12	35.3	1	10.0	16	29.6
Low	94	10.7	25	7.0	6	15.4	12	23.5	5	14.7	2	20.0	9	16.7
Medium to high	19	2.2	3	.8	1	2.6	1	2.0	1	2.9	—	—	3	5.6
Low to medium	11	1.3	4	1.1	2	5.1	2	3.9	—	—	—	—	—	—
Total	876	100.0	356	99.8	39	100.1	51	100.0	34	100.0	10	100.0	54	100.0

TABLE G-15 Physicians' Opinions of the Effectiveness of Their Own Genetic Counseling

	Pediatricians		Obstetricians		Family Practitioners		Total	
Belief about Own Counseling	*N*	%	*N*	%	*N*	%	*N*	%
Highly effective	90	24.9	84	35.6	24	18.0	198	27.1
Partially effective	200	55.2	111	47.0	64	48.1	375	51.3
Ineffective	7	1.9	7	3.0	16	12.0	30	4.1
Cannot estimate	65	18.0	34	14.4	29	21.8	128	17.5
Total	362	100.0	236	100.0	133	100.0	731	100.0
No response	106	—	104	—	151	—	361	—

TABLE G-16 Perceived Importance of Detecting Potential or Actual Genetic Disorders, by Specialty

	Pediatricians		Obstetricians		Family Practitioners		Total	
Importance of Detection	*N*	%	*N*	%	*N*	%	*N*	%
Extremely important	239	51.7	155	46.5	84	30.2	478	44.5
Important	204	44.2	169	50.8	175	62.9	548	51.1
Unimportant	7	1.5	2	0.6	15	5.4	24	2.2
Other	12	2.6	7	2.1	4	1.4	23	2.1
Total	462	100.0	333	100.0	278	100.0	1073	100.0
No response	6	—	7	—	6	—	19	—

TABLE G-17 Beliefs about Whether Screening for Particular Traits or Conditions Should Be Encouraged

	Pediatricians		Obstetricians		Family Practitioners		Total	
Should Screening Be Encouraged?	*N*	%	*N*	%	*N*	%	*N*	%
Yes	379	83.5	245	77.3	136	51.7	760	73.5
No	21	4.6	16	5.0	30	11.4	67	6.5
No opinion	54	11.9	56	17.7	97	36.9	207	20.0
Total	454	100.0	317	100.0	263	100.0	1034	100.0
No response	14	—	23	—	21	—	58	—

TABLE G-18 Opinions about the Desirability of Screening for Genetic Disorders

	Pediatricians		Obstetricians		Family Practitioners		Total	
Preferences for Screening	*N*	%	*N*	%	*N*	%	*N*	%
Community-wide campaigns	178	38.4	134	39.9	111	39.8	423	39.2
Physician or hospital service	260	56.0	175	52.1	134	48.0	569	52.7
Both community programs and medical service	9	1.9	14	4.2	5	1.8	28	2.6
No opinion	9	1.9	11	3.3	22	7.9	42	3.9
Opposed to screening	8	1.7	2	0.6	7	2.5	17	1.6
Total	464	100.0	336	100.0	279	100.0	1079	100.0
No response	4	—	4	—	5	—	13	—

TABLE G-19 Beliefs about the Relative Benefits of Screening for PKU over the Past Few Years

	Pediatricians		Obstetricians		Family Practitioners		Total	
Beliefs about Benefits	*N*	%	*N*	%	*N*	%	*N*	%
Screening has been beneficial	129	28.9	90	28.4	53	19.9	272	26.4
Screening has not been beneficial	159	35.7	89	28.1	88	33.1	336	32.7
Don't know	158	35.4	138	43.5	125	47.0	421	40.9
Total	446	100.0	317	100.0	266	100.0	1029	100.0
No response	22	—	23	—	18	—	63	—

TABLE G-20 Beliefs about the Relative Benefits of Screening for Sickle Cell Trait over the Past Few Years

	Pediatricians		Obstetricians		Family Practitioners		Total	
Beliefs about Benefits	*N*	%	*N*	%	*N*	%	*N*	%
Screening has been beneficial	119	26.7	107	33.6	53	20.3	279	27.2
Screening has not been beneficial	107	24.0	60	18.9	37	14.2	204	19.9
Don't know	219	49.2	151	47.5	171	65.5	541	52.8
Total	445	100.0	318	100.0	261	100.0	1024	100.0
No response	23	—	22	—	23	—	68	—

TABLE G-21 Beliefs about the Medical Significance of Carrying the Sickle Cell Trait

	Pediatricians		Obstetricians		Family Practitioners		Total	
Medical Significance	*N*	%	*N*	%	*N*	%	*N*	%
Harmless	61	14.1	49	15.9	35	14.1	145	14.6
Rarely causes problems	198	45.6	90	29.1	62	25.0	350	35.3
Occasionally causes problems	160	36.9	147	47.6	114	46.0	421	42.5
Frequently causes problems	15	3.5	23	7.4	37	14.9	75	7.6
Total	434	100.0	309	100.0	248	100.0	991	100.0
No response	34	—	31	—	36	—	101	—

TABLE G-22 Sources of Medical Information and Perceived Importance of Detecting Genetic Disease

	Perceived Importance of Detection										
	Extremely Important		Important		Un-important		Other		Total		
Proxy Measure of Knowledge	*N*	%	*N*	%	*N*	%	*N*	%	*N*	%	No Response
Reads at least two journals containing genetic information and regularly attends out-of-state professional meetings	190	50.7	169	45.1	9	2.4	7	1.9	375	100.0	6
Does one of above	215	45.2	249	52.3	4	0.8	8	1.7	476	100.0	7
Does neither	73	32.9	130	58.6	11	5.0	8	3.6	222	100.0	6
Total	478	44.5	548	51.1	24	2.2	23	2.1	1073	100.0	19

TABLE G-23 Perceived Risk of Four Genetic Diseases[a] and Perceived Importance of Detecting Genetic Disease

	Perceived Importance of Detection										
	Extremely Important		Important		Un-important		Other		Total		
Perceived Risk of Four Genetic Diseases	*N*	%	*N*	%	*N*	%	*N*	%	*N*	%	No Response
All four are high risk	51	62.2	29	35.4	2	2.4	0	0	82	100.0	1
Three are high risk	87	58.0	60	40.0	1	0.7	2	1.3	150	100.0	2
Two are high risk	258	45.9	281	50.0	6	1.1	17	3.0	562	100.0	4
One is high risk	65	33.5	116	59.8	9	4.6	4	2.1	194	100.0	1

[a] See question 17 of questionnaire.

TABLE G-24 Experience with Genetic Disease and Perceived Importance of Detecting Genetic Disease

	Experience with Genetic Disease					
	Frequent		Occasional		Rare or None	
Importance of Detection	*N*	%	*N*	%	*N*	%
Extremely important	158	58.1	283	40.0	31	36.9
Important	108	39.7	387	54.7	50	59.5
Unimportant	2	0.7	19	2.7	3	3.6
Other	4	1.5	19	2.7	0	—
Total	272	100.0	708	100.0	84	100.0
No response	4	—	9	—	4	—

TABLE G-25 Perceived Impact of Genetic Disease on Affected Families and Perceived Importance of Detecting Genetic Disease

	Impact on Affected Families							
	Extremely Serious		Moderately Serious		Not Serious		No Opinion	
Importance of Detection	*N*	%	*N*	%	*N*	%	*N*	%
Extremely important	287	59.8	125	35.6	7	12.1	50	31.1
Important	175	36.5	218	62.1	43	74.1	100	62.1
Unimportant	4	0.8	5	1.4	7	12.1	7	4.3
Other	14	2.9	3	0.9	1	1.7	4	2.5
Total	480	100.0	351	100.0	58	100.0	161	100.0
No response	7	—	3	—	0	—	7	—

TABLE G-26 Perceived Benefits of PKU Screening and Perceived Importance of Genetic Screening

	Benefits of PKU Screening					
	Beneficial		Don't Know		Not Beneficial	
Importance of Detection	*N*	%	*N*	%	*N*	%
Extremely important	140	51.9	192	46.6	124	37.5
Important	118	43.7	207	50.2	188	56.8
Unimportant	5	1.9	8	1.9	10	3.0
Other	7	2.6	5	1.2	9	2.7
Total	270	100.0	412	100.0	331	100.0
No response	2	—	—	—	5	—

MEDICAL OPINIONS AND EXPERIENCES CONCERNING GENETIC DISORDERS

Please return completed questionnaire in the enclosed stamped, self-addressed envelope to:

Commission on Human Resources - JH 638
National Research Council
2101 Constitution Avenue, Washington, D.C. 20418

A. BACKGROUND INFORMATION

1. Are you currently engaged in medical practice?

   1 ☐ YES ↓ 2 ☐ NO, please return the questionnaire in the enclosed envelope (7)

   1 ☐ Solo practice
   2 ☐ Group practice - fee for service
   3 ☐ Group practice - prepaid
   4 ☐ Other (please specify)________________________________ (8)

2. What is the nature of your practice?

   1 ☐ Specialty practice ↓ 2 ☐ General practice (Go to Q.6) (9)

3. Which speciality? 1 ☐ Pediatrics
   2 ☐ Obstetrics-Gynecology
   3 ☐ Other (please specify)________________________ (10)

4. Do you have board certification in your specialty?

   1 ☐ YES 2 ☐ NO (11)

5a. Is your major employment in an academic institution?

   1 ☐ YES ↓ 2 ☐ NO (Go to Q.6) (12)

b. Are you responsible for the care of patients?

   1 ☐ YES (Go to Q.6) 2 ☐ NO, please return the questionnaire in the enclosed envelope (13)

6. When did you receive your medical degree?

   1 ☐ 1970 or later 3 ☐ 1960-1964 5 ☐ 1940-1949
   2 ☐ 1965-1969 4 ☐ 1950-1959 6 ☐ Prior to 1940 (14)

7. How long have you been in medical practice, i.e., since completion of your house staff experience?

   1 ☐ Less than 2 years
   2 ☐ 2-5 years
   3 ☐ 6-10 years
   4 ☐ 11 years or longer (15)

8. Do you regularly participate in medical school or hospital educational functions such as grand rounds?

   1 ☐ YES 2 ☐ NO (16)

9. What are your most frequent sources of information about new medical problems and practices? (check all that you use regularly) (17-22)

1 ☐ Discussion with other practitioners
2 ☐ Medical journals (which ones?) 1.________________

2.________________

3.________________ (23-28)

3 ☐ Regular attendance at in-state professional meetings
4 ☐ Regular attendance at out-of-state professional meetings
5 ☐ Participation in continuing education courses
6 ☐ Literature from pharmaceutical firms
7 ☐ Drug detail men
8 ☐ Other (please specify)________________

10. When you were in medical school, did your school offer one or more courses in genetics?

1 ☐ YES (Go to Q.11) 2 ☐ NO (Go to Q.12) (29)

11. Did you take one or more courses in genetics?

1 ☐ YES 2 ☐ NO (Go to Q.12) (30)

1 ☐ a required course
2 ☐ an elective course
3 ☐ both a required and an elective course
4 ☐ neither
5 ☐ other (please specify)________________ (31)

B. CHARACTERISTICS OF PRACTICE

QUESTIONS 12 AND 13 ARE DIRECTED TOWARD PHYSICIANS WHOSE PRACTICE INCLUDES A SUBSTANTIAL PROPORTION OF ADULT PATIENTS.

12. How frequently would you estimate your practice has involved potential genetic disorders, that is, adults at greater risk than that of the normal population of having offspring with genetic disorders? (32)

1 ☐ I have never had such high risk patients (Go to Q.14)
2 ☐ I have rarely had such high risk patients
3 ☐ I have occasionally had such high risk patients
4 ☐ I have had quite a few high risk patients
5 ☐ I have had a great many high risk patients
6 ☐ Not applicable; I see relatively few or no adults (Go to Q.14)

13. Please indicate in descending order of frequency the genetic problems confronted (e.g., Sickle Cell), listing the most frequent first.

1.________________ 4.________________

2.________________ 5.________________

3.________________ (33-42)

QUESTIONS 14 AND 15 ARE DIRECTED TOWARD PHYSICIANS WHOSE PRACTICE INCLUDES A SUBSTANTIAL PROPORTION OF PEDIATRIC PATIENTS.

14. How frequently would you estimate your practice has involved actual genetic disorders in children? (43)

1 ☐ Never (Go to Q.16) 3 ☐ Infrequently
2 ☐ Extremely infrequently 4 ☐ Significantly frequently

15. Please indicate in descending order of frequency the genetic problems confronted (e.g., PKU, Down's Syndrome), listing the most frequent first.

1.________________ 4.________________

2.________________ 5.________________

3.________________ (44-53)

16. Within the last five years have you referred any of your patients or parents of your patients for determination of possible genetic disorders? (54)

1 ☐ YES 2 ☐ NO (Go to Q.17)

Which conditions? 1.________ 3.________ 5.________

2.________ 4.________ (55-64)

17. This question attempts to define your professional opinions about what constitutes high, low or medium risk of genetic disorders in offspring. For each of the four hypothetical situations described please indicate whether you would consider the risk of genetic disease in an offspring to be high, medium or low. The question concerns probability of occurrence, not seriousness of the condition.

	Risk of Disease in an Offspring			
	High	Medium	Low	
a) A female patient is known to be a carrier for hemophilia. The probability of her bearing a child with the disease is 1/4; if the child is male, the probability is 1/2.	☐	☐	☐	(65)
b) A husband and wife are each known to be carriers for the Tay-Sachs gene. The probability of their having a child with the disease is 1/4.	☐	☐	☐	(66)
c) A female patient, aged 30, has had a previous child with Down's Syndrome. If the usual incidence of Down's Syndrome for a mother of 30 years of age is about 1/1200, her probability of having a second affected child is about 1/100.	☐	☐	☐	(67)
d) A couple has had one child with cleft lip/palate. The risk of their having another child with this condition is about 1/25.	☐	☐	☐	(68)

C. OPINIONS ABOUT GENETIC SCREENING AND GENETIC DISEASE

18. Generally speaking, how important do you believe it is to attempt to detect potential or actual genetic disorders? (69)

1 ☐ Extremely important 2 ☐ Important 3 ☐ Unimportant 4 ☐ Other (please specify)

____

19. Specifically, are there any genetic traits or conditions for which you believe either antenatal or postnatal screening should be encouraged? (70)

1 ☐ YES 2 ☐ NO (Go to Q.21) 3 ☐ No opinion (Go to Q.21)

Please list those you are thinking of 1.________ 4.________

2.________ 5.________

3.________ (71-80)

20. For each condition listed above indicate the kind of management, if any, that you would recommend and your opinion about how effective that treatment is likely to be.

	Conditions (as you listed them above)	Recommended treatment (e.g., counseling, abortion, therapy)	Probability of successful counseling or therapy (high, medium, low)
1.			
2.			
3.			
4.			
5.			

(6-15)

21. Should genetic screening be required by law?

1 ☐ YES, for all testable conditions 2 ☐ NO 3 ☐ No opinion (16)

4 ☐ YES, but only for the following conditions:

1.__________________ 4.__________________

2.__________________ 5.__________________

3.__________________ (17-26)

22. Some recent literature suggests that many metabolic disorders associated with enzymatic deficiencies are genetically determined. Which single statement best describes your opinions on this matter? (27)

1 ☐ I believe the assertion is true and expect even more such metabolic disorders will be shown to have genetic determinants in the future.
2 ☐ I believe the assertion is true but have no clear opinions about what future research will show.
3 ☐ I am not certain about the truth of the assertion.
4 ☐ I believe that the role of genetic influences as causes of metabolic disorders has been somewhat exaggerated.
5 ☐ I believe that the role of genetic influences as causes of metabolic disorders has been greatly exaggerated.

QUESTIONS 23 AND 24 ARE HYPOTHETICAL AND HAVE NO CLEAR-CUT "CORRECT" ANSWERS. WE DO, HOWEVER, WISH TO ELICIT YOUR OPINIONS. IF YOU WISH TO QUALIFY ANY ANSWER IN TERMS OF CONDITION, TYPE OF PATIENT, ETC., PLEASE WRITE YOUR ANSWER IN THE SPACE PROVIDED FOR COMMENTS.

23. In your view, if treatment for all genetic disorders of metabolism were discontinued, how serious, in general, would the impact be on affected children and their families?

1 ☐ Extremely serious COMMENTS (if any)__________________
2 ☐ Moderately serious
3 ☐ Not serious __________________
4 ☐ Of unknown severity
5 ☐ No opinion __________________ (28)

24. In your view, if treatment for all genetic disorders of metabolism were discontinued, what would be the general financial and social impact on society?

1 ☐ Extremely serious COMMENTS (if any)__________________
2 ☐ Moderately serious
3 ☐ Not serious __________________
4 ☐ Of unknown severity
5 ☐ No opinion __________________ (29)

25. In general, do you approve of a) organized, community-wide campaigns for screening for the carrier state in genetic disease, b) do you prefer such tests to be offered only as a service through physicians or hospitals, or c) do you prefer such tests not to be given at all?

1 ☐ Prefer community campaigns ↓ 2 ☐ Prefer physician service or hospital (Go to Q.26) 3 ☐ Am opposed to genetic screening (Go to Q.28) 4 ☐ No opinion (Go to Q.28) (30)

Who should organize such campaigns? (check one or more)

1 ☐ Voluntary health organizations 4 ☐ Medical societies (31-35)
2 ☐ State or local health departments 5 ☐ Others (please specify)
3 ☐ The federal government

____

26. Who should pay for the service? (check all that apply)

1 ☐ The individual screened (or his third-party payer) 3 ☐ The federal government
2 ☐ The state, city or county 4 ☐ Voluntary agencies
5 ☐ Other (please specify) (36-40)

____

27. Do you have general criteria for referral of patients for genetic screening? (41)

1 ☐ YES   2 ☐ NO (Go to Q.28)   3 ☐ Don't know (Go to Q.28)

What are your criteria? ______________________________

____

______________________________ (42)

28. Do you favor screening for genetic disorders to increase scientific knowledge, even when there is no treatment for the disorder?

1 ☐ YES   2 ☐ NO (44)

29. Have you ever had occasion to provide genetic counseling for any patients?

1 ☐ YES   2 ☐ NO (Go to Q.32) (45)

For which conditions? 1.____________

2.____________

3.____________ (46-51)

30. In general, how effective do you believe your genetic counseling to have been?

1 ☐ Highly effective   3 ☐ Ineffective (52)
2 ☐ Partially effective   4 ☐ Cannot estimate effectiveness

31. Have you experienced any significant difficulty in communicating genetic information to high risk parents?

1 ☐ YES   2 ☐ NO (Go to Q.33) (53)

What problems have you experienced? (check all that apply)

1 ☐ Communicating the concept of probability of disease in subsequent children (54-57)
2 ☐ Communicating the concept of severity and impact of disease
3 ☐ Communicating the proper preventive or remedial actions that may be required
4 ☐ Other (please specify) 1.____________

2.____________

3.____________

32. In your opinion, are the difficulties in genetic counseling great enough to warrant more widespread development of specialized genetic counseling centers, or are physicians adequately equipped to provide genetic counseling? (58)

1 ☐ Most physicians are competent to provide needed counseling.
2 ☐ Most physicians, with some additional training, would be competent to provide needed counseling.
3 ☐ Most physicians should be competent to provide most needed counseling, but should have genetics counseling clinics available for complicated cases.
4 ☐ Most counseling should be done by trained genetic counselors in special clinics.
5 ☐ Genetic disorders are so infrequent that no special provisions for counseling are necessary.
6 ☐ No opinion.

33. In your opinion, have the benefits of screening for PKU over the past few years outweighed the costs?

1 ☐ YES   2 ☐ NO   3 ☐ Don't know (Go to Q.34) (59)

Please explain______________________________

____

____

34. In your opinion have the benefits of detection of the Sickle Cell carrier over the past few years outweighed the costs?

1 ☐ YES   2 ☐ NO   3 ☐ Don't know (Go to Q.35) (60)

Please explain______________________________

____

35. In your opinion, have the benefits of screening for any other genetic conditions over the past few years outweighed the costs? (61)

1 ☐ YES → Which ones?
2 ☐ NO (Go to Q.36)
3 ☐ Don't know (Go to Q.36)

____

____

______________________________ (62-67)

36. In your opinion, what is the <u>medical</u> (in contrast to genetic) significance of being a sickle cell trait carrier? (68)

1 ☐ harmless
2 ☐ causes medical problems exceedingly rarely
3 ☐ causes medical problems occasionally
4 ☐ causes medical problems frequently

37. Do you favor the idea of listing persons with genetic disease in a national or regional registry which would be available to physicians for rapid identification of high risk relatives so as to prevent new cases of genetic disease? (69)

1 ☐ I am opposed to such registers
2 ☐ I favor such registers without qualification
3 ☐ No opinion
4 ☐ I would favor such registers with the following qualifications: ______________________________

____

____

____

38. In your opinion, how frequent are genetic defects among live births? (70)

1 ☐ Less than 1% of live births
2 ☐ 1-5% of live births
3 ☐ 6-10% of live births
4 ☐ More than 10% of live births

39. In your opinion, are inborn errors of metabolism occurring with sufficient frequency to warrant <u>each</u> of the following special actions?

	YES	NO	
a) Placing more emphasis on metabolic errors in medical education?	☐	☐	(71)
b) Providing continuing medical education on the topic?	☐	☐	(72)
c) Instituting community-wide screening programs for selected genetic conditions?	☐	☐	(73)
d) Instituting prenatal screening programs for inborn metabolic errors for which there are no postnatal therapies?	☐	☐	(74)
e) Other (please specify) ______________________________	☐	☐	(75)

____

____

APPENDIX

H Screening for PKU in the United Kingdom

When treatment for PKU became available—and screening of newborns therefore appeared beneficial—the National Health Service was already in existence in the United Kingdom. Lines of communication between the central government and local health personnel existed, and health services were comprehensive and coordinated. This report considers how these factors influenced the development, operation, and effectiveness of the PKU program.

STRUCTURE OF THE NATIONAL HEALTH SERVICE

The National Health Service was established by Parliament in 1946. "The Secretary of State for Social Services is responsible to Parliament for seeing that health services of all kinds and of the highest possible quality are available to all who need them."[1] Approximately 95% of all health services are financed by tax revenues and insurance contributions. The Department of Health and Social Security (DHSS) and, for Scotland, The Scottish Home and Health Department disperse most of the funds. They communicate to hospitals through 20 Regional Boards, to practitioners through 157 Executive Councils, and to health professionals engaged largely in preventive medicine (health visitors and domiciliary midwives) through 231 Local Health Authorities, supervised by Medical Officers of Health. There is at least one teaching hospital in each Region. (The numbers do not include Northern Ireland.)

The organization of the health sector is not, however, as tight as this makes it sound. A Local Health Authority may straddle the jurisdiction of two or more Regional Boards. And the DHSS does not have the power to specify the lines of communication between regions, or between practitioners, hospitals, and local authorities. The reorganization of the National Health Service, which became effective April 1, 1974, should remedy these problems.

DEVELOPMENT OF PKU SCREENING AND MANAGEMENT POLICIES

History

In 1960 the Ministry of Health suggested to the Medical Research Council (MRC) that a conference committee be appointed and a conference be held to consider the detection and management of PKU.[2] As a result of the conference the Ministry asked Medical Officers of Health "to consider undertaking routine screening tests of infants aged 4–6 weeks" using the Phenistix method on urine.

The Conference report noted "the importance of using standardized methods of biochemical control and mental testing" and suggested that "full opportunity should be provided for the collection of complete data on the progress of all cases reported in Britain." Consequently, in 1964 the MRC's Working Party on Phenylketonuria (a continuation of the conference committee) and the DHSS organized a register for phenylketonuria that was to include all phenylketonurics diagnosed after January 1, 1964.

Today, the Register is notified of new patients by two sources: the screening laboratory and the pediatric consultant, who is asked to complete a follow-up form once a year on each patient in whom the diagnosis is confirmed. Conscientious and complete reporting requires pediatricians to standardize, to some extent, their management of children with PKU because specific psychometric and behavioral assessments, physical measurements and developmental evaluations at designated ages, and monitoring of the blood phenylalanine concentration are all requested. In addition, a provocation test with normal food is recommended 4 and 9 months after treatment starts.

Only through compliance with the Register are standardized management procedures approached. Legitimate disagreement regarding optimal management hampers further standardization. A Working Party subcommittee, established in 1968, is considering "the feasibility of initiating a study to determine the optimum duration of treatment of patients suffering from phenylketonuria." In the absence of a formal protocol it is anticipated that some pediatricians will terminate the diet at a specific age while others will continue it. By comparing results, which will be reported to the Register on the standard forms, it is hoped that some conclusion regarding optimum duration of therapy will emerge.

The Register records were incomplete for the first few years. They did indicate, however, that the Phenistix test was not detecting all infants who were tested and later turned out to have PKU. Of the 71 PKU infants reported to the Register who were born in 1964 and 1965 and screened before 3 months of age, 24 had a negative Phenistix on the first test. Fourteen of the 24 missed were tested after 4 weeks of age, as recommended.[3,4]

The Working Party then coordinated a study to determine whether better methods of detection were available and at what age they should be employed. Urine and blood from newborn siblings of known phenylketonurics and infants with positive screening tests (usually the Guthrie) were tested by four different screening methods at designated ages between 5 and 28 days (a few determinations were performed earlier). In 21 infants, a diagnosis of PKU was established and the age at which each test first became positive was compared. On the basis of the results, the Working Party recommended use of either the Guthrie test on blood or the urine *o*-hydroxyphenylacetic paper chromatographic method[3]; and suggested that the Guthrie test be performed at 5 days of age or later and the urine *o*-hydroxyphenylacetic acid test at 10 days or later (fluorometric and chromatographic procedures for the detection of blood phenylalanine were not evaluated).

In recommending the age at which screening should be performed, the Working Party took into consideration a personal communication from Robert Guthrie, in which he estimated that at least 11% of infants with PKU would be missed if the Guthrie test was performed only during the first 3 days of life, and a report published by Hsia[5] showing that blood phenylalanine rose significantly during the first week of life in infants with PKU.

In September 1969, the DHSS notified appropriate components of the health delivery system that it had accepted the recommendation of the Working Party "that Phenistix testing of infants for phenylketonuria should be replaced by the Guthrie test on blood specimens . . . between the 6th and the 14th day of life."[6] The circular made the following points: (a) Infants still in the hospital on the sixth day were to be tested by the hospital but infants discharged by then were the responsibility of the Local Authority's Medical Officer of Health. (b) "An adequate recording and tracing system [should] be organized to insure that all babies are tested, their results made known and further investigation and therapy instituted at the earliest date." (The circular advised that a standard request form was available.) (c) The laboratory procedures should be "concentrated to the greatest possible extent." (Implementation was left to the Regional Hospital Boards.) (d) Other methods could be used, but parallel studies with the Guthrie test would be valuable. (e) Infants with positive tests "should be referred immediately to the consultant pediatric service which will advise on the diagnosis and treatment." (f) "Special advisory centers, with the necessary facilities for the biochemical control of treatment, psychometric testing and expert dietary advice could with advantage be associated with the designated laboratory." (g) "Where a diagnosis of phenylketonuria has been made the general practitioner will have to play a part in the further management of the patient." (The relation between the general practitioner, consultant pediatrician, and special advisory centers was not stipulated.)

Major Attributes of the British Policy Development

Policy Formation Policy regarding PKU screening was established but not mandated by the DHSS. Medical and scientific expertise was sought, and utilized, in the formulation of this policy. The continuing operation of the MRC's Working Party facilitates the research necessary to improve detection and management of PKU. (However, progress on a prospective study on dietary management has been slow.) Input on non-health professionals is negligible.

Policy Implementation Policy is disseminated to hospitals, practitioners, and Local Authorities through established channels, although there is no legal enforcement of the policy. The participation of health professionals who are involved in screening for, and management of, PKU in the formulation of policy (by membership on the MRC's Working Party) improves the likelihood that the policy will be accepted at the operating level. The only centralized effort at quality control is through the PKU Register, which, if fully utilized, would indicate whether infants were being missed by screening and would also yield information regarding the outcome of treatment. Since 1970 reporting has probably been virtually complete.

Policy Review A number of people were asked under what circumstances Parliament might intervene in the establishment of policy. Parliament has in the past, through legislation, specifically asked the DHSS to look into particular health problems (hearing loss). Generally, it was believed that if a health need were not being met, intervention might be forthcoming, but that this would not necessarily take the form of legislation. The Secretary of State for Social Services could be asked to explain the DHSS policy and perhaps be given time to formulate one.

OPERATION OF PKU PROGRAMS

This section considers the extent to which the various programs reflect the objectives stipulated in the 1969 DHSS circular.[6] Information was collected from interviews with screening center directors and data provided by them. Directors of only 10 of the 37 screening centers were interviewed, but these centers performed over 60% of all tests.[7] (It should be noted that the interviewees, who are listed in Table H-8, included those most intimately involved in the development of PKU screening, and hence their programs may reflect the objectives to a greater than average degree.) Directors of eight PKU clinics were also interviewed. They care for well over half of all phenylketonuric children discovered as a result of screening.

Completeness of Screening

Implementation of Phenistix testing was rapid. Although the Medical Officer of Health was not compelled to institute the tests, by May of 1962 they were done routinely in 131 of 145 Local Health Authorities. Usually a health visitor went to the home and performed the test in a urine-soaked diaper.[2]

None of our sources was aware of any Local Authority that was not testing in 1973. It is not possible, however, to determine for the country as a whole what proportion of live-born infants are screened, because in some regions infants with negative tests are not reported to the Local Authority, which keeps a record of live births. In addition, as some babies are residents of one Region but are born in another, so the precise proportion of babies screened cannot be determined by dividing the number of tests by the number of live births in a specific region.* Minimum estimates are possible, however, and it appears likely that well over 90% of all live-born infants surviving past the first week are screened.

* The proportion could be obtained from a future British Birth Survey. The last survey collected information on each of the births occuring in the United Kingdom in one week in 1970. The survey asked, among other things: "Was the baby tested for phenylketonuria?" However, the forms were completed on the 7th day so that babies screened later would not be covered.

Age at Time of Screening

Four centers (London, 1972; Bristol, 1970; Cardiff, 1973; and Cambridge, 1973) provided data that enabled us to determine the number of infants tested by a blood phenylalanine method on each day of life. The vast majority of infants are being screened between 6 and 14 days as recommended, in striking contrast to the pattern in the United States[8] and in Ireland[9] (Figure H-1). In the centers still determining urine *o*-hydroxy-

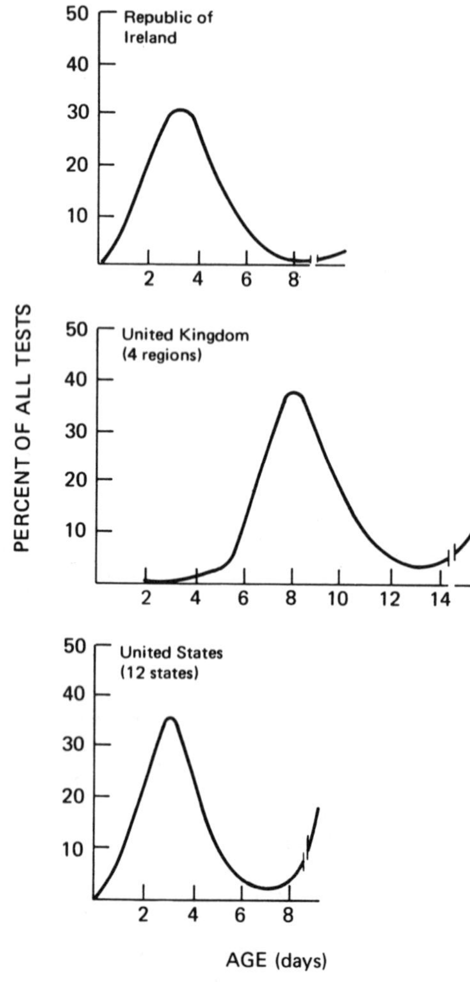

FIGURE H-1 Age distribution of blood phenylalanine screening in the United Kingdom, Republic of Ireland, and the United States.

phenylacetic acid by paper chromatography fewer than 2% of tests were performed before the tenth day, again in accordance with the recommendation of the MRC's Working Party.

Unfortunately, the National Register does not include the age of PKU infants at the time of first screening. Six clinics, however, provided these data on 118 infants in whom a diagnosis of PKU was later esablished, showing that 90 were screened on the sixth day of life or later (Table H-1). (Screening appears to be slightly earlier in Scotland.) Four screening centers provided the age distribution of all infants with positive tests, showing that 80% of positives were screened on or after the sixth day (Table H-2). If Scotland is excluded, 91% were screened on or after the sixth day.

Recording and Tracing

Each screening center has its own system for collecting specimens, recording results and returning them to the appropriate parties. As already indicated, not all centers return negative results to the Medical Officer of Health (this was not required in the 1969 circular).

Northern Ireland has the most sophisticated recordkeeping system. The name, address, date of birth, sex, and date of test of every baby screened is entered into the computer, together with the results of the phenylalanine, tyrosine, and methionine determinations. Each Medical Officer of Health receives a printout containing all of this information for all of the babies born in his district. He also receives individual printouts for inclusion in each baby's chart. Information on infants with positive tests is retained in the computer until a follow-up is obtained. A program exists to print out the names of infants whose first test was positive but who have not had a repeat within a specified interval. Information concerning any infant can be retained on the computer tape.

In England and Wales in the first 6 months of 1971, 38.3% of newborns were discharged from the hospital before they were 6 days old.[10] The trend continues toward earlier discharge. As fewer than 5% of babies are screened by 6 days (Figure H-1), many specimens must be obtained in the home. The Scotland laboratory reported that only 3% of infants are screened before they leave the hospital.

The domiciliary midwife has statutory responsibility for the newborn up to 10 days of age, at which time the health visitor assumes it. The specimen for the PKU test is obtained by the midwife or the health visitor in the home. For babies still in the hospital after 5–6 days, the blood sample is obtained in the hospital; repeat tests are avoided because the hospital informs the Local Authority of the screening tests that have been performed.

TABLE H-1 Age at Time of First Screening of Infants Proved To Have Phenylketonuria [a]

Clinic	Years	Age (Days) at Time of Screening 0–4	5	6	7	8–10	11–14	15–21	>21	Total
Bristol	1970–1973	0	0	1	8	4	0	0	0	13
Cardiff[a]	1968–1973	0	1	0	0	1	1	3	0	6
East Anglia[b]	1970–1973	0	0	0	0	5	0	0	0	5
Glasgow	1966–1973	14[c]	12	4	5	4	5	1	1	46
Great Ormond Street	1971–1973	0	0	8	6	2	0	1	0	17
Manchester	1969–1973	1	0	0	2	5	12	9	2	31
Total		15	13	13	21	21	18	14	3	118

[a] With the exception of Cardiff, which determines urine *o*-OH-phenylacetic acid as the screening procedure, all other centers screen blood for phenylalanine elevations, Bristol by the fluorometric method, East Anglia and Manchester by paper chromatography, and Glasgow and Great Ormond Street by the Guthrie test.
[b] 3 clinics follow 1 patient each and 1 follows 2. Screening done at Cambridge.
[c] Includes 6 younger sibs of known phenylketonurics.

TABLE H-2 Age at Time of First Screening of Infants with Positive First Test

Screening Center [a]	Year	Age (Days) at Time of Screening 0–4	5	6	7	8–10	11–14	15–21	>21	Total
Bristol	72	0	5	48	328	501	82	40	11	1015
Carshalton	72	0	82	140	41	12	1	4	1	281
Scotland (Stobhill)	72	53	135	56	28	15[b]	—	—	50[b]	337
Sheffield	72	1	87	122	17	17	3	3	1	251
Total		54	309	366	414	545	86	47	63	1884

[a] All centers screen blood for phenylalanine elevations, Bristol and Sheffield by the fluorometric method and Carshalton and Scotland by the Guthrie method.
[b] Stobhill General Hospital performs screening for most of Scotland. The number of infants with positive first test was provided for each of the first 9 days and, after that, for all days combined.

These procedures point out the advantage of the availability of Local Authority personnel who assume the responsibility for health care in the community as well as of the Maternity Liaison Committees, which coordinate the activities of hospitals, Local Authorities, and practitioners. Positive results are reported to the Medical Officer of Health (and often to the general practitioners as well) and to the hospital staff if the specimen was obtained in the hospital. The screening laboratory often provides specific instructions regarding follow-up (see the section on effectiveness and efficiency, below).

Centralization

With only one exception, all screening laboratories are located in hospitals. In some Regions one laboratory performs all tests; in others, several laboratories are involved. The number of tests performed in any one laboratory varies between 700 and 117,000 per year.[7] Many interviewees felt that further centralization was possible. To our knowledge there is no centralized quality control whereby unknown specimens are circulated to different laboratories for comparative testing.

Although five hospital centers in the United Kingdom care for about half of all phenylketonurics, there are several pediatric consultants who care for only one or two phenylketonurics. Most interviewees believe that each patient with PKU should be evaluated, at least on some occasions, by a pediatrician who has considerable experience with the disorder. On the other hand, many consultants recognize the financial and time constraints in transporting patients to distant centers.

There is no consistent policy regarding the relation between referring physicians and the specialized centers. In some areas the practitioner prescribes the low-phenylalanine formulas (although the center suggests what to prescribe), while in others the specialized center assumes the financial burden of providing the diet. Some centers will also provide transportation for some patients.

Method Evaluation

In addition to the Guthrie bacterial inhibition assay for blood phenylalanine,[11] fluorometric[12] and chromatographic[13-15] methods for blood phenylalanine determination are currently being used.[7] A number of investigators have compared different methods.[12,16,17] Although not rigorously evaluated, the chromatographic methods on blood appear to be capable of detecting phenylalanine concentrations if they are greater than 4–6 mg%. Thus, if they are employed after 6 days of age, they are probably as reliable as the Guthrie method. They have the advantage of detecting other amino acids as well. Several patients with histidinemia have been discovered with this method of screening.

EFFECTIVENESS AND EFFICIENCY

Some measures of effectiveness, such as completeness of screening, have already been discussed. In this section we consider another measure—namely, whether, among babies screened by methods currently in use, all those with PKU are detected and how long it takes to obtain follow-up. A highly efficient program would yield very few false positives, and this problem is also considered.

False Negatives

We are not aware of any infants screened for blood phenylalanine elevation in the United Kingdom whose result was negative but in whom a diagnosis of PKU was subsequently established. The two centers still employing the urine *o*-hydroxyphenylacetic acid method reported two false negatives. The first was screened at approximately 2 months of age and the second at 12 to 14 days.

The high effectiveness of blood screening (with the absence of any false negatives) contrasts with the situation in the United States and, to a lesser extent, with that in the Republic of Ireland (Table H-3). We believe that this difference is due to the later age at the time of screening in the United Kingdom than in either of the other two countries (Figure H-1). Seventeen of the twenty-four (71.9%) false-negative infants in the United States and the Irish Republic were screened on or before the fourth day of life.

Fourteen of the twenty-four phenylketonurics missed by screening were females, and there is evidence to suggest that the rise of blood phenylalanine in female phenylketonurics during the first week of life is delayed compared to that in males.[8] Further support for this hypothesis comes from a comparison of the number of infants of each sex discovered at different ages during the first week of life (Table H-4). On the first 3 days of life, there is the least probability of detecting an infant with PKU but the probability is equal in males and females. On the fourth day there is a significantly higher probability of detecting PKU in males than in females, but after the fourth day the probability for detecting PKU in both sexes is again equal and considerably higher than earlier. Recently, Hawcroft and Hudson reported that of the 377 babies with PKU born between 1964 and 1972 in the United Kingdom and reported to the Register, 189 were males.[18]

TABLE H-3 Sensitivity of Phenylketonuria Detection

Country	Year	Source of Data	Number Missed by Screening	Number Discovered	Percent Missed
Republic of Ireland	1966–1972	Entire program[9]	1	73	1.4
United Kingdom	1964–1972	Blood assays (Register)	0	251	0
	1968–1972	Urine assays (2 centers)	2	7	22.2
United States	1962–1971	16 states[19]	23	253	8.3

TABLE H-4 Neonatal Screening for Phenylketonuria: Sex Differences among Infants with Phenylketonuria

	Age (Days) at Time of Screening					
	0–3		4		>4	
Country	Males	Females	Males	Females	Males	Females
Republic of Ireland [9]	13	9	9	3	17	22
United Kingdom [a]	2	3	1	0	47	61
United States [8]	96	97	50	30	76	64
Total	111	109	60	33	140	147

[a] PKU Register patients reported for 1971–1972. Three of the five infants screened on the first 3 days of life were siblings of known phenylketonurics.

Because of the rise of phenylalanine during the first week of life in infants with PKU, those screened later should present with higher levels. Thus, in the United Kingdom, where infants are screened late, only two infants with PKU were found to have blood phenylalanine concentrations of less than 10 mg% on the initial test (both were females with levels between 8 and 10 mg% at 6 and 7 days of age, respectively). This contrasts sharply with the situation in the United States and the Republic of Ireland (Table H-5).

Efficiency of Follow-up

A very small proportion of infants with transient phenylalanine elevations present with blood phenylalanine concentrations on initial screening of 10 mg% or higher, whereas (as discussed above) infants in whom the diagnosis of PKU is subsequently established almost always present with concentrations above 10 mg%. This fact greatly facilitates follow-up. When

TABLE H-5 Screening Blood Phenylalanine Concentrations in Infants with Phenylketonuria[a]

		Initial Phenylalanine (mg%), Percent of Total Infants		
Country	Number of PKU Infants	4–10	11–20	>20
Republic of Ireland[9]	73	21	15	64
United Kingdom[a]	116	2	9	89
United States[20]	338	27	31	42

[a] Data supplied by screening centers at Bristol (1970–1972), Cambridge (1970–1973), Glasgow (1966–1973), Great Ormond Street (1970–1973), Manchester (1969–1973), and Sheffield (1972). Only the first 6 months of 1973 are included.

an infant is discovered to have a blood phenylalanine concentration on screening of 20 mg% or higher, the Medical Officer of Health is notified and the baby is immediately referred for hospitalization without a repeat test at home. For concentrations between 8 and 20 mg%, the Medical Officer of Health is usually notified by phone and a repeat test is obtained. A more leisurely approach is taken for infants whose initial screening level was elevated, but to less than 8 mg%; some centers will delay follow-up for 4–6 weeks. Most centers still request repeat tests for any concentration higher than 4 or 6 mg%.

The mean time between screening test and follow-up for PKU infants in the United Kingdom is 7 days. This includes infants who were immediately referred into the hospital (Table H-6). The mean time for infants whose screening test was positive but in whom a diagnosis of PKU was not necessarily established by follow-up was 12 days (Table H-7; centers intentionally delaying follow-up are not included).

CONCLUSIONS

The development of policy by a central health agency, and communication of this policy to local providers of health services, facilitates, but does

TABLE H-6 Interval between Screening Test and Follow-up Test in Infants with Phenylketonuria

Country	Years	Days			Mean Number of Days
		0–14	15–30	>30	
Republic of Ireland[9]	1966–1972	64	5	0	5 ± 5
United Kingdom[a]	1971–1972	98	10	1	7 ± 7[a]
United States (18)	1968–1970	285	72	31	12 ± 19[a]
		$\chi^2 = 25.0243$			$t = -2.7783$[a]
		$p < .001$			$p < .005$

[a] Data from PKU Register.

TABLE H-7 Interval between Screening Test and Follow-up Test in Infants with Elevated Screening Phenylalanine[a]

Country	Years	Number	Mean Number of Days
United Kingdom[b]	1971–1972	736	12
United States 18	1968–1970	1283	25

[a] Excluding infants with phenylketonuria.
[b] Data supplied by screening centers at Carshalton, Great Ormond Street, Manchester, and Sheffield.

TABLE H-8 Interviewees in the United Kingdom

Department of Health and Social Services	John S. Stevenson (Scotland)
Margaret Bell[a] (Scotland)	Richard Wilkinson (Oxford)
Eileen Ring	
Sheila Waiter	PKU Clinics
J. M. G. Wilson[a]	David Burman (Bristol)
	Nina Carson (Northern Ireland)
Medical Research Council	Hugh Ellis (Oxford)
Ashley Miller[a]	Peter Harper (Cardiff)
Ian Sutherland[a]	Freddie Hudson[a] (Liverpool)
	George Komrower[a] (Manchester)
PKU Register	Sandra McBean (Glasgow)
Janet Hawcroft	Otto Wolff[a] (London)
Freddie Hudson[a]	
	Medical Officers of Health
Screening Centers	Trevor Evans (Camden, London)
Nina Carson (Northern Ireland)	Dr. Langton (Edinburgh)
Barbara Clayton[a] (London)	
A. F. Heeley (Cambridge)	British Birth Survey
John B. Holton (Bristol)	Roma Chamberlain
George Komrower[a] (Manchester)	
R. Mahler (Cardiff)	Republic of Ireland
R. J. Pollitt (Sheffield)	Seamus Cahalane
Jan Stern (Carshalton)	Thomas Fitzgerald
	Doreen Murphy
	Louis Wolff (Visiting)

[a] Member, MRC Committee on PKU.

not assure, an effective screening program. The experience with Phenistix testing is illustrative. The fault was not with the system but with the screening test. And the presence of the centrally organized PKU Register, and the ability to utilize information fed back from it, facilitated rectification of the problem.

When an effective procedure became available, the existence of health services of wide scope and their coordination through a central health agency enhanced the efficiency with which it was used. Thus, the fact that every baby is visited by a midwife or health visitor greatly improves the likelihood that testing will be complete. The Local Authority provides a focal point from which specimens can be sent and to which results can be returned. Established channels of communication between the Health Visitors and the Medical Officer of Health on the one hand and screening laboratories, referral centers, and practitioners on the other, improve the likelihood of rapid and adequate follow-up of infants with elevated tests.

The availability of the midwife or health visitor to collect specimens in the home, given the risks of early screening,[3] must have been a key determinant in the decision to defer screening until 6 days of age or later. The evidence on which the late screening decision was based was available in the United States (in fact, it came from the United Kingdom), but there was (and is) no system in the United States for assuring testing of every baby after discharge from the hospital.

The procedures for collection and reporting are fairly consistent across the United Kingdom, but there are certain components of the PKU screening and management program that vary among Regions. Different screening laboratories employ different tests and handle different numbers of specimens; and some PKU patients are referred to centers that manage many patients, while others are treated by pediatricians without any extensive experience with the disorder. Unless one procedure can be shown to be superior to another, there is no justification for demanding uniformity.

NOTE ON SCREENING IN THE REPUBLIC OF IRELAND

Following a pilot study of the Guthrie test, conducted by Cahalane at the Children's Hospital, Dublin, screening was instituted throughout Ireland on February 1, 1966. The program was financed by the Department of Health. Local Health Authorities disseminated information to practitioners, and the public was informed through press and television coverage. From 1966 through April 1973, 93.6% of live births were tested. There were 29,000 infants not screened, among whom 5 infants with PKU have been discovered. These were between 10 and 33 months old at the time of diagnosis and all were already retarded. The incidence of approximately 1 in 6,000 is the same as that among infants discovered by screening. This high degree of ascertainment speaks very well for the organization of consultative care in the Republic. The very short interval between screening and follow-up (Table H-6) for infants with PKU is also impressive.

Infants are screened at an earlier age in Ireland than in the United Kingdom (Figure H-1). Thus far only one infant who was screened has been missed, and he was screened at 7 days of age.

REFERENCES

1. The National Health Services. Survey of Early History and Main Features. NHS Note 1, October 1971. London: Department of Health and Social Security, 1971.
2. Treatment of phenylketonuria. Report to the Medical Research Council of the Conference on Phenylketonuria. Brit. Med. J. 1:1691–1697, 1963.

3. Moncrieff, A. Present status of different mass screening procedures for phenylketonuria. Brit. Med. J. 4:7–13, 1968.
4. Hawcroft, J., and F. P. Hudson. Personal communication, 1974.
5. Hsia, D. Y-Y. Screening tests for the detection of phenylketonuria homozygotes and heterozygotes. In J. A. Anderson and K. F. Swaiman, eds. Phenylketonuria and Allied Metabolic Diseases. Washington, D.C.: U.S. Department of Health, Education, and Welfare, Children's Bureau, 1967.
6. National Health Service. Screening for Early Detection of Phenylketonuria. London: Her Majesty's Stationery Office, 1969, p. 72.
7. Medical Research Council. Screening Centers. London: Medical Research Council, October 1972.
8. Holtzman, N. A., A. G. Meek, E. D. Mellits, and C. H. Kallman. Neonatal screening for phenylketonuria. III. Altered sex ratio: Extent and possible causes. J. Pediat. 85:175–181, 1974.
9. Cahalane, S. Personal communication, 1973.
10. Medical Research Council. On the State of the Public Health. Annual Report of the Chief Medical Officer of the Department of Health and Social Security for the Year 1971. London: Her Majesty's Stationery Office, 1972, p. 104.
11. Newman, R. L., and D. J. T. Starr. Technology of a regional Guthrie test service. J. Clin. Pathol. 24:564–575, 1971.
12. Holton, J. B. A large scale comparison of the bacteriological inhibition assay and the automated fluorimetric method for phenylketonuria screening. Ann. Clin. Biochem. 9:118–122, 1972
13. Ireland, J. T., and R. A. Read. A thin layer chromatographic method for use in neonatal screening to detect excess amino acidaemia. Ann. Clin. Biochem. 9:129–132, 1972.
14. Raine, D. N., J. R. Cooke, W. A. Andrews, and D. F. Mahon. Screening for inherited metabolic disease by plasma chromatography (Scriver) in a large city. Brit. Med. J. 3:7–13, 1972.
15. Sardharwalla, I. B., G. M. Komrower, C. Bridge, and D. B. Gordon. One-dimensional chromatography of plasma in Manchester. Ann. Clin. Biochem. 9:126–128, 1972.
16. Baker, J. R., C. Yi-Ming, H. J. Liebeschuetz, and M. Sandler. A comparison of two blood phenylalanine assay procedures in the diagnosis of phenylketonuria. J. Ment. Defic. Res. 8:176–182, 1964.
17. Belton, N. R., J. D. Crombie, S. P. Robins, R. Stephen, and J. W. Farquhar. Measurement of phenylalanine in routine care of phenylketonuric children. Arch. Dis. Child. 48:472–475, 1973.
18. Hawcroft, J., and F. P. Hudson. Sex ratio among phenylketonuric infants in the United Kingdom. Lancet 2:702–703, 1973.
19. Holtzman, N. A., A. G. Meek, and E. D. Mellits. Neonatal screening for phenylketonuria. I. Effectiveness. JAMA 229:667–675, 1974.
20. Holtzman, N. A., E. D. Mellits, and C. H. Kallman. Neonatal screening for phenylketonuria. II. Age dependence of initial phenylalanine in infants with PKU. Pediatrics (In press).

APPENDIX

I Screening Practices in Canada

This Appendix has two parts. The first is a survey of government-sponsored resources for screening, counseling, and treatment of hereditary metabolic disease and other types of genetic disease. The second is a description and analysis of the Quebec Network of Genetic Medicine.

Canada occupies 3.8 million square miles of North America, largely north of the 49th parallel. Its population in 1974 was slightly more than 23 million. The population density is highest in a 100-mile band along the Canadian–American border. Significant population density north of this band occurs only in the Lac St.-Jean region of Quebec and in the Edmonton region of Alberta. The far north has only two population settlements of more than 2,500 persons, one on Baffin Island at Frobisher Bay, the other in the Peace River Valley at Yellowknife. The principal race is Caucasian, of many ethnic subdivisions; Mongols, as native Inuit (Eskimo) and Indian and as immigrant Chinese and Japanese, comprise no more than 1 percent of the Canadian population; the Negro contributes an even smaller fraction.

Canada has a federal parliamentary system that is replicated at the provincial level. There are 10 provinces. The federal Ministry of National Health and Welfare is responsible for a national tax-supported health care program (valued at about $2.3 billion in 1974) that consumes over half of the NH&W budget. Over 90% of the federal disbursements are in payments to the provinces for Medicare and for hospital insurance programs. The extramural federal health research program in 1973–1974 was valued at about $90 million and comprised about 85% of the combined funds from federal and voluntary sources for this purpose.

Health care delivery is the responsibility of the provinces, except in the Northwest Territories, where it is under a federal agency. The combined federal and provincial health budgets bring the national total to $6–7 billion; only about $10 million is allocated by the provinces for extramural health research. Therefore, the combined extramural health research program in Canada is equivalent to about 1.5% of the total cost of the health industry. Genetics (basic and applied) at all levels of jurisdiction in Canada consumes no more than 2% of the total health research budget, or 0.03% (at most) of the budget for the health care industry.

SURVEY OF GOVERNMENT-SPONSORED RESOURCES FOR SCREENING, COUNSELING, AND TREATMENT OF GENETIC DISEASE

The federal government has no sector devoted to genetics in the Ministry of National Health and Welfare. Any "responsibility" for genetics is found mainly in the Medical Research Council (MRC), a Crown corporation that reports through the Ministry to the Cabinet. The MRC is responsible for 55% of extramural medical research at the federal level; the funds available to MRC in 1973–1974 were $40.36 million.

The MRC established a review committee (study section) in 1968 for handling grant applications in "basic" genetics. Awards to investigators for genetic research were valued at $1 million in 1973, and they include support of one MRC Group in Medical Genetics. "Applied" research in genetics is largely the responsibility of the National Health Grant program in the Ministry, which has no study section for genetics as such. The Long Range Planning Program in NH&W sponsored a questionnaire on genetic counseling to arrive at a consensus for developing counseling services as a National Resource. The Medical Research Council has fostered an interprovincial program to evaluate research and its application in the area of prenatal diagnosis; MRC publishes the *Prenatal Diagnosis Newsletter* twice yearly.

The provincial governments, through their respective Ministries of Health, are responsible for programs of diagnosis and treatment in medical genetics. These programs operate in various patterns (see below); they largely reflect the initiative of individuals or groups of persons who, more often than not, hold no position in government but who act as advisors to the genetics program.

There are several voluntary national organizations interested in genetics. The Genetics Society of Canada has a membership of 470, with an additional 50 student members. It meets annually and publishes a journal and bulletin. The Canadian Society for Clinical Investigation has an active membership of 630 scientists and physician investigators. The Society holds an annual meeting, at which about 160 papers are selected for presentation; one section of the "specialty program" is now devoted to genetics. Among other societies with an interest in genetics are the Canadian Federation of Biological Societies and the Canadian Pediatric Society. The Royal College of Physicians and Surgeons, the principal agency in Canada for certification in the medical specialties (equivalent to board qualification in the United States), sponsors symposia and brief presentations on genetic topics at its annual and regional meetings and requires a knowledge of genetics for a number of its accreditation examinations.

An *ad hoc* group called the Committee for Improvement of Hereditary Disease Management, comprising about 50 scientists and laymen, was formed in 1970. It has sponsored various publications relating to the frequency of genetic admissions among children and to the diagnosis of hereditary aminoacidopathies. A newly established national "food bank" to facilitate treatment of patients with inborn errors of metabolism is the result of this *ad hoc* group's action.

GENESIS AND METHODS OF THE SURVEY

A previous report by the Committee for Improvement of Hereditary Disease Management[1] showed that, in recent years, changing patterns of major illness in early life have been associated with an increased proportion of children admitted to hospital due to diseases of genetic origin. In a survey of 12,801 admissions conducted in a large Canadian children's hospital in 1969–1970, it was found that 11.1% of all admissions were for patients with "genetic" disease; another 18.5% of admissions could be attributed to abnormal gene–environment interaction during development. It was estimated from these findings that about 4,000 families whose children were cared for at the hospital in question could benefit from the services of personnel with special skills in diagnosis, counseling and management of genetically allied health problems. Other reports have also described the high proportion of pediatric medical admissions,[2,3] total community pediatric bed occupancy,[4] potential and declared morbidity at birth,[5,6] and pediatric mortality[7,8] that may be ascribed to genetic disease.

The provincial governments, through their respective Ministries of Health, are largely responsible for existing programs of diagnosis and treatment of genetic diseases in Canada. The survey described here was made with the hope that the resulting interprovincial comparisons might catalyze improvements in existing programs and thereby eventually enhance the development of more extensive genetic services throughout Canada.

The Health Minister, or his deputy, in each province was first approached in 1971 by letter and also by telephone in several instances. Information was obtained from each province about its screening program for inherited metabolic disease, the compliance rate, the diseases screened for, the facilities for confirmatory diagnostic testing, and the methods of funding. Details were also obtained about facilities and funding for the counseling and treatment of patients with genetic disease. The information was updated in 1973.

Results

Services for Diagnosis Table I-1 gives an overview of the situation in Canada with regard to diagnostic facilities for genetic disease. Nine of the ten provinces have screening programs for the detection of hereditary metabolic diseases in the newborn. The first was initiated in 1963, the latest in 1969. There are no equivalent federal programs, except for pilot studies funded under the National Health Grants Program of the Ministry of National Health and Welfare.

The principal objective of the screening programs is to detect diseases amenable to medical intervention. In most provinces, this objective is confined to phenylketonuria and other hyperphenylalaninemic states. Capillary blood samples collected, on filter paper, from the infant's heel are most commonly used for the screening tests.

Two provinces (Manitoba[9] and Quebec) elected a broader mandate for disease diagnosis when they established their programs, and a third, Prince Edward Island, has recently expanded its program to embrace other aminoacidopathies. One program (in Quebec) is continually revising its technology and currently espouses three types of screening: for the purpose of intervention; for reproductive counseling; and for enumeration and surveillance.

The facilities for screening are largely centralized for technical reliability, accuracy, and uniformity. In Ontario, however, 25% of the Guthrie tests used for detection of hyperphenylalaninemia are analyzed in local institutions. In Newfoundland, all screening is done on an *ad hoc* basis at local hospitals. Regionalized backup facilities to investigate patients with positive tests and to confirm diagnoses are available in the major population centers of all provinces. In the Maritimes, one center in Halifax (at the I. W. Killam Hospital for Children) served Nova Scotia, New Brunswick and Prince Edward Island.

The cost of genetic screening in the newborn is borne by the provincial departments of health; families do not pay directly for the service.

Compliance with the government programs exceeds 83% and, with only two exceptions, is greater than 90%. The high rate reflects the nature of the population being served; provincial screening is largely directed at the newborn infant. In programs directed at other populations —for example, at persons in the childbearing age group for purposes of heterozygote detection and reproductive counseling, or at postnewborn infants for urine screening—the rates of participation are usually lower.

Counseling Services

Table I-2 lists the genetic counselors operating in the various provinces. In addition, as shown in Table I-3, each provincial screening program for hereditary metabolic disease has access to persons who have experience with the target traits or diseases and who can offer the appropriate genetic counseling to families of probands. It should be noted that these additional persons, who are largely pediatricians, do not usually consider themselves genetic counselors in the broad sense of the term. Certain provincial centers (particularly Quebec) can also rely on allied health personnel to provide continuous counseling and supervision of treatment of patients with hereditary metabolic disease. These two types of resource personnel augment counseling facilities for inborn errors of metabolism *per se* by about twofold.

Medical geneticists, with the customary credentials that permit them to handle the broad spectrum of genetic counseling, are found in all but two provinces. They are few, however, probably not many more than one per million population, for the nation as a whole. Classification of genetic counselors is a sensitive area, and Dr. Hauser of the Long Range Planning Program of the Federal Ministry of National Health and Welfare is attempting to define a consensus on the qualifications for genetic counseling and on the question of whether accreditation of counselors should be developed in Canada. An earlier and cautious survey of genetic counselors was published by the Genetics Society of Canada[10] in an effort to define this resource.

Treatment Services

Table I-4 gives an overview of the treatment facilities available in Canada, by province. The provincial services are least uniform in their commitment to systematized medical care of patients with hereditary metabolic disease. Treatment in nearly all provinces is delegated to a regional medical center at which there is the necessary expertise in per-

TABLE I-1 Facilities for Diagnosis of Genetic Disease in Canada, by Province

	British Columbia	Alberta	Saskatchewan	Manitoba	Ontario
Mass screening					
Date instituted	1964	1969	1965	1965	1965
Trait(s) screened for	PKU	PKU	PKU	Aminoacid-opathies, galactosemia, fructose intolerance	PKU
Percent of live births screened	95.0	66.5 in 1969 and 1970; perhaps 83.1 in 1971	96.0	98.5	96.0
Agency responsible	← Provincial departments of health [a] →				
Location of screening laboratory	Central labs in Vancouver and Victoria	Central lab at University of Alberta	Provincial lab	Provincial lab	75% in Central Public Health lab; 25% in local hospital
Backup facilities (confirmation, work-up, etc.)	In Children's Hospital, Vancouver and UBC	At University Hosp.	Mental Retardation Unit, Univ. of Sask., and South Sask. Hosp., Regina	At Children's Hospital, Winnipeg	PKU Centres in Toronto, Kingston, London, and Hamilton
Funding	By govt., for diets through Woodlands School for Dietary Management	By govt., for diet, Public Health Nurses	Diet provided free by Dept. of Health	By govt., for diet, transport, Public Health Nurses	By govt., for diet and transport
Special testing and other facilities	—	Considering extension for galactosemia	—	Plans to extend program to screen follow-up blood and urine samples	(Pilot program, Toronto, Tay-Sachs heterozygote)

[a] Provincial Network of Genetic Medicine.

sonnel and technology. In Quebec, the Ministry of Health and Social Affairs has appointed four university-based genetic centers to form the Quebec Network for Genetic Medicine, to which all patients in its program are referred.* The emphasis in this program is on ambulatory care, with

* The Quebec Network for Genetic Medicine is described in detail later in this Appendix.

Quebec	New Brunswick	Nova Scotia	Newfoundland	Prince Edward Island
1969	1966	1966	No provincial program	1963
Aminoacidopathies (urine), PKU, tyrosinemia (plasma), galactosemia, hyperuricacidurias	PKU	PKU	—	All aminoacidopathies since 1973
92.0	"Almost all"	Near 100	20.0 in St. John's only	95.7
←Provincial departments of health[a]→				
Childrens Hosp., Université Laval (Main), Childrens Hosp., Université Sherbrooke, Montreal Childrens Hosp., Ste-Justine Hosp.	Regional lab at St. John	Central lab at Killam Hospital	Hospitals	Provincial lab
At Network Centres noted in above category	Regional lab at St. John	Presumably at Killam Hospital	—	I. W. Killam Hospital at Halifax
Special grant to network (all Rx)	Govt. pays if patient not able to afford	Diet provided free by Dept. of Health	No special provisions but services available on request	Provincial government
Tay-Sachs screening program (Montreal region), cytogenetics register, tissue culture bank, blood thyroxine (exp.), Prenatal Dx, Lysosomal enzyme	—	—	—	—

a minimum of hospitalization for treatment and supervision. Delivery of care, and monitoring of the response to treatment, is performed largely by allied health personnel.

In several provinces, the government pays for the special diets required for treatment of genetic disease; the government may also facilitate and pay for the distribution of diets to patients. Manitoba, British Columbia,

TABLE I-2 Counseling Resources—Genetic Counselors for Medical Genetic Problems

Province	Counselors	Location
British Columbia	J. R. Miller P. A. Baird	Dept. of Medical Genetics, Medical Genetics Unit, University of British Columbia, Vancouver 8
	R. B. Lowry P. MacLeod	Dept. of Medical Genetics, Clinical Genetics Unit, University of British Columbia, Vancouver 9
	S. Styles	Royal Jubilee Hospital, Victoria
Alberta	P. Bowen	4-120 Clinical Sciences Bldg., Dept. of Pediatrics, University of Alberta, Edmonton
Saskatchewan	E. J. Ives	Dept. of Pediatrics, University Hospital, Saskatoon
Manitoba	W. D. MacDiarmid	Dept. of Medicine, St. Boniface Hospital, University of Manitoba, St. Boniface
	J. L. Hamerton M. H. K. Shokeir	Dept. of Pediatrics, (Division of Medical Genetics), Children's Hospital, Health Sciences Centre, Winnipeg
Ontario	J. M. Berg D. W. Cox N. L. Ruddy M. W. Thompson	Dept. of Genetics, Hospital for Sick Children, Toronto
	I. Uchida	Dept. of Pediatrics, McMaster University, Hamilton
	H. C. Soltan	Dept. of Pediatrics, University Hospital, London
	N. E. Simpson	Dept. of Pediatrics, Queen's University, Kingston
	M. H. Roberts	Dept. of Pediatrics, University of Ottawa
Quebec	F. C. Fraser	Dept. of Medical Genetics, Montreal Children's Hospital
	L. Pinsky	Lady Davis Institute, Jewish General Hospital, Montreal
	L. Dallaire	Medical Genetics Section, Dept. of Pediatrics, Ste Justine Hospital, Montreal
	C. Laberge	Division of Medical Genetics, Centre Hospital, Université Laval, Ste-Foy

TABLE I-2 (*Continued*)

Province	Counselors	Location
	P. L. Delva	Centre Hospital, Université Sherbrooke
Novia Scotia and the Maritimes	J. P. Welch	Dept. of Pediatrics, I. W. Killam Hospital, Dalhousie University, Halifax
Newfoundland	G. Fraser	Janeway Hospital, Memorial University, St. John's

and Quebec appear to have the most liberal policies in this regard, and in these provinces there is no direct cost to any patient for treatment of the diseases of interest to the screening program. Equivalent program-derived arrangements for treatment do not prevail in all provinces. In some they exist only for one disease, usually phenylketonuria; in others, they are confined to a particular treatment item (e.g., a low-phenylalanine milk substitute).

Most provinces maintain an index of patients who have hereditary metabolic disease. This simple facility is used for enumeration and for coordination of regional services. Two provinces (British Columbia and Alberta) have an extensive registry of handicapping diseases (including inborn errors of metabolism). The British Columbia registry is part of the Department of Vital Statistics; it honors confidentiality and provides a means for planning medical resources in the community for patients with many forms of genetic disease.

The relationship between research in health care delivery and development of new resources is tenuous or nonexistent in many provinces. In most cases, new developments are dependent on the initiative of individuals working in the field. In only one province (Quebec) does the Ministry formally espouse research and development as an essential part of its program; in that province, several of its current service activities have emanated from earlier research work, and all of its service programs were preceded by carefully evaluated pilot projects.

Discussion of Survey Findings

Genetic screening programs in Canada are voluntary; there are no health laws or regulations that enforce screening for genetic disease. The viability of various provincial programs more often than not reflects the initiative of individuals or groups outside government who act as advisors to government programs. The diverse nature of the provincial programs un-

TABLE I-3 Supplementary Counseling Resources—Consultants for Patients with Hereditary Metabolic Disease Referred by Various Testing and Screening Programs

Province	Resource Person	Location
British Columbia	B. Tischler	Woodlands School, New Westminster
	G. Davidson	Dept. of Pediatrics, University of British Columbia, Vancouver
Alberta	E. McCoy	Dept. of Pediatrics, University of Alberta, Edmonton
Saskatchewan	W. Zaleski	Alvin Buckwold Centre, Saskatoon
Manitoba	J. C. Haworth	Dept. of Pediatrics, Children's Hospital, Health Science Centre, Winnipeg
Ontario	T. A. Doran A. H. Gardner	Antenatal Genetics Clinic, Toronto General Hospital
	E. H. Hutton L. Stevens	Dept. of Genetics, Hospital for Sick Children, Toronto
	W. B. Hanley A. Sass-Kortsak	Hospital for Sick Children, Toronto
	D. T. Whelan	Dept. of Pediatrics, McMaster University, Hamilton
	M. R. F. Jenner	Dept. of Pediatrics, University Hospital, London
	R. Gatfield F. Sergovitch	Children's Psychiatric Institute, London
	M. Partington	Dept. of Pediatrics, Queen's University, Kingston
Quebec	C. R. Scriver R. J. M. Gold	Dept. of Biochemical Genetics, Montreal Children's Hospital
	F. H. Glorieux	Genetics Unit, Shriners Hospital, Montreal
	J. Letarte J. B. Melancon	Dept. of Pediatrics, Ste Justine Hospital, Montreal
	R. Gagne	Division of Medical Genetics, Centre Hospital, Université Laval, Ste-Foy
	B. Lemieux	Dept. of Pediatrics, Centre Hospital, Université Sherbrooke
Nova Scotia and the Maritimes	M. Spence R. B. Goldbloom	Dept. of Pediatrics, I. W. Killam Hospital, Dalhousie University, Halifax
Newfoundland	A. Davis	Dept. of Pediatrics, Janeway Hospital, Memorial University, St. John's

doubtedly reflects the interests of their advisors. The trend toward comprehensive medical insurance systems, which characterizes medicine in Canada, offers an advantage for the initiation and maintenance of programs in medical genetics. The emphasis on the prevention of hereditary metabolic disease is appropriate, considering that technology for diagnosis and treatment is more readily available for this fraction of genetic disease than for the remainder. The cost-effectiveness in the management of this form of potentially expensive chronic disease has not escaped the interest of health care planners.[11,12] Costs of the programs are relatively modest; for example, Manitoba invests about $1.50 per birth and Quebec $3 per birth for its Network for Genetic Medicine, which embraces screening, treatment, and genetic counseling for over 30 diseases. Current estimates indicate a favorable cost–efficiency ratio in these programs.[11,12]

The foregoing description of services does not emphasize the many special genetics programs that serve the Canadian public. Some are found in the provincial programs, while others are under various independent agencies. For example, the Rh Blood Grouping Laboratory in Winnipeg is probably the oldest functioning genetics testing unit in Canada, and there are also special programs for typing of pseudocholinesterase mutants and alpha-1-antitrypsin deficiency at two laboratories in the University of Toronto. Several regional programs are concerned with diseases with high frequency in subisolates: for example, Tay-Sachs testing and counseling programs serving the many geographic regions in Canada where Ashkenazi Jews live and the Fabry's disease testing program now under development in Nova Scotia. Quebec added thyroid hormone screening[13] to its newborn screening program after development of the technology at Laval University. These programs are run largely by community or university resources, but they could be incorporated into government programs for disease prevention.

Prenatal diagnosis and amniocentesis, as a mode of diagnosis and reproductive counseling in certain high-risk situations, has developed as a series of intraprovincial regional programs, sometimes under the auspices of the government (Quebec), more often based in universities or hospitals. Long-term evaluation of results and of possible hazards is being made by an interprovincial working group[14] and reports are issued through the MRC-sponsored *Prenatal Diagnosis Newsletter*. A standard for the service has been defined, and emphasis has been placed on centralization of activities at genetic centers. Some prenatal diagnosis centers have developed their own periodic newsletter to inform physicians in their orbit of the emerging role of medical genetics in general, and of prenatal diagnosis in particular; these efforts provide a form of continuing education for the busy physician.

TABLE I-4 Treatment Facilities for Hereditary Metabolic Disease, by Province

	British Columbia	Alberta	Saskatchewan	Manitoba	Ontario
Recordkeeping	Central Registry for Handicapping Disease in the Division of Vital Statistics	Registry similar to BC model	PKU and cystic fibrosis cases recorded centrally in Saskatoon or Regina	Index of patients identified with HMD kept by Director Clinical Health Services and University Department of Pediatrics	Central Registry for PKU patients kept by Ministry of Health
Location of facilities	At Woodlands Hospital and in Genetics Department UBC	At University Hospital	At University Hospital and Alvin Buckwold Centre, Saskatoon	At Children's Hospital	For PKU, at provincial centers. (Toronto, Kingston, London, Hamilton)
Personnel Used	Professional (genetic and medical) and public health nurses	Professional and public health nurses	Professional	Professional (genetic and medical); public health nurses	Professional (genetic and medical) and support staff

A tissue culture bank, designed initially for regional needs but now serving international clients, was established at McGill University in the Quebec system; this facility provides reference material and receives "deposits" from other genetic centers in Canada and abroad.

Collaboration between the Division of Nutritional Research of the Health Protection Branch, Ministry of National Health and Welfare, and sixteen participating provincial genetic centers has led to the establishment of the National Food Distribution Centre for Management of Patients with Hereditary Metabolic Disease. The "Food Bank" is managed as a public service by a large food retailer (Steinberg's Ltd.) on behalf of the genetic centers. Authority and responsibility for treatment rests solely with the genetic centers, which instruct the Bank; the latter has an overview of the national cumulative caseload of patients with treatable hereditary metabolic diseases.

It is not the purpose of this survey to be exhaustive. As stated earlier, its objective is only to provide some interprovincial comparisons that might catalyze expansion of genetic screening programs where advisable. There are deficiencies by present international standards, especially an overall deficiency in the number of genetic counselors. The World Health Organization[6] recommends a minimum of 5 professional counselors per million population; the average in Canada is a little more than 1 per million. The situation is improved somewhat by the availability of

Quebec	New Brunswick	Nova Scotia	Newfoundland	Prince Edward Island
Data Bank for Quebec Network for Genetic Medicine	Centralized Index of PKU patients	Centralized register of patients identified by screening	No central registry	Partial registry
4 regional centers: Childrens Hospital, Université Laval, Childrens Hospital, Université Sherbrooke, Ste-Justine, Montreal Children's Hospital	Dept. of Health Headquarters Centennial Building, Fredericton	At I. W. Kiliam Hospital, Halifax	Special services developing at Janeway Hospital	Referral to Halifax
Professional (genetic and medical), allied health personnel, and public health nurses	Public health services	Professional (medical) and public health nurses	Not specified	General medicine and public health staff

experts in the area of most effort in genetic screening, namely for hereditary metabolic disease. Physicians, specialists, and allied health personnel offer an important resource for these activities, and these programs may provide models to be emulated in other areas of medical genetics.

The survey found less than optimal communication between the provinces regarding their genetic screening programs. Many of the government representatives contacted seemed to have little or no knowledge of programs existing in other provinces, even in those that were geographically adjacent. At least one representative requested guidance in setting program objectives for his province.

The survey found that provinces, with the exception of Quebec, had little or no funds for research and development in applied medical genetics. Research is largely a federal responsibility; but little provincial or federal money is specified for medical genetic research or health care delivery in medical genetics. In 1973–1974, the total extramural program at the federal level for grants in aid and for personnel support was valued at about $58 million; about another $10 million was allocated by the provinces for this purpose. As mentioned at the beginning of this Appendix, the total health research program in Canada is estimated to be about 1.5% of the total cost of its health industry.[15] Genetic research (basic and applied), at all levels of jurisdiction consumes about 2% of the nation's health research budget. In other words, only 0.03%

of health funds are spent to do research on the mechanisms of disease and its prevention for an area that represents up to 30% of the disease burden in some sectors of the industry.

The genetic services available to Canadians are quite good compared to those in other countries. But the survey points up deficiencies, even in the area of genetic screening, where there is considerable strength, foresight, and potential. We have much more to accomplish before Canada's health systems can come to grips with genetic disease as a total problem.

Summary

Government-sponsored resources in Canada, for diagnosis and treatment of genetic disease, were surveyed in 1973. The major emphasis of government programs is on hereditary metabolic disease; relatively little effort has yet been invested on the very large fraction of genetic disease remaining.

All provinces but one have voluntary mass screening programs to detect inherited metabolic diseases in the newborn for the purpose of medical intervention. In most provinces the programs are directed toward hyperphenylalaninemia case-finding alone; a few provinces (Quebec and Manitoba in particular) provide multiphasic screening, sometimes at several postnatal ages. The average compliance rate in the newborn screening programs is 94.9% (ranging from 83% to more than 99%). The Quebec government also sponsors screening for the purpose of reproductive counseling in populations at high risk for untreatable genetic disease, such as Tay-Sachs disease.

All provinces have facilities for confirmatory diagnosis. Genetic counseling resources comprise two types: individuals skilled in the full spectrum of medical genetic counseling and persons who by experience or by preference restrict their effort to specific subgroups of genetic disease. In Quebec, there is an additional systematized program that utilizes trained allied health personnel to provide counsel in the provincial network of genetic referral centers. No province meets the World Health Organization recommendation of at least 5 professional counselors per million population.

Services for treatment are less uniformly established than those for screening. Some provinces have a broadly structured prepaid treatment network with emphasis on ambulatory care of patients. Others limit their service to the provision of a low-phenylalanine product for treatment of phenylketonuria. British Columbia and Alberta maintain registries of handicapping disease that serve as resources for the planning of services for patients with genetic disease of all types.

Prenatal diagnosis is offered as a component of reproductive counseling at many genetic centers across the country. Ongoing evaluation of the risks and benefits of the procedure is accomplished through the interprovincial cooperation of several centers under the administrative sponsorship of a Medical Research Council committee.

Special interjurisdictional activities are found either as centralized intramural or extramural projects; these include "typing" (for example, of blood groups and of mutational variants of serum pseudocholinesterase or alpha-1-antitypsin activity); and "banking" of skin fibroblasts that express mutant phenotypes and of special foods for treatment of hereditary metabolic diseases.

THE QUEBEC NETWORK FOR GENETIC MEDICINE

The Quebec Network provides screening and diagnosis, genetic counseling, and treatment for over thirty hereditary conditions. It is operated by four university medical centers for the Ministry of Social Affairs. The budget for the Network is provided by the Ministry.

The Network observes two dominant working principles: (a) integrated communication among its regional centers, the central laboratories and the patients and (b) the use of mandatory pilot studies before implementation of a new service.

History

Genetic screening was initiated by the province in 1969 on the recommendation of the heads of the pediatric departments at the four provincial medical schools (Laval, McGill, Montreal, and Sherbrooke). A pilot study[16] had demonstrated the feasibility of screening for purposes of medical intervention in the province.

The initial Working Committee included two representatives from each university and appropriate representation from the Ministry. Their first task was to organize screening for neonatal hyperphenylalaninemia; this program began in February 1970. The committee designed the subsequent Network program by delegating separate tasks to its four different centers and by integrating the existing regional systems for follow-up, diagnosis, counseling, and treatment of patients with genetic disease.

The committee selected two problems for initial emphasis: (a) hereditary tyrosinemia, an important hereditary illness of French-Canadians[17,18]; and (b) the evaluation of ambulatory care of hereditary metabolic disease by allied health personnel.[19,20] The Ministry agreed that operational research for purposes of disease prevention was in its own best interest at a time when a universal prepaid medicare system was being inaugurated. The committee found the formalized relationship between research and service a stimulating opportunity, and research and development has remained a cornerstone of the Network program.

In 1972, the Network for Genetic Medicine was created to encompass a range of interrelated activities. The objective was to coordinate applied medical genetics related to disease prevention. The responsibility for the operation of the Network was vested in the universities; financial support and final approval of the programs resided with government.

Services Offered by the Network

Mass Screening

On Blood Capillary blood from the heel is collected on filter paper at 5–7 days of age. Phenylalanine is estimated in the material by the automated fluorometric method of McCaman and Robins[21]; tyrosine is measured simultaneously by Hochella's method as modified by Grenier and Laberge[22]; galactose is also determined by the automated method of Grenier and Laberge.[23] Most recently, thyroxine (T_4) determination by the method of Dussault and Laberge[13] has been added to the repertoire of tests applied to whole blood spots received on the filter paper kits.

On Urine The sample is collected from the infant on filter paper at 5 days of age in the hospital and again at 14 days by the parents in the home. Chemical tests for reducing substances, cystine and keto acids are performed on eluted material and after spotting by a semiautomatic device,[24] amino acids are determined by one-dimensional partition chromatography on thin layer; the uric acid:creatinine ratio is also measured on the eluted sample by an automated method.[25]

High-Risk Screening The following tests are provided under appropriate circumstances. Cytogenetic screening of referred patients*; modified assay for serum hexosaminidase A and B[26] and two-test discrimination of heterozygotes[26,27] in the Ashkenazi community; prenatal diagnosis at two centers in the Network for selected indications[14]; chemical and chromatographic screening for aminoacidopathies and other disorders[28-31]; assays of hexosaminidase arylsulfatase, β-galactosidase,

* Karyotyping and Barr body determination are provided by pathologists in the medicare system.

sphingomyelinase, and acid phosphatase in leukocytes, cultured skin fibroblasts, and cultured amniotic fluid fibroblasts.

Confirmatory Diagnosis Initial positive screening tests are verified on a second sample. Confirmatory diagnosis is then pursued at one of the regional centers.

Counseling Services Genetic counseling is provided for all patients identified in the newborn screening program; counseling for reproductive options is offered in conjunction with prenatal diagnosis and is also offered to heterozygotes identified in the Tay-Sachs testing program; and continuous counseling is provided in the treatment programs. The counselors are professional medical geneticists, pediatricians with expertise in the relevant care, and allied health personnel trained for the role.

Treatment Treatment resources include diets and medications, continuous monitoring of treatment effect, and evaluation of clinical progress.[20] Ambulatory methods are emphasized and in-home care is provided for patients with hereditary metabolic disease.

Repositories The Network maintains two repositories: one for screening and demographic data, the other for cultured skin fibroblasts.[32]

Research and Development within the Network

Applied research for purposes of helping the patient with genetic disease has been a consistent concern of the Network.[12] Many developments in the laboratory have since been incorporated into the regular service activities of the Network. Ongoing pilot studies embrace screening for thalassemia minor in the Montreal Greek community, blood lipid analysis in children, and a Food Bank to facilitate the use of semisynthetic diets for treatment of patients with hereditary metabolic disease.[33] A series of publications describes new methods for diagnosis, counseling, and treatment and reports the results of clinical investigation sponsored by the Network.

Cost of Network

The provincial government provides $3–4 per live birth (the Canadian birth rate is 15.9 per 1,000 population) to support the service functions of the Network and another $1–1.50 per birth for research and development. The Network has been fortunate in capitalizing on existing facilities, including laboratories, medical services, and medical genetics programs within the Quebec medicare system. It also benefits from university-derived support of several committee members and from the academic programs in genetics. The budget of the Network, therefore, represents an amount added to the existing costs of medical service and education within the province.

The cost of the Network can be evaluated in terms of the benefits it brings to an integrated prepaid system of health care delivery. For example, there has been a reduction in the prevalence of mental retardation and morbidity due to phenylketonuria, homocystinuria, and maple syrup urine disease. Admission rates of patients to institutions for the retarded have fallen, and no patient with phenylketonuria is known to have been missed in the screening program. The Tay-Sachs testing program, coupled with the prenatal diagnosis service, has prevented the birth of four Tay-Sachs infants in 2 years, thus relieving the state and family of the burden of their care had they been born. The treatment program has kept patients in the home and at school and has significantly reduced the costs required for in-hospital and outpatient care.[12]

Results of Screening

Compliance rates in the blood-testing program and the 5-day urine test are 92% of live births; compliance in the 14-day urine-testing program is better than 80%. Ninety-seven percent of hospitals with obstetric services participate in the voluntary program.

The incidence of phenylketonuria in Quebec province is 1:23,000 live births; the incidence is similar for nonphenylketonuric hyperphenylalaninemia. Among the French-Canadians in the Province, the incidence of phenylketonuria is about 1:35,000 births and of hyperphenylalaninemia, 1:24,000 births, conforming to the relative frequencies for these traits in continental France. Hereditary tyrosinemia affects 1:8,000 live births in the province. Nearly all of these patients are born in the Lac St.-Jean district, where the frequency of the disease is 1:650 live births. The screening program as it pertains to tyrosinemia serves several purposes, namely, (a) to enumerate the relative frequencies of hereditary tyrosinemia[17,18] and neonatal tyrosinemia[16,34]; (b) to introduce genetic counseling into the region at high risk for hereditary tyrosinemia; (c) to facilitate research on the disease; and (d) to stimulate research into the causes of a relatively high rate (1%) of neonatal tyrosinemia in the French-Canadian population.

Galactosemia caused by uridyltransferase deficiency (1:120,000) and galactokinase deficiency (1:120,000) has been detected in the blood screening program. The urine screening programs (at birth and in hospital patients) have identified persons with histidinemia, cystinuria, isolated glutamicaciduria, renaliminoglycinuria, maple syrup urine disease, the Fanconi syndrome, and argininosuccinicaciduria.

Communication of Information

Role of the Network The two central laboratories are responsible for all communications related to mass screening of the newborn population (blood screening at Laval; urine screening at Sherbrooke). Each center is responsible for communication in its special projects—for example, Tay-Sachs heterozygote detection, prenatal diagnosis, cytogenetics, high-risk urine screening on hospitalized patients.

Normal test results are computerized in a data bank. Trimestrial printouts are returned to the 135 hospitals participating in newborn screening. Since almost all births in the province take place in hospitals (96% of the births take place in the participating hospitals), the Ministry fulfills its obligation to retain the patients' data while obviating the burden of mailing and filing a large volume of normal test results. When abnormal test results or technically unsatisfactory samples are identified, the Network contacts the parents directly for a second sample.

Studies performed in 1972 revealed that compliance rates for follow-up samples improved greatly when the parent instead of the physician was asked to obtain the repeat test. Only when a positive test result has been confirmed is the patient's physician involved directly.

The Quebec Corporation of Physicians has agreed that direct communication between the Network and the patient is in the best interest of all concerned. As a result, the average elapsed time between birth and initiation of treatment of patients with phenylketonuria is only 17 days (range 13–20 days) in the provincewide program, and as low as 12 days at one center with a largely urban referral region. When the diagnosis is established, the Network plays a consultative role. The physician takes charge of the patient's health care; the Network center supervises only the management of the particular genetic disease.

Consent for participation in the program is implied by voluntary compliance of the client in screening, counseling, and treatment. Since the Network is operated as a public health program within medicare, the onus is on the client if he chooses not to participate. A survey of mothers at the time of delivery revealed virtual unanimity in favor of preventive screening, the purpose of the Network program, and the need for them as parents to participate in the urine-testing program. This opinion was offered even though only 10% of parents were previously aware of the existence and scope of the program.

Role of the Physician The physician receives help for the care of his patient from his regional center, where the responsibility for follow-up and confirmatory diagnosis has been placed. In Quebec province, the physician is a resource person for patients seeking medical services. It is assumed that most practicing physicians at present have little experience with the diagnosis, counseling, and treatment of the majority of genetic disease. Consequently, centralization of special resources and regionalization of centers at which expertise with rare disease exists can aid the physician and his patient. Regional centers for management of genetic disease comply with current recommendations of the World Health Organization.[6]

Summary

The Quebec Network for Genetic Medicine is a voluntary program operated by four university-based genetic centers within the Quebec medicare system. Its purpose is to apply knowledge to the patient with genetic disease[12] and its major effort at present is the provision of screening and diagnosis for a broad spectrum of mendelian inborn errors of metabolism.

Samples for mass screening are analyzed in central laboratories, and all participating hospitals are monitored through a computerized data bank. Screening projects for high-risk groups are carried out at the individual regional centers.

The Network operates mass screening programs in the newborn as well as several high-risk screening projects. Genetic counseling and treatment, where appropriate, are provided by the program.

Research and development is an important activity in the Network program. Many services have originated from the pilot research projects component of the program.

The program utilizes the four genetic centers, each situated at a university medical center, to centralize its activities and to regionalize its influence. The Network relies heavily on the patients (and parents) as the primary respondent(s) for compliance. Consent for participation is a function of the medicare system. Physicians assume responsibility for the general health care of patients with genetic disease. The regional genetic centers assist the physician in a consultative capacity and provide resources for detailed counseling, monitoring, and treatment.

REFERENCES

1. Scriver, C. R., J. L. Neal, R. Saginur, and A. Clow. The frequency of genetic disease and congenital malformation among patients in a pediatric hospital. Can. Med. Assoc. J. 108:1111–1115, 1973.
2. Childs, B., S. M. Miller, and A. G. Bearn. Gene mutation as a cause of human disease, pp. 3–14. In H. E. Sutton and M. I. Harris, eds. Mutagenic Effects of Environmental Contaminants. New York: Academic Press, 1972.
3. Day, N., and L. B. Holmes. The incidence of genetic disease in a university hospital population. Amer. J. Hum. Genet. 25:237–246, 1973.
4. Miller, J. R. Human genetics in public health research and programming, p. 21. In L. E. Schacht, ed. Human Genetics in Public Health. St. Paul, Minn.: Minnesota Department of Health, 1964.
5. Stevenson, A. C. Frequency of congenital and hereditary disease. With special reference to mutation. Brit. Med. Bull. 17:254–259, 1961.
6. World Health Organization. Genetic Disorders: Prevention, Treatment and Rehabilitation. WHO Tech. Rep. Ser. No. 497. Geneva: World Health Organization, 1972.
7. Carter, C. O. Changing patterns in the causes of death at the Hospital for Sick Children. Great Ormond Street J. No. 11:65–68, 1956.
8. Roberts, D. F., J. Chavez, and S. D. M. Court. The genetic component in child mortality. Arch. Dis. Child. 45:33–38, 1970.
9. Fox, J. G., D. L. Hall, J. C. Haworth, A. Maniar, and L. Sekla. Newborn screening for hereditary metabolic disorders in Manitoba, 1965–1970. Can. Med. Assoc. J. 104:1085–1088, 1971.
10. Miller, J. R. Survey of genetic counselling. Genet. Soc. Bull. 3:21–24, 1972.
11. Webb, J. F. PKU screening—Is it worth it? Can. Med. Assoc. J. 108:328–329, 1973.
12. Clow, C. L., F. C. Fraser, C. Laberge, and C. R. Scriver. On the application of knowledge to the patient with genetic disease. Prog. Med. Genet. 9:159–213, 1973.
13. Dussault, J. H., and C. Laberge. Dosage de la thyroxine (T4) par méthode radio-immunologique dans l'éluat de sang séché: Nouvelle méthode de dépistage de l'hypothyroïdie néonatale? Union Med. Can. 102:2062–2072, 1973.
14. Hamerton, J. L. The Medical Research Council Working Group on Prenatal Diagnosis of Genetic Disease. MRC Prenatal Diagnosis Newsletter 1:2–3, 1972.
15. Phillipson, D. Medical research policy in Canada: The evaluation and convolution of policy, politics and $. Can. Med. Assoc. J. 110:1388–1394, 1974.
16. Clow, C., C. R. Scriver, and E. Davies. Results of mass screening for hyperaminoacidemias in the newborn infant. Amer. J. Dis. Child. 117:48–53, 1969.
17. Laberge, C. Hereditary tyrosinemia in a French Canadian isolate. Amer. J. Hum. Genet. 21:36–45, 1969.
18. Scriver, C. R., M. Partington, and A. Sass-Kortsak, eds. Conference on Hereditary Tyrosinemia. Can. Med. Assoc. J. 97:1045–1101, 1967.
19. Clow, C. L., and C. R. Scriver. Hereditary metabolic disease, pp. 650–659. In M. Green and R. J. Haggerty, eds. Ambulatory Pediatrics. Philadelphia: Saunders, 1968.

20. Clow, C., T. M. Reade, and C. R. Scriver. Management of hereditary metabolic disease. The role of allied health personnel. N. Engl. J. Med. 284:1292–1298, 1971.
21. McCaman, M. W., and E. Robins. Fluorimetric method for the determination of phenylalanine in serum. J. Lab. Clin. Med. 59:885–890, 1962.
22. Grenier, A., and C. Laberge. A modified automated fluorimetric method for tyrosine in blood spotted on paper: A mass screening procedure for tyrosinemia. Clin Chim. Acta (In press).
23. Grenier, A., and C. Laberge. Rapid method for screening for galactosemia and galactokinase deficiency by measuring galactose in whole blood spotted on paper. Clin. Chem. 19:463–465, 1973.
24. Shapcott, D., B. Lemieux, and A. Sahapoglu. A semi-automatic device for multiple sample application to thin-layer chromatography plates. J. Chromatogr. 70:174–178, 1972.
25. McInnes, R., P. Lamm, C. L. Clow, and C. R. Scriver. A filter paper sampling method for the uric acid:creatinine ratio in urine. Normal values in the newborn. Pediatrics 49:80–84, 1972.
26. Delvin, E., A. Pottier, C. R. Scriver, and R. J. M. Gold. The application of an automated hexosaminidase assay to genetic screening. Clin. Chim. Acta 53:135–142, 1974.
27. Gold, R. J. M., U. R. Maag, J. L. Neal, and C. R. Scriver. The use of biochemical data in screening for mutant alleles and in genetic counselling. Ann. Hum. Genet. 37:315–326, 1974.
28. Scriver, C. R., C. L. Clow, and P. Lamm. On the screening, diagnosis and investigation of hereditary aminoacidopathies. Clin. Biochem. 6:142–188, 1973.
29. Davies, E., and C. R. Scriver. Laboratory Manual of Screening Methods. Montreal: Montreal Children's Hospital.
30. Thomas, G. H., and R. R. Howell. Selected Screening Tests for Genetic Metabolic Diseases. Chicago: Yearbook Medical Publishers, 1973.
31. Mamer, O. A., W. J. Mitchell, and C. R. Scriver. Application of gas chromatography–mass spectrometry to the investigation of human disease. Proceedings of a Workshop. Published privately by McGill Univ.–Montreal Children's Hospital Research Institute. Montreal, 1974.
32. Goldman, H. The repository for mutant human cell strains. MRC Prenatal Diagnosis Newsletter 1:5–8, 1972.
33. Clow, C. L., H. Ishmael, C. R. Scriver, K. Murray, H. Campeau, D. Long, and H. A. Steinberg. The National Food Distribution Centre for Management of Patients with Hereditary Metabolic Disease. Bull. Genet. Soc. Can. (In press).
34. Avery, M. E., C. L. Clow, J. H. Menkes, A. Ramos, C. R. Scriver, L. Stern, and B. P. Wasserman. Transient tyrosinemia of the newborn: Dietary and clinical aspects. Pediatrics 39:378–384, 1967.

Index